Exploring the Pressures of Medical Education From a Mental Health and Wellness Perspective

Christina Ramirez Smith
University of the Bahamas, Bahamas

A volume in the Advances in Medical Education, Research, and Ethics (AMERE) Book Series

IGI Global
DISSEMINATOR OF KNOWLEDGE

Published in the United States of America by
IGI Global
Medical Information Science Reference (an imprint of IGI Global)
701 E. Chocolate Avenue
Hershey PA, USA 17033
Tel: 717-533-8845
Fax: 717-533-8661
E-mail: cust@igi-global.com
Web site: http://www.igi-global.com

Library of Congress Cataloging-in-Publication Data

Names: Smith, Christina Ramirez, 1958- editor.
Title: Exploring the pressures of medical education from a mental health and wellness perspective / Christina Ramirez Smith, editor.
Description: Hershey, PA : Medical Information Science Reference, [2018] | Includes bibliographical references.
Identifiers: LCCN 2017010737| ISBN 9781522528111 (hardcover) | ISBN 9781522528128 (ebook)
Subjects: | MESH: Students, Medical--psychology | Burnout, Professional--prevention & control | Health Promotion | Mental Health--education | Self-Injurious Behavior--prevention & control
Classification: LCC RC459 | NLM WM 172 | DDC 616.890071/1--dc23 LC record available at https://lccn.loc.gov/2017010737

This book is published in the IGI Global book series Advances in Medical Education, Research, and Ethics (AMERE) (ISSN: 2475-6601; eISSN: 2475-661X)

British Cataloguing in Publication Data
A Cataloguing in Publication record for this book is available from the British Library.

All work contributed to this book is new, previously-unpublished material.
The views expressed in this book are those of the authors, but not necessarily of the publisher.

For electronic access to this publication, please contact: eresources@igi-global.com.

Advances in Medical Education, Research, and Ethics (AMERE) Book Series

ISSN:2475-6601
EISSN:2475-661X

MISSION

Humans are living longer now than ever as a result of advances in the medical field. Having the tools available to train knowledgeable and ethical future generations of doctors and medical researchers is essential to continuing to advance our understanding of the human body and develop new ways of treating and curing sickness and disease.

The **Advances in Medical Education, Research, and Ethics (AMERE)** book series highlights publications pertaining to advancements in pedagogical practice for developing future healthcare professionals, research methods, and advancements in 10 the medical field, as well as moral behavior and practice of healthcare professionals, students, and researchers. Featuring research-based book publications that are highly relevant to the healthcare community, this series is ideally designed for library inclusion at medical universities and research institutions as well as personal use by medical professionals, researchers, and upper-level students entering the field.

COVERAGE

- Clinical Research
- Conflicts of Interest
- Ethics in Medicine
- Healthcare Pedagogy
- Medical Curricula
- Medical Simulation
- Patient Data
- Professional Development
- Research Methods
- Scientific Misconduct

IGI Global is currently accepting manuscripts for publication within this series. To submit a proposal for a volume in this series, please contact our Acquisition Editors at Acquisitions@igi-global.com or visit: http://www.igi-global.com/publish/.

The Advances in Medical Education, Research, and Ethics (AMERE) Book Series (ISSN 2475-6601) is published by IGI Global, 701 E. Chocolate Avenue, Hershey, PA 17033-1240, USA, www.igi-global.com. This series is composed of titles available for purchase individually; each title is edited to be contextually exclusive from any other title within the series. For pricing and ordering information please visit http://www.igi-global.com/book-series/advances-medical-education-research-ethics/132365. Postmaster: Send all address changes to above address.

Titles in this Series

For a list of additional titles in this series, please visit:
https://www.igi-global.com/book-series/advances-medical-education-research-ethics/132365

Impact of Medical Errors and Malpractice on Health Economics, Quality, and Patient Safety
Marina Riga (Health Economist-Researcher, Greece)
Medical Information Science Reference • © 2017 • 334pp • H/C (ISBN: 9781522523376) • US $200.00

Advancing Medical Education Through Strategic Instructional Design
Jill Stefaniak (Old Dominion University, USA)
Medical Information Science Reference • © 2017 • 349pp • H/C (ISBN: 9781522520986) • US $205.00

Organizational Culture and Ethics in Modern Medicine
Anna Rosiek (Nicolaus Copernicus University in Toruń, Collegium Medicum in Bydgoszcz, Poland) and Krzysztof Leksowski (Nicolaus Copernicus University in Toruń, Collegium Medicum in Bydgoszcz, Poland)
Medical Information Science Reference • © 2016 • 448pp • H/C (ISBN: 9781466696587) • US $225.00

Handbook of Research on Advancing Health Education through Technology
Victor C.X. Wang (Florida Atlantic University, USA)
Medical Information Science Reference • © 2016 • 588pp • H/C (ISBN: 9781466694941) • US $335.00

Optimizing Medicine Residency Training Programs
Jayita Poduval (Pondicherry Institute of Medical Sciences, India)
Medical Information Science Reference • © 2016 • 300pp • H/C (ISBN: 9781466695276) • US $220.00

For an enitre list of titles in this series, please visit:
https://www.igi-global.com/book-series/advances-medical-education-research-ethics/132365

IGI Global
DISSEMINATOR OF KNOWLEDGE

701 East Chocolate Avenue, Hershey, PA 17033, USA
Tel: 717-533-8845 x100 • Fax: 717-533-8661
E-Mail: cust@igi-global.com • www.igi-global.com

Editorial Advisory Board

Table of Contents

Preface xv

Acknowledgment xxviii

Introduction xxxii

Section 1
Overview

Chapter 1
Medical Students' Quest Towards the Long White Coat: Impact on Mental Health and Well-Being 1
Christina Ramirez Smith, University of the Bahamas, Bahamas

Section 2
Problems, Issues, and Controversies

Chapter 2
Medical Students' Perceived Stigma in Seeking Care: A Cultural Perspective 44
Virginia Joseph, Spartan Health Science University, Saint Lucia
Jozelle M Miller, Milton Cato Memorial Hospital, Saint Vincent and the Grenadines

Chapter 3
Perfectionism: Addressing Lofty Expectations in Medical School 68
Samantha Ilia Smith, West Virginia School of Osteopathic Medicine, USA
Mitchell Dandignac, West Virginia School of Osteopathic Medicine, USA

Chapter 4
Medical Student Burnout: A Social Cognitive Learning Perspective on Medical Student Mental Health and Wellness 92
Robert Lubin, Technion – Israel Institute of Technology, Israel
Michael D. Hamlin, Touro University Worldwide, Israel

Chapter 5
Deliberate Self-Harm and Suicide Ideology in Medical Students 122
Vinod Gopalan, Griffith University, Australia
Erick Chan, Griffith University, Australia
Debbie Thao Thanh Ho, Griffith University, Australia

Section 3
Graduate Medical Education

Chapter 6
From Medical Student to Medical Resident: Graduate Medical Education and Mental Health in the United States 145
Warren G. McDonald, Methoodist University, USA
Matt Martin, Southern Regional Area Health Education Center, USA
Lenard D. Salzberg, Southern Regional Area Health Education Center, USA

Section 4
Solutions

Chapter 7
Resident Physician and Medical Academic Faculty Burnout: A Review of Current Literature 171
Emma A. Omoruyi, University of Texas Health Science Center at Houston, USA
Fehintola Omidele, Johns Hopkins Bloomberg School of Public Health, USA

Chapter 8
Developing a Comprehensive Wellness Program for Medical Students............190
LaTanya Love, The University of Texas Health Science Center at Houston, USA
Dana McDowelle, The University of Texas Health Science Center at Houston, USA

Chapter 9
Medical School Wellness Initiatives 209
Lynda Tierney Konecny, A. T. Still University, USA

Section 5
The Future

Chapter 10
Essentials for Education and Training for Tomorrow's Physicians 230
Timothy Edward A. Barrett, University of the West Indies, Bahamas

Conclusion 253

Appendix 263

Glossary 270

Compilation of References 297

About the Contributors 340

Index 346

Detailed Table of Contents

Preface xv

Acknowledgment xxviii

Introduction xxxii

Section 1
Overview

Chapter 1
Medical Students' Quest Towards the Long White Coat: Impact on Mental Health and Well-Being 1
Christina Ramirez Smith, University of the Bahamas, Bahamas

Every year across the globe, thousands of students begin the quest towards becoming a medical doctor and donning a long white coat. Global research indicates that after beginning medical education, medical students' mental health and well-being dramatically declines. The loss of well-being continues into the residency and practice of medicine. The aim of this chapter is to broadly examine the pressures unique to medical students within the context of medical education training, higher education, and the general population. A call for medical education to adopt innovative policy, plans, and administrative and curricular changes designed to foster a culture conducive to the long-term positive mental health and well-being of medical students during training and into the internship and long-term practice of medicine concludes the chapter.

Section 2
Problems, Issues, and Controversies

Chapter 2
Medical Students' Perceived Stigma in Seeking Care: A Cultural Perspective 44
Virginia Joseph, Spartan Health Science University, Saint Lucia
Jozelle M Miller, Milton Cato Memorial Hospital, Saint Vincent and the Grenadines

This chapter discusses the stigma and the barriers, which hinder medical students from seeking help for both physical and mental health conditions. Stigma will also be explored from a cultural perspective; the authors will demonstrate how it is embedded in help seeking behaviour. The authors will explore the existing literature to highlight these issues, and demonstrate how negative help seeking behaviour contributes to the poor academic performance of the students, as well produces chronic mental and physical health conditions. Solutions and interventions to address this perceived stigma will also be discussed. The authors will emphasise the importance of educators and staff of medical schools taking a more proactive role, in providing the necessary environment to facilitate such change in behaviour, by implementing some of these interventions.

Chapter 3
Perfectionism: Addressing Lofty Expectations in Medical School 68
Samantha Ilia Smith, West Virginia School of Osteopathic Medicine, USA
Mitchell Dandignac, West Virginia School of Osteopathic Medicine, USA

Perfectionism is the refusal to accept any standard short of perfect. Perfectionist students might strive for 'faultless performance, meticulous attention to detail and high levels of competency'. In a field as complex and advanced as medicine, faultless performance is unrealistically expected. This chapter will discuss how the rigours of medical school promote perfectionistic behaviours in students. What is perfectionism? How does perfectionism in medical school affect students? How can educators and administrators identify perfectionism, provide psychoeducation, or address maladaptive perfectionism? How can students address perfectionism? It is essential to recognise perfectionism in medical students as research has shown that maladaptive perfectionism has been correlated to physician suicide. The chapter concludes with recommendations on how students and medical educators can employ strategies to promote sound mental health and wellbeing during medical school.

Chapter 4
Medical Student Burnout: A Social Cognitive Learning Perspective on Medical Student Mental Health and Wellness 92
Robert Lubin, Technion – Israel Institute of Technology, Israel
Michael D. Hamlin, Touro University Worldwide, Israel

Medical students' mental health is a topic of great interest as it has implications not only for medical students but also for the patients of these future doctors. Medical students face many academic pressures and burnout is one possible consequence of these stressors with some studies suggesting that burnout affects up to 50% of medical students. Our own study of American students in a medical programme located outside of the U.S. showed that student perceptions of the medical learning environment were linked with burnout suggesting that reducing burnout requires a pedagogical approach that addresses academically related stress factors. This chapter contends that one institutional strategy to prevent problems such as burnout is to adopt a theory-based approach to instructional design that addresses the causes of medical student stress and burnout from the instructional side.

Chapter 5
Deliberate Self-Harm and Suicide Ideology in Medical Students 122
Vinod Gopalan, Griffith University, Australia
Erick Chan, Griffith University, Australia
Debbie Thao Thanh Ho, Griffith University, Australia

The risk of deliberate self-harm (DSH) and suicide ideology in medical students is a pertinent issue that has received a surge in attention over recent years. Medical students are at risk of normalisation of DSH and suicide ideology despite their mental health literacy levels and are still susceptible to the stigma of help-seeking for their mental wellbeing. This chapter will explore assessment, preventative and management strategies to improve education, awareness and ultimately reduce the rates of DSH and suicide risk. A comprehensive review of practices and techniques that medical training community and their family members could utilise to aid medical students to adequately and safety manage DSH and suicide ideology. This will assist in identifying crucial areas for future research to aid students, professionals, family and friends in supporting medical student health to optimise mental health overall wellbeing of medical students.

Section 3
Graduate Medical Education

Chapter 6
From Medical Student to Medical Resident: Graduate Medical Education and Mental Health in the United States 145
Warren G. McDonald, Methoodist University, USA
Matt Martin, Southern Regional Area Health Education Center, USA
Lenard D. Salzberg, Southern Regional Area Health Education Center, USA

The transition from medical school to board-certified medical practice includes a period of intense, practical training known as medical residency. Medical residents are at risk for greater mental health distress than the general population. Interns, which are first year residents, are most at risk for, at worst, depression and suicidal ideation, and, at best, negative outlooks on the medical profession. Risk factors include role transition, decreased sleep, relocation, isolation, stigma toward mental health problems and treatment, and health care industry changes. Untreated mental health problems can lead to burnout later during a physician's career. Residents thrive on social and organisational support which can include systematic screening and treatment of mental health problems. Although research regarding best practices for addressing mental health problems during residency is limited, we offer four core strategies for preventing and addressing mental health problems in medical residents: education, screening, treatment, and support.

Section 4
Solutions

Chapter 7
Resident Physician and Medical Academic Faculty Burnout: A Review of Current Literature 171
Emma A. Omoruyi, University of Texas Health Science Center at Houston, USA
Fehintola Omidele, Johns Hopkins Bloomberg School of Public Health, USA

Physician burnout finds its roots in both undergraduate and graduate medical education and has emerged as an important cause of academic faculty turnover. Recognition of the need for resiliency training has led to the development and implementation of wellness programmes throughout the country and world. This chapter examines the causes and potential solutions of combating resident physician and academic faculty burnout in medical education. The authors reviewed current literature on wellness programmes in medical education, including both traditional and curricular approaches and provide a template for creating a well-rounded wellness programme to promote resident physician and academic faculty wellness.

Chapter 8
Developing a Comprehensive Wellness Program for Medical Students............190
LaTanya Love, The University of Texas Health Science Center at Houston, USA
Dana McDowelle, The University of Texas Health Science Center at Houston, USA

This chapter addresses the various components that go into the development of a comprehensive wellness programme. Medical school can be a difficult time for students and some will experience an increase in burnout, stress, and anxiety that can lead to less empathetic physicians, decline in professionalism, and ultimately impact the quality of healthcare. Increased stress, burnout, and anxiety can lead to less empathetic doctors, decline in professionalism, and ultimately impact the quality of healthcare. One way to address these issues is through the development of a comprehensive wellness programme that addresses both academic and non-academic contributing factors. Prior to the development of a comprehensive wellness programme one must identify key stakeholders and assess the factors that are contributing to medical student well-being. Equal consideration must be given to both academic and non-academic factors that contribute to overall student well-being and incorporated into the design of a comprehensive wellness programme.

Chapter 9
Medical School Wellness Initiatives..209
Lynda Tierney Konecny, A. T. Still University, USA

In this chapter, wellness, and the importance of balance among wellness dimensions for medical students will be defined based on information found in relevant peer-reviewed and/or professional literature. Practical, evidence-based examples of wellness programme and initiatives within medical schools will be discussed. Benefits and challenges of the wellness program examples will be presented; limitations to programme results will be provided. Health education models and/or theory applicable to the needs assessment, development, implementation, and evaluation of medical school wellness programmes will be explored. Recommendations and best practices will be suggested to facilitate the practical implementation of wellness initiatives. A discussion of emerging trends will also be presented for future consideration.

Section 5
The Future

Chapter 10
Essentials for Education and Training for Tomorrow's Physicians 230
Timothy Edward A. Barrett, University of the West Indies, Bahamas

Education and training of medical students and postgraduate residents must undergo a critical review in light of the changing times and attitudes. The demands of life in general are enough to provide significant stressors for today's students in addition to coping with pressures of balancing passing exams with meeting the expectations of family and instructors. This chapter will highlight the realities of the effect of the pressures of study on the students' mental health and well-being. It will then describe several changes that can be made to the way medical students are trained which then shifts the focus to personal growth and development and away from the traditional goals of knowledge, skills and competencies for the goal of passing the exams. In the end, this chapter will challenge readers and institutions to pause and reconsider the current approach to training of medical students.

Conclusion 253

Appendix.. 263

Glossary 270

Compilation of References 297

About the Contributors 340

Index... 346

Preface

AN OVERVIEW OF THE SUBJECT MATTER

The central theme of this book is the exploration of the pressures medical students experience during medical school and the impact of these stressors upon their mental health and well-being during medical training and beyond. Physicians withstand one of the longest and most gruelling training processes in the world. Kathleen Franco (2013) shared results from a research study by the Association of American Medical Colleges which found that 6% of medical students are unsuccessful at 'achieving their dream in seven years'. A myriad of professional and personal developmental milestones during the pursuit towards achieving the status of wearing a 'long white coat', are encountered. For some students, these obstacles and challenges negatively impact medical students' mental health.

This book attempts to conceptualise various pressures that contribute to what is now recognised worldwide as a crisis in medical education: medical student, resident, and physician mental health problems affecting the ability of this group to maintain sound well-being. Evidence of this crisis has been documented in academic journals, social media, blogs, and top media and newspapers, all of which report the high rate of physician suicides in America—400 per year. This alarmingly high incidence of suicide is the equivalent of a medical school freshman class in some instances.

Issues such as relocation, which results in fewer support systems, feelings of isolation, sleep deprivation, and transitions in role, in addition to the large financial cost of medical education, are cited as common causes of stress associated with medical training (Dyrbye et al., 2010, 2011; Noori et al., 2017). Such stressors associated with medical training are purported to involve numerous risks for mental illness. Evidence-based research reported that medical students have higher incidences of ill health than students of the same age range and that of the general population. Issues common within the general population also impact medical students and include eating disorders, substance abuse, learning disabilities, depression and anxiety-related disorders, obsessive-compulsive disorder, and post-traumatic stress disorder. A unique characteristic found in medical students and doctors is the spectrum of the behaviours associated with perfectionism and neuroticism. These characteristics for high-achieving medical students may serve positively in helping them to manage tasks but may also work against them as a negative source of stress.

Becoming a physician is difficult, and once a medical student, the training is filled with specific challenges that confront students' abilities to withstand the pressures of long hours of study, constant academic evaluation of a massive amount of medical education, perceived peer competition, a medical school culture that is a system of formal structures (academic), informal structures (how the faculty and staff interact with students), and hidden curriculum, where the unspoken rules of engagement are either learned quickly, missed, or result in extra burdens upon medical students' abilities to maintain the resilience, persistence, and tenacity needed.

Issues such as stigma still pervade the culture of medical education, and although it is fading, most medical programmes are not yet equipped with faculty, staff, and administrators trained to recognise the negative impact stigma has on the medical school learning environment. The stigma associated with mental health is a powerful barrier to students seeking support. Barriers include the systems designed to assist students in distress. For example, the role a student affairs division plays within the medical school, although designed to assist with concerns related to personal and/or academic distress, is sometimes perceived by students to lack the confidentiality needed because staff might play a dual role in the institution. The time and number of staff needed to handle immediate situations might not be available, and the student might have to wait for an appointment (3 months or more).

There is insufficient time to seek off-campus help due to the demands of the academic day, studying, family commitments, or students' inabilities to establish a primary care physician in a new location. Oftentimes, the wait period for getting an appointment takes too long or is too far away from the medical programme location. Many medical students believe that there is a stigma associated with experiencing stress and distress because of the myths pervading the medical school culture, such as 'If I have a mental health condition, then it will damage my career prospects', 'seeking help is a sign of weakness', or 'I cannot take time off from my medical studies'. The invisible nature of mental illness might account for the stigma associated with seeking treatment or even the lack of recognition by professionals, families, and friends that something is wrong or 'off' in the student's behaviour. Unlike a physical illness that is more apparent, illnesses such as depression and anxiety frequently go untreated because there is an expectation that if a student gets into medical school, then, automatically, the ability to handle the stress is present.

Sometimes, students are barriers to themselves as they attempt to treat their own symptoms or do not even recognise that something is seriously amiss. Subtle behaviours amongst faculty and staff where poor self-care is the model students observe may result in an unintended message that incites copying of bad habits. The influence of academic faculty, staff, and administrators self-sacrificing behaviours warrants further research as to the impact on medical student choices in making their own well-being a priority. Added to the unintended messages in the hallways of medical schools, students recognise similar patterns of the lack of self-care found within environments such as hospitals, clinics, and the health profession. The modelling of healthy self-care and management is a systemic problem, and it is time for the medical culture to embrace its own oath of care by practising what they preach.

Research and researchers like Slavin (2016) shows that medical education training programmes have responded to the mental health crisis of medical students with implementation of wellness-type programmes aimed at the student's ability to provide self-help through engaging in mindfulness training, yoga, peer interactions, and some physical education or extracurricular activities. Despite the fact that the wellness movement has been positive, the underlying problems, issues, and controversies associated with medical students receiving the type of professional, confidential, expedient, and useful help needed to prevent mental health problems continues to be a challenge for medical education programmes worldwide (Hafferty, 1998; Rubin, 2014; Schwenk, 2010).

The time is upon medical schools to change the type of wellness activities from a reactive mode to a preventive mode, whereby, from day one, students are taught how to make their own mental health and well-being a priority. This means that the (formal) aspects of the programme's structure must be reformed to allow students, faculty, staff, and administrators to foster self-care habits in a positive and confidential environment. Medical education has a responsibility to practise what they teach.

BACKGROUND OF THE PROBLEM

The enormity of the problems associated with mental health issues in societies across the globe has seen a rise in international, national, and regional efforts to address the issue. The World Bank, the United Nations' sustainable development agenda to transform the world by 2030, and The World Health Organisation (WHO) comprehensive mental health action plan for 2013–2020 adopted by the 66th World Health Assembly are viewed as landmark achievements. For example, the WHO plan calls for changes in the attitudes that perpetuate stigma and discrimination that have isolated people for decades, and it calls for an expansion of services in order to promote greater efficiency in the distribution and use of resources needed to integrate and increase investments in the mental health budgets of countries (high-income to low-income societies).

Globally, the importance of the promotion of mental well-being is fundamental to the quality of life and productivity of nations. Currently, the hidden problem of mental illnesses affects more than 300 million people worldwide, and studies such as Rotenstein et al. (2016) have reported that greater than 600 million suffer from depression and anxiety disorders. Depression is cited as the leading cause of disability world-wide. Results from systematic reviews of the literature on mental health and meta-analyses indicated that 1 in 5 adults suffer from some type of distress, feelings of being unable to cope, and missing work because of a mental disorder and or mental distress. The prominence of the mental health global problem is linked by the commonality of issues across types of countries where high- versus low-income countries were found to have similar levels of people suffering with mental disorders. For instance, females were more likely to experience a mood or anxiety disorder and males were more likely to experience an alcohol or other substance use disorder.

Therefore, it is no surprise that institutions of higher education are experiencing a crisis with the traditional student body who are also subjected to stress and inimitable pressures of pursuing higher education. Diagnoseable mental health and student distress have risen dramatically on university campuses around the world. In the United States, the Jed Foundation (2014), an organisation that promotes mental health and suicide prevention, noted that more institutions of higher education are starting to prioritise student wellness. In September 2016, the Jed Foundation partnered with the Clinton Foundation Health Matters Initiative to create the 'Campus Programme'. More than 65 colleges are currently participating in the programme, which is designed to help colleges and universities promote emotional and mental well-being and includes reducing substance abuse and preventing suicide.

Examples of similar initiatives are also occurring in countries such as the United Kingdom, where a survey of more than 1,000 students (YouGov, 2014) documented the extent of mental health problems in UK universities. According to the survey results, more than a quarter of students (27%) reported having a mental health problem of one type or another. A significant finding emphasised that female students are more likely to admit to having mental health problems than males (34% vs. 19%), and LGBT students have a particularly high likelihood of mental health problems compared to their heterosexual counterparts (45% vs. 22%). Outcomes of surveys like YouGov reveal similar incidences of depression and anxiety disorders amongst young people globally, although there are countries with pressures and issues unique to the particular cultural environment and academic settings thus representing the values of that society.

Around the world, the mental health picture has changed dramatically in the past 20 years, and scholars, universities, medical schools, and governments are grappling with and racing to figure out how to handle this troubling international situation as we move towards universal health and well-being for all people. Higher education stakeholders who, by law, must provide high-quality academic experiences for their students are challenged to do the same in supporting students with mental health issues on campus.

There are lessons to be shared, innovative strategies, and international movements led by policymakers and organisations, including WHO, the World Bank, and the United Nations, to promote the mental health problem as an international policy matter that must be at the centre of a global agenda. The outcomes designed must help countries create health policies, increase health budgets, and provide treatment and services aimed at prevention and restoration of mental health.

WHO IS THIS BOOK FOR?

The philosophy underlying the promotion of health and well-being is based upon the concept of prevention, even though many healthcare systems appear to be disease-oriented. The aim of this book is to (1) bring awareness to the general public about the plight faced by medical students and students in higher education settings; (2) illustrate how the pressures associated with the pursuit of a medical education require a different kind of teaching and learning environment than the outdated structures in most medical schools today; (3) highlight in lay terms examples from the practitioners who prepare medical students for all aspects of training through a comprehensive examination of how medical education is addressing the crisis through the development of best practices in wellness programming on campus; (4) highlight several critical distresses—stigma in seeking help, suicide, and burnout in medical students, residents, and academic faculty—and examine the traits and life of a typical medical student; and (5) offer solutions and recommendations useful to a plethora of stakeholders concerned about the welfare of medical students: medical educators, health professionals, higher education administrators, counselling departments, student affairs divisions, medical student recruiters, admissions departments, mental health practitioners, primary care physicians, academic advisors, medical school boards, medical school faculty, staff, and administrators, policy officials, governments, families and friends of medical students, prospective medical students, current medical students, medical interns and residents, preceptors, physicians, and anyone who cares about the mental health and well-being not only of society at large but also, in particular, of medical students' and physicians' abilities to take care of themselves, and as a result, render quality care.

ABOUT THIS BOOK

The overall intention of this book is to advance the awareness of the problems that affect and impact medical students' mental health and well-being in an adverse way by presenting key issues, controversies and solutions to these hindrances. Some of the shortcomings of information available on the topic and the debate surrounding the pressures medical students, residents and physicians face are steeped in statistical and professional jargon. The book is meant to be informative so that the lay person connected to an existing medical student or prospective student may garner useful tips on how to support the quest of these hard-working learners.

The reader should know that several foundational premises underlie this book. First, the assumption is that not all medical students experience mental health and well-being problems after beginning medical school. However, the medical literature around the world agrees that the pressures of medical school significantly impact more than a quarter of any given student body. Thus, the problems some students face may be life-threatening.

Second, the focus of this work is on improving the teaching and learning environments in medical schools and at the graduate levels of medical education to promote a culture whereby doctors can get help for problems experienced without personal sacrifice to health and well-being or the ability to practise medicine. Reading this book as set forward will provide the reader with a comprehensive exploration of the book's subject matter beginning with chapter 1 in which an overview of medical education and the pressures associated with its system are explored.

Section 1: Overview

Chapter 1 'Medical Students' Quest Towards the Long White Coat: Impact Upon Mental Health and Well-Being', presents a general overview of the medical student and common pressures associated with the pursuit of a medical education. Findings from the literature in higher education, mental health, and medicine inform this chapter's objectives. Five questions are presented as a means of discussing the chapter's topics. Medical training is a long and arduous journey for students worldwide. An international crisis impacting the mental health and well-being of medical students has been associated with the pressures experienced after matriculating into medical educational programmes. The pressures commonly researched and reported on in the medical arena over the past 8 decades noted unusually high incidences of depression, anxiety, and related disorders in addition to myriad problems such as academic performance, isolation, sleep deprivation, fear of failing, and peer competition, to name just a few. Pressures such as these that result in an extraordinary rate of burnout and suicide are now globally recognised as major threats to healthcare systems.

The chapter presents several definitions to establish what it means to have good mental health and what well-being attributes contribute to sound mental health. Additionally, a general scan of the literature on the problems associated with mental health in society in general and their trickle-down effects on students pursuing higher and medical education is presented as a means of putting the problem of medical students' mental health in context. The author briefly discusses some of the prevalent characteristics commonly associated with medical students and offers a profile of what a typical medical student life looks like. The chapter concludes with solutions and recommendations for stakeholders directly involved in the training, guidance, and hiring of future doctors.

Section 2: Problems, Issues, and Controversies

Section 2 of this book is comprised of four chapters that focus upon hot-button problems associated with medical students' mental health and well-being: stigma, perfectionism, burnout, and suicide.

Stigma

Stigma is cited most often in medical and mental health literature as a barrier preventing people with mental health problems from seeking help. Research about medical students specifically reports that there is a major problem facing medical students as they seek help for their mental and medical health issues, which impacts both their well-being and their academic performance. Chapter 2 will highlight and discuss some of these major barriers that influence students seeking help, such as the stigma towards mental health, student culture, and issues around confidentiality and trust. Importantly, the authors make recommendations and propose solutions aimed at fostering changes in the attitudes of medical students towards seeking help. Emphasis is placed on the importance for medical school educators and staff to take a more proactive role in providing and facilitating the necessary environment pivotal for such change in behaviour through the implementation of some of these interventions. The authors hope this chapter will not only shed light on an important phenomenon but also allow for behaviour change and tolerance as it relates to a patient's (be it a medical student or not) human right to seek out needed care in a safe, confidential, and equipped environment.

Perfectionism

Chapter 3 describes the impact of a common characteristic seen in the medical profession and in medical students: perfectionism. The stressors associated with this personality trait are presented from two authors' perspectives, one a learning specialist who works with medical students and one from a third-year medical student. Perfectionism is the refusal to accept any standard short of flawless. Perfectionistic students might strive for 'faultless performance, meticulous attention to detail and high levels of competency' (Humphris & Kaney, 1998). This may seem like a noble idea, but there are several potential pitfalls to this approach. In a field as complex and advanced as medicine, faultless performance is usually not an option. Mistakes are bound to be made, and part of gaining mastery of the material is learning from those mistakes and through trial and error. Why do we strive for perfection? Is it to satisfy the expectations of others? Is it to satisfy our expectations of ourselves? Why do some of us hold such expectations? These are just a few of the questions explored in Chapter 3. The authors of the chapter present suggestions and recommendations for medical students, medical academic faculty and administrators from their personal experiences as well as from the evidenced-based literature on how to address this characteristic.

Burnout

Chapter 4 deals with the topic of medical students' mental health, which has implications not only for medical students but also for patients of these future doctors. Academic pressures, including overwhelming amounts of material to learn in short periods of time, unclear expectations, and the current shift from mostly didactic instruction to one that is focused on patient care, contribute to excessive stresses during medical school. Burnout is one possible consequence of these stressors, and studies suggest that burnout affects up to 50% of medical students. The authors' study of American students in a medical programme located outside the United States showed that the majority of learning environment domains were associated with burnout, suggesting that reducing burnout requires a pedagogical approach that addresses academically related stress factors. This chapter introduces a theory-based approach to instructional design that addresses the causes of medical student stress and burnout from the curricular perspective of medical training.

Suicide

This chapter (5) deals with the most difficult and sad issue of suicide. Stress and anxiety resulting from the competitiveness of medical school are possible causes of depressive and suicidal symptomatology in medical students, and the authors contend that restructuring medical school curricula and student evaluations could ameliorate the medical school experience. The risk of deliberate self-harm and suicide ideology in medical students is a pertinent issue that has received a surge of attention in recent years. Medical students are at risk of normalisation of deliberate self-harm and suicide ideology despite their mental health literacy levels and are still susceptible to the stigma of help-seeking for their mental well-being. This chapter explores assessment, preventive, and management strategies to improve education and awareness and ultimately to reduce the rates of deliberate self-harm and suicide risk. The authors provide a comprehensive review of practices and techniques that the medical training community and its family members could utilise to aid medical students to adequately and safely manage deliberate self-harm and suicide ideology. The chapter provides a definition of deliberate self-harm and suicide ideology as well as their relation to each other and the impact of these behaviours on medical students. This chapter will assist in identifying crucial areas for future research to aid students, professionals, families, and friends in supporting medical student health to optimise mental health and the overall well-being of medical students. The chapter concludes with pertinent information on current screening methods and recommendations for clinical practise, medical educators, and administrators.

Section 3: Graduate Medical Education

This section of the book is composed of one chapter that offers insight into a critical transition in the life of medical students who, after graduation, progress to the internship and residency. This passage represents a major life shift for medical students who, on the day of graduation from undergraduate medical education, are deemed ready to assume the full rights and responsibilities of a physician. An important discussion in Chapter 6 is the imperative need to address the high-stress environment under which medical residents work.

Residents and Graduate Medical Education

The residency represents passage into the graduate medical education phase of a physician's training, and the newly minted doctor is referred to as the 'resident'. The transition from medical school to board-certified medical practice includes a period of intense, practical training known as medical residency. Medical residents are at risk for greater mental health distress than the general population. Interns, who are first-year residents, are most at risk for, at worst, depression and suicidal ideation and, at best, negative outlooks on the medical profession. Risk factors include role transition, decreased sleep, relocation, isolation, stigma towards mental health problems and treatment, and healthcare industry changes. Untreated mental health problems can lead to later burnout during a physician's career. Residents thrive on social and organisational support, which can include systematic screening and treatment of mental health problems. Although research regarding best practises for addressing mental health problems during residency is limited, the authors offer four core strategies for preventing and addressing mental health problems in medical residents: education, screening, treatment, and support.

Section 4: Solutions

This section of the book contains three chapters, each presenting solutions and recommendations based upon lessons learnt in medical education. The information herein is particularly suited for those faculty and other stakeholders responsible for preparing medical students. Guidelines are shared on how to prevent many of the pressures experienced during medical education by teaching future doctors how to take care of themselves first and creating twenty-first century curricula that teaches to the whole student and extends the traditional science-based teaching methods that only academically teach future doctors about medicine. Chapter 7 provides instruction on how medical educators can develop programmes to promote positive mental health and well-being. Chapter 8 is a primer on how to develop a comprehensive wellness programme. Chapter 9 completes the section with a discussion that challenges how medical students are taught and presents a paradigm for restructuring medical education to focus on preparing physicians who are trained from a curricular perspective that extends beyond the traditional medical academic curriculum. Instead, medical education ought to reconsider what components of the curriculum should be reformed to enhance the essential training required to produce 'good doctors'. The synopsis of these four chapters which follows describes the content in more detail.

Resident Physician and Medical Academic Faculty Burnout and Wellness

Chapter 7 introduces this section with a discussion of the role burnout plays on physicians, residents and academic faculty in the medical education environment. The impact of stress on the teaching faculty in medical education has not been researched widely, and the authors a practising paediatrician and a medical school administrator, present a meaningful discussion on how faculty burnout negatively influences medical students. A brief review of the extant literature on this topic concludes the chapter, along with solutions and recommendations for medical educators to consider when developing a well-rounded wellness programme to meet the mental health and well-being needs of these senior doctors, faculty and residents.

Developing Comprehensive Wellness Programmes

The subject of Chapter 8 reports on the components that are fundamental in the development of a comprehensive wellness programme. Medical school can be a difficult time, and some students will experience an increase in burnout, stress, and anxiety that can lead to declines in professionalism and decreased empathy, which ultimately impact the quality of healthcare (Muzafar et al., 2015). Doctors are expected to be expert caregivers to their patients, but little emphasis is placed on the well-being of future physicians. Medical schools should consider ways to be more proactive in addressing the various factors that contribute to the decline in well-being experienced by many medical students. One way to address these issues is through the development of a wellness programme that focusses on academic and non-academic factors and is integrated into the formal curriculum. For sustainability of a comprehensive wellness programme, there must regular programme evaluation.

Wellness Initiatives

In Chapter 9, wellness and the importance of balance among wellness dimensions for medical students will be defined based on information found in relevant peer-reviewed and/or professional literature. Practical, evidence-based examples of wellness programmes and initiatives within medical schools are discussed. Benefits and challenges of the wellness programme examples are presented, and limitations to programme results are provided. Health education model and/or theory applicable to the needs assessment, development, implementation, and evaluation of medical school wellness programmes are explored. Recommendations and best practices are suggested to facilitate the practical implementation of wellness initiatives. A discussion of emerging trends is also presented for future consideration.

Section 5: The Future

Chapter 10 proposes curricular changes that will ignite a cultural and systemic change in how future doctors are prepared for practice. What should the medical education of twenty-first century physicians look like? Medical schools worldwide are still in the throes of re-engineering archaic teaching strategies based on outdated curricular in many instances. Dr. Tim Barrett, the author of this chapter, a practising psychiatrist, outlines the essentials for preparing future physicians. The majority of the chapter is based upon the author's experiences as a medical educator for the University of the West Indies medical programme based in the Bahamas in the roles of faculty and preceptor. The author contends that medical education must go beyond the traditional academic preparation and train medical students capable of practising from all a holistic perspective which encompasses academic and personal development training.

After reading this book, it is hoped that medical students, prospective medical students, and all stakeholders involved before, during, and after the medical education of future doctors will participate in the promotion of healthy medical education, residency, and ultimately, practitioners' well-being. Medical students are the caretakers of our health in the future, and it is imperative that support for self-care is taught, fostered, and modelled from day one of medical school training.

REFERENCES

Dyrbye, L. N., Power, D. V., Stanford Massie, F., Eacker, A., Harper, W., Thomas, M. R., & Shanafelt, T. D. (2010). Factors associated with resilience to and recovery from burnout: A prospective, multi-institutional study of US medical students. *Medical Education*, *44*(10), 1016–1026. doi:10.1111/j.1365-2923.2010.03754.x PMID:20880371

Dyrbye, L. N., & Shanafelt, T. D. (2011). Commentary: medical student distress: a call to action. *Academic Medicine: Journal of the Association of American Medical Colleges*, *86*(7), 801–803. doi:10.1097/ACM.0b013e31821da481 PMID:21715992

Franco, K. (2013). *Understand Common Reasons Students Leave Medical School*. Retrieved from news.com/education/blogs/medical-school-admissions-doctor/2013/10/22/understand-common-reasons-leave-medical-school

Hafferty, F. W. (1998). Beyond curriculum reform: Confronting medicines hidden curriculum. *Academic Medicine*, *73*(4), 403–407. doi:10.1097/00001888-199804000-00013 PMID:9580717

Humphris, & Kaney, S. (1998). The encouragement of perfect health professionals. *Medical Education, 32*(5), 452-455.

Muzafar, Y., Khan, H. H., Ashraf, H., Hussain, W., Sajid, H., Tahir, M., & Ahmad, W. (2015). Burnout and its Associated Factors in Medical Students of Lahore, Pakistan. *Cureus, 7*(11). .10.7759/cureus.390

Noori, S., Blood, A., Meleca, J., Kennedy, V., & Sengupta, D. (2017, March 6). Current directions in medical student well-being. *Col Med Rev.*, *1*(2), 10–19.

Rotenstein, L.S., Ramos, M.A., Torre, M., Segal, J.B., Oeluso, M.J., Guille, C., … Mata, D.A. (2016). Prevalence of Depression, depressive symptoms, and suicidal ideation among medical students: A systematic review and meta-analysis. *JAMA, 316*(21), 2214-2236. doi:10.1001/jama.2016.17324

Rubin, R. (2014). Recent suicides highlight need to address depression in medical students and residents. *Journal of the American Medical Association, 312*(17), 1725–1727. doi:10.1001/jama.2014.13505 PMID:25369478

Schwenk, T. L., Davis, L., & Wimsatt, L. A. (2010). Depression, stigma, and suicidal ideation in medical students. *Journal of the American Medical Association, 304*(11), 1181–1190. doi:10.1001/jama.2010.1300 PMID:20841531

Slavin, S. J. (2016). Medical Student Mental Health Culture, Environment, and the Need for Change. *Retrieved from JAMA., 316*(21), 2195–2196. doi:10.1001/jama.2016.16396 PMID:27923076

Steel, Z., Marnane, C., Iranpour, C., Jackson, J. W., Patel, V., & Silove, D. (2014). The global prevalence of common mental disorders: A systematics review and meta-analysis 19802013. *International Journal of Epidemiology, 43*(2), 476–493. doi:10.1093/ije/dyu038 PMID:24648481

The Jed Foundation. (2014). *The Comprehensive Approach to Mental Health Promotion and Suicide Prevention on College and University Campuses.* JED Foundation and the Suicide Prevention Resource Center. Retrieved from https://www.jedfoundation.org/what-we-do/

The World Health Organisation Mental Health Action Plan 2013 – 2020. (n.d.). Retrieved from http://www.who.int/mental_health/action_plan_2013/en/

YouGov. (2014). *One in four students suffer from mental health problems*. Retrieved from https://yougov.co.uk/news/2016/.../quarter-britain-students-are-afflicted-mental-hea/ https:/

Acknowledgment

There are many people who collaborated to make this project a reality, working across time zones, through personal setbacks and problems in addition to carrying on with daily work and family responsibilities, thank you for an outstanding and supportive experience during the writing of this book.

Chapter Contributors: Composed of extraordinary collaborators from several countries: Australia, The Bahamas, Israel, St. Lucia, St. Vincent and The Grenadines, and the United States of America. The insightful chapters are based upon the combined years of experience of this groups' work with medical students, residents, and from their own backgrounds as practicing physicians, medical school faculty, administrators, learning specialists, counsellors, and current medical students:

Chapter 2: Ms. Virginia Joseph of St Lucia and Dr. Jozelle Miller from St. Vincent and the Grenadines whose compelling chapter on stigma from a cultural perspective will enhance the literature on this taboo subject in medical education.

Chapter 3: The voices from the field represented by Mitchell Dandignac and Samantha Smith of West Virginia School of Osteopathic Medicine, who were determined to see the writing of the chapter about the topic of perfectionism to its conclusion despite challenges of serious time constraints and long periods where it was simply impossible to connect.

Chapter 4: Drs. Michael Hamlin and Robert Lubin worked together through two time zones between California and Israel to complete the chapter on medical students' burnout.

Chapter 5: Dr. Vinod Gopalan with current medical students Debbie Ho and Erick Chan, representing The School of Medicine at Griffith University, Australia penned the chapter on Suicide.

Chapter 6: Drs. Warren McDonald, Matthew Martin, and Lenny Salzberg's informative chapter on residents and graduate medical education provides a candid look into the experience of residents.

Chapter 7: Drs. Emma A. Omoruyi, University of Texas Health Science Centre and Fehintola Omidele, Johns Hopkins School of Public Health chapter offers a look into the specific nature of resident physician burnout and addresses a topic of concern 'medical faculty burnout.'

Chapter 8: Drs. LaTanya Love, a practicing paediatrician, and Dana McDowelle, Medical Admissions Officer at The McGovern Medical School at the University of Texas Health Science teamed-up to write a thorough chapter designed to help the lay person understand the intricacies of medical education as students' progress through training from the first year of medical school to graduation.

Chapter 9: Dr. Lynda Tierney Koency, Professor at A.T. Still University, presents a comprehensive chapter about innovative wellness initiatives in the United States as well as a framework for medical educators to consider in the design of wellness programmes.

Chapter 10: Dr Tim Barrett wrote the final chapter in the book while serving as a consultant on the project by clarifying many details pertaining to the differences between medical education in the Caribbean, Europe, and United States.

Again, each contributor is acknowledged for the valuable contributions to the book. The dual roles of authors and service as peer-reviewers enabled the process of writing the book to flow easily. The completion of these double tasks are truly a mark of professionalism and service.

Editorial Advisory Board (EAB) and Reviewers: A specialised project such as this book would have been impossible without the support of experts in the fields of medical education, higher education, medicine, teaching, and psychology. The Editorial Advisory Board is composed of a team of experts who served as peer-reviewers through several rounds of peer reviewing activities. An extra commendation to the (EAB) whose members include: Drs. Calhoun Cunningham, III, Colleen Halupa, Richard Handel, Michael Hamlin, Harry Munnings, Vincent Nwosa and Samantha Smith, a current medical student.

Students and Educators: The editor is grateful to the medical and doctoral students as well as colleagues in the medical education community with whom the privilege of learning and teaching has been possible over these past 38 years. Knowing you, if only briefly, has made the difference in my learning, my work, and hope for a bright future.

Curiosity has led me to writing about subjects that I am passionate about and medicine is one of those areas that continues to hold my attention especially as it relates to the personal and professional development of future physicians. This book is a tribute in particular to medical students Samantha, Dan, Jena, Will, Clint, Bethany, Sara, Kevin, Julie, Megan, Shcarry, first through third year students at several United States medical schools with whom intimate conversations about successes, struggles, worries, and plans for the future amid daily pressures of doing well in classes, staying connected to people outside of school while working through the ever-present tasks associated with being a medical student occurred. Those talks, inspired the writing of this book along with information collected from residents, doctors, admissions officers, medical school student affairs officers, academic medical faculty, and other health professionals who answered a myriad of questions. The transparent exchange of ideas served as a rich source of learning for the editor. Without these forthright conversations, my curiosity would remain unfulfilled. To these professionals an extra round of thanks is expressed. A special note of thanks to Dr. Molly Zhou, a colleague at Dalton State University in the United States. Dr. Zhou managed to check in throughout the process and offered help at just the right time.

Finally, to Samantha Smith, a heartfelt note of thanks for your conscientiousness in completing the duties accepted to ensure that this project was accomplished. Your words of encouragement, 2-minute texts and WhatsApp consultations during your demanding days of third year are appreciated more than any words could express. Sam, your unflinching determination inspires me every day. Thank you so much.

The University of The Bahamas: The work of writing a book requires many hands and without the patient and kind smile of Mrs. Rosalie Sands at The University of The Bahamas, this work would have been insurmountable some days. The Librarian, staff and students at the University of The Bahamas' Law Library are especially noted for consenting to the use one of the few quiet study rooms for an extended period during the preparation of this work. Thanks again!

IGI Global: To the team at IGI Global Publishing, especially my publisher Marianne Caesar for understanding the technology glitches that occurred periodically while posting the work and for always promptly answering questions. Marianne, thanks for the outstanding work.

Family: My deepest gratitude is saved for my family: my daughter Samantha, who shares intimate joys and pains on her quest towards fulfilling one of her life-time goals of becoming a physician. Since the since the age of 8 with profound love of science and a level of commitment untouchable despite a number of setbacks along the way. Samantha encouraged the research for the book by providing a look into the customary and usual existence of medical students. Exposure to peers on a 'quick' Monday night supper of homemade lasagne presented a time for relaxation, laughter and a look at the tenacity, persistence and ability to delay gratification seen amongst her peers. These students stuck together to create a semblance of normal life amidst long hours of isolation and study. My son Sean, an amazing "thinker" who consistently reminds me that students today are wired differently than those of the past and respond best to teaching and learning environments that are directly related to something they can "apply" immediately. To my Mum, Leanna Ramirez-McGoran, a life–long learner, lover of knowledge, and the best teacher I know and my sister, Tasha Etter, for always believing in me no matter what the situation and motivating me to finish the book. These words of recognition barely express how the love and support of family empowers dreams. Being married to an explorer is not an easy task and may be challenging on many levels for my husband, Rodney. Thanks for letting me do what I love; learn, solve problems, make teaching and learning better for students, faculty and ultimately for society. This book would not be completed without his support.

To the readers, I hope that you find many ideas that you can use and share to make the lives of our future doctors fulfilling both personally and professionally.

Christina Ramirez Smith
University of the Bahamas, Bahamas

Introduction

The pressures of medical school can wreak havoc on medical students' mental health and well-being. Although mental health has become more widely discussed in recent times and is gradually becoming less stigmatised, the case is not the same for medical students worldwide. The fact that almost 200 medical studies have documented the serious effects of medical training on medical students' mental health provides serious pause for global concern and action. The impact of depression, anxiety, and suicide in medical school and the profession in general suggests that the underlying causes need to be examined so that the problems, issues, and controversies resulting in medical student distress may proactively be addressed.

Discussions about medical students' depression, anxiety, and suicide are most often presented in statistics and percentages that may be unknown outside the medical environment. For example, when numbers such as one in five medical students suffer from depression are reported, a comparison against the population may not be common information. However, upon careful analysis of the surveys and studies over the past years reporting on these problems, the truth is that medical students' depression is at a rate 15–30% greater than the general population.

An attempt to understand the problem of medical students' distress, as a phenomenon, may be viewed through an examination of the current state of affairs of mental health and well-being internationally, considerations of students pursing a first university degree, and students situated in professional educational pursuits such as doctoral and graduate degrees. Furthermore, upon observation of medical students lived experiences, the nature of medical education is exceptionally longer than the pursuit of other degrees, and this fact warrants further exploration.

Although medical students are reported to be healthy at the beginning of medical school, the demands and adjustments result in mental and physical health declines. What may not be common knowledge to the lay person is how intense the process of attaining a medical education remains from the beginning of medical school, through residency, and into practise. The amount of time to become a licensed physician varies around the world, but the lived experiences of medical students show a commonality in the massive amounts of medical information learned over the course of medical education. Some researchers report that more than ten thousand new words are learned by the time a student becomes a physician. Other stressors include constant evaluation of learning, lectures, participation in laboratories, hospital rotations, and being sleep deprived while living in fear of failing to accomplish the academic requirements necessary to transition through the various stages of medical education. Students in the first two years of training are self-reportedly stressed out, and many assume that the extraordinary amount of distress experienced is normal because of the demands of medical school. Unfortunately, as medical students' progress into the third and fourth year of medical school, the stress does not dissipate.

Like many high achieving students, medical students' manifest perfectionist and obsessive characteristics, which may make them more emotionally receptive to failure. The culture of medical education as perceived by some students may cause them to downplay health problems when they arise for fear of professional repercussions. As a result, self-care is ignored, a mental attitude of toughness is displayed, and self-sacrifice is endured. Unfortunately, medical students and even seasoned physicians are generally slow to recognise or acknowledge the anguish in which they find themselves whilst in the midst of medical school culture and medicine in general. The arduous journey and extended exposure to prolonged stress might provide some information on why medical students are increasingly presenting with mental ill health.

Medical school culture comprised of a formal curriculum, an informal curriculum, and a hidden curriculum (Hafferty, 1998, p. 404), along with the perceptions medical students hold about the nature of medical education, may contribute to the barriers encountered in self-seeking behaviour and self-care. Twenty-seven per cent of medical students around the world reported depression or depressive symptoms, and 11% experienced thoughts of suicide during medical school, according to recent research (Rotenstein et al., 2016). Upon recognition that medical education is challenging, it is imperative to also recognise that the stress some students experience is related to personal expectations for performance.

In addition to the traditional medical school population, there are subsets of students who have been found to be more vulnerable to mental health problems than usual. Minority students are most likely to report other stress-related issues outside the usual academic stressors. These problems have been attributed to negative experiences in relation to ethnicity and race. LGBT students suffer from problems of low self-esteem, feelings of harassment, and more feelings of isolation. Rampant in medical literature are findings from studies that show female medical students to be the most distressed, but minority females are the most stressed of all medical students.

The culture of medicine appears to silently endorse characteristics of perfectionism, strength, and overall ability to carry on no matter what personal discomforts may be experienced. The lived experiences of medical students necessitate a deeper understanding by society of exactly what medical school is like for some students and how it may negatively impact well-being. Because it is unclear from research studies how depression levels in medical students compare with those in nonmedical undergraduate students and professional graduate level students, in this book, any discussion of nonmedical students is offered as a context for understanding what pressures impact medical students' mental health, causing a degeneration after beginning medical studies.

The goal of this book is to offer information, increase awareness and understanding, and present guidance and solutions that will move the discussion of this serious threat to future doctors' mental health from a statistical assessment to a massive global restructuring of medical education designed to prepare doctors who are complete people.

Reading this book will:

- Provide a basic understanding of the meaning of mental health, well-being, and wellness.
- Provide a context for understanding who medical students are and what their lives are like during the process of medical education and residency.
- Provide a context for understanding issues of burnout and suicide as two foremost problems faced by medical students.
- Provide a context for thinking about stigma aside from its general definition by delving into the cultural perspectives that impede some students from seeking help.
- Provide solutions and recommendations for approaching the development of wellness programmes within medical schools.
- Introduce a framework for the preparation of doctors in the twenty-first century.

Why this book is needed today? This book is about the pressures medical students feel that are both real and imagined. As a veteran professor, educational administrator, leadership and professional development consultant an intimate awareness of the levels of depression and anxiety and related disorders in the doctoral students was not uncommon. At the graduate school level such as doctorate level, a heightened level of despondency was noticeable in candidates who otherwise seemed to have everything going for them both personally and professionally. In many cases, students were struggling with completing the long, difficult, and lonely task of researching a topic of choice, writing and defending a dissertation proposal in order to conduct research and complete the dissertation process which culminates in the achievement of receiving a doctoral degree (PhD). An inability to finish the programme of study became a colossal problem for some of these students. Issues of perfectionism, competitiveness, worry about debt, and struggles with isolation wore heavily on the student-teacher relationship and ultimately explains some of the low graduation levels from doctoral programmes.

While visiting a medical school and interacting with first, second year medical students, faculty and staff, the idea of exploring the parallels between the lived experiences of doctoral and medical students emerged. Observing a dedicated space called the 'Mindfulness Room' ignited a series of questions as to why such a room was necessary. Earlier during the same visit, a trip to the library rendered packed chairs with students hunched over wads of books, papers, and ears covered by sound blocking earphones. To the curious, at first, the students seemed immersed in studying. Upon closer inspection, some students were actually asleep, steering into space or surfing on cell phones. Body language was stressful and the atmosphere thick with tension. In the hallway, students taking breaks were eager to chat with a stranger and it was there that the conversations brought to light how pressured each day in the life of a medical student comes to pass. The memory of observing a medical student sitting in the semi-darken room, taking a break and relaxing on a bean bag, evoked thoughts of peacefulness.

It became apparent how the similarities in the doctoral and medical student academic experiences are and how both groups of students were pursuing courses of professional education requiring the ability to delay gratification and immersed themselves in an experience very few people would understand. Though, the educational pathway to these advanced degrees is teeming with long periods of isolation necessary to study while living in a state complicated by feelings of mental exhaustion and sleep deprivation. Observations of these students showed that many of these problems were confounded by very little time for socialisation or down time.

These experiences coupled with the memory of how calm that one medical student looked on a sunny day in the basement of a medical school triggered action into the examination of the reasons students partaking in arduous academic pursuits were at some point likely to encounter bouts of depression, anxiety and other ill health issues. A scan of the educational literature on graduate level and professional degree seeking student mental health and wellbeing related issues materialised. The information, though, was in the form of dated research studies, student blogs (medical student) and journal articles. A complete reference source offering an exploration of these issues, problems and controversies was unavailable.

The need for an examination of these issues became imperative and this book is a result of these experiences. A work of this nature would not be possible without a team of experts. This book is written by myriad higher education professionals, medical practitioners, and physicians and also includes the voices of three medical students. It is not intended to answer in any scientific way the questions of why medical student distress persists. Instead, the book is meant for the general public as well as those stakeholders vested in the education and well-being of medical students around the world to embrace the notion that the promotion and well-being of physicians impacts everyone on the planet in some way, and as a result, medical students' mental health issues are a global policy matter. Solutions to the problems and pressures are offered in layman's terms and call for reforms that must entail dramatic changes at the curricular and environmental levels of medical education.

HOW TO USE THIS BOOK

You do not have to be a medical doctor or have any background in medicine, mental health, well-being, or higher education to use this book. It weaves together information about the problems, issues, and controversies experienced by medical students around the world and offers solutions, recommendations, and a toolkit that anyone who is concerned about the mental health and well-being of medical students, residents, and physicians may find useful.

The book is comprised of 10 chapters divided into five sections to organise the thinking on the subject matter: pressures associated with medical education and how these stressors impact medical students. Chapter 1 commences the book with a general overview of the pressures commonly found in medical students' experiences during medical school and provides several viewpoints on definitions of mental health and well-being to establish a context for reading the book.

Section 2 of the book includes Chapters 2–5 and is intended to provide insights into the problems of stigma, perfectionism, burnout, and suicide. The authors of these chapters include medical educators from Australia, Israel, the United States, and St. Lucia who work first-hand with medical students on a daily basis as well as two student authors currently enrolled in the School of Medicine at Griffith University in Australia. The issues and controversies associated with the stigma perceived and experienced by students seeking help is discussed through the lens of a cultural perspective that adds another dimension to the problem causing medical students to avoid getting help when issues arise with mental health. Stigma exists in what is termed the hidden curriculum of medical school and follows students into residencies and practice. The authors of Chapter 3 provide a compelling discussion of the characteristics and pressures associated with being perfectionistic, a trait commonly found in high achievers, notably in the medical profession. Chapters 4 and 5 discuss two of the most prevalent problems faced by medical students: burnout and suicide. The long hours of study, prolonged evaluation of academic performance, exposure to death and dying amongst myriad physical issues including lack of sleep, poor eating and exercise habits, diminished self-esteem, and a loss of support from friends and family due to a lack of time or relocation to engage in personal and social activities have been shown to lead to a build-up of stress and anxiety. In turn, these feelings lead to depression and even suicidal consideration, known as suicidal ideation. The solutions and recommendations in this part of the book are based upon both best practises for preparing future doctors and the authors experiences.

Section 3 of the book contains Chapter 6 and addresses the problems and pressures experienced by residents at the graduate level of medical education commonly referred to as the residency. The poor mental health of residents is also characterised by high rates of burnout, depression, and suicide ideation. The authors are intimately aware of these issues confronted by medical residents and contribute significantly to a deeper understanding of how the transition from medical school to residency poses a crisis in graduate medical education. While this topic warrants more research to gain an understanding of the causes of mental ill health in residency, the authors combined experiences as medical educators and a physician venture to provide solutions and recommendations to help inform the philosophy needed to promote healthy resident well-being.

Section 4 of the book is comprised of Chapters 7 -9. These chapters offer the reader an opportunity to learn about the preeminent approaches medical schools and medical arena are taking to radically change the culture of medicine to one of well-being and well-ness. To that end, Chapter 7 offers a literature review on the problem of burnout in resident physicians, and an issue that warrants further study, the burnout of medical school faculty. The roles and responsibilities of medical faculty, in addition to research, may include long hours of teaching, preparation to teach, student advisement, and maintaining one's clinical practice. Many medical faculty are expected to conduct research in addition to general teaching duties. Faculty burnout may impact how they interact with students (informal curriculum) and ultimately negatively add to some of the pressures perceived by students who watch faculty work through sickness and respond to students' interactions, requests, and needs in a less sensitive or compassionate manner. The chapter concludes with a template for developing wellness programmes to meet the distress needs of physicians, residents and faculty. Chapters 8 and 9 add to the literature the depth and breadth of issues that ought to be considered when developing wellness programmes for medical students. Examples from medical schools that have introduced innovative intervention and services to combat the pressures medical students experience are included to aid in the understanding of the role adult learning theory and innovation play in changing the culture of medical education.

Section 5 concludes the book with Chapter 10 and is a proposal for addressing the core of medical school culture by asking the question: 'What are the essential facets of preparing physicians for the twenty-first century?' The chapter's author, who trained in medicine in the United Kingdom, contends that medical education must address the training and preparation needs of medical students beyond the traditional academic format.

The information in this book is intended to increase awareness and to provide an educational perspective and resources that might help current medical students, their families and friends, prospective medical students, and everyone who is associated with the training of future doctors. Read the individual chapters, book sections, or better yet, the entire book, and share your insights with other concerned citizens.

Be aware that this book is not a substitute for scientific research or a definitive resource on the topics presented. It is, however, written to focus attention on a global crisis impacting our future physicians. Educating and promoting good mental health and well-being is of concern to everyone. Taking charge of the education of medical students so they learn from day one how to take care of themselves first could impact the care you receive in the future.

Section 1
Overview

Chapter 1
Medical Students' Quest Towards the Long White Coat:
Impact on Mental Health and Well-Being

Christina Ramirez Smith
University of the Bahamas, Bahamas

ABSTRACT

Every year across the globe, thousands of students begin the quest towards becoming a medical doctor and donning a long white coat. Global research indicates that after beginning medical education, medical students' mental health and well-being dramatically declines. The loss of well-being continues into the residency and practice of medicine. The aim of this chapter is to broadly examine the pressures unique to medical students within the context of medical education training, higher education, and the general population. A call for medical education to adopt innovative policy, plans, and administrative and curricular changes designed to foster a culture conducive to the long-term positive mental health and well-being of medical students during training and into the internship and long-term practice of medicine concludes the chapter.

INTRODUCTION

The 'long white coat' is the symbol of the medical profession and universally worn by physicians (Lippman, 2016). Patients, physicians themselves, medical and health professionals, and the community at large maintain some idea of what it represents. Each year across the world, new medical students slip on a short white coat and begin what the author terms a quest towards the achievement of wearing a long

DOI: 10.4018/978-1-5225-2811-1.ch001

white coat, symbolising to everyone the successful completion of training at the undergraduate medical education level, followed by an internship and residency leading to practice as a doctor. Along the way, evidence-based research over the past eight decades (Rotenstein et al., 2016; Strecker, 1936) has revealed that the prevalence of stress, anxiety, and depression among medical students is higher than the general population (McManus et al., 2009).

Studies highlight medical students' mental health deterioration over time (Slavin, 2016; Wasson et al., 2016). Clearly, it has been established that the pressures of pursuing a medical degree have a negative impact upon some medical students' mental health and well-being. The problem is considered to have reached an epidemic level (Gunderman, 2016; Hafferty, 1998; Mousa et al., 2016; Slavin, 2016). Given what is known about the academic competencies and personality traits necessary for students to succeed in medical education (Abbiati et al., 2016; Gunderman, 2016; Rotenstein et al., 2016), this chapter offers a brief examination through five general questions of the problems, issues, and controversies contributing to the persistence of the crisis regarding student mental health and well-being during medical school.

- Who are medical students?
- What is the meaning of mental health and well-being and the significance of the long white coat?
- Globally, what pressures contribute to college students' mental health crises?
- What is medical student life like, and what pressures encountered during medical education negatively impact mental health and well-being?
- How can the culture of medicine and medical education create policy, planning, and administrative and curricular innovations to improve the mental health and well-being of future physicians?

BACKGROUND

Who Are Medical Students?

Across the globe, medical students generally have attained an undergraduate degree at a university or college followed by a medical programme of study of 4 to 5 years of medical school (GKEN, 2009). Upon completion of the medical school curriculum, which can include a couple of years of classroom instruction followed by another 2 years of practical experiences, the student is awarded a Doctor of Medicine (MD) or Doctor of Osteopathic Medicine (DO) degree. Graduation from medical school is followed by the residency, with the length of time and training varying according to the chosen speciality. Clinical speciality training can be as little as 3 years and up to

8 years and culminates with board certification. In the United States, medical school training includes a period of 10 to 16 years of higher education, and postgraduate training defines the pathway to becoming a doctor (American Medical Association, 2014).

Medical Student Characteristics

There is current debate on which personal competencies are important for students entering medical school (Abbiati et al., 2016) and which of these characteristics could predict future success as caring, efficient, professional, and empathic doctors (Koenig et al., 2013; Mahon et al., 2013). While the academic requirements necessary to handle the rigour of medical education training are well documented (Monroe et al., 2013; Povis, 2015; Richardson et al., 2013) and include standardised examinations such as the Medical School Admission Test (MCAT), high school GPA, and undergraduate GPA, how to assess the personality characteristics for handling stress, motivation, and learning traits is not a standard process.

Although there is no single answer to the question of what it takes to be a successful medical student, medical school admissions website list many of the following characteristics deemed desired and essential for students to be successful:

- Strong academic background. Students must possess knowledge of the basic scientific model, biology, and possess scores from college grades and medical school admissions tests indicating the potential to succeed.
- Time management skills. The daily schedule of attending classes, labs, and related requirements is incredibly time-consuming in addition to the long hours of study. These activities pull students in many directions at once, and the ability to prioritise, plan, and stick to a schedule is vital.
- Personal motivation and ambition. Students must be able to persist and persevere through the long and exhausting routines of medical education.
- Interpersonal skills. Students must demonstrate the ability to collaborate with peers, faculty, and staff and to work with healthcare teams. Oral and written communication skills are needed to share information and to convey empathy.
- Professional conduct. This is assessed by personal integrity, honesty, and ethical behaviour. Students must be aware of their own strengths and weaknesses and know when to ask for help. Owning prior experiences where compassion was evident and a commitment to improving the human condition are essential components of professional conduct.
- Genuine interest. This is the ability to delay gratification in social and personal areas of life in order to put in the long hours of work necessary to learn volumes of information. A love of the material and a sense of curiosity

are needed to sustain the difficult and sometimes overwhelming challenges encountered.

- Stress management skills. Stress in medical school is a constant. An essential quality for navigating the process is students' abilities to take care of themselves when being intellectually pushed to their limits while being deprived of sleep and exercise. The ability to ask for help is crucial. Psychological resilience demonstrated through emotional stability, coping skills, maturity, an ability to endure hardship and sacrifice, and good judgement are fundamental skills.

In the United States, Belgium, and Canada, admissions departments have added strategies to evaluate personality traits of perspective students by use of the personal statement, letters of recommendation, involvement in extracurricular activities, on-campus interviews, and multiple mini-interviews. Situational judgement tests as well as psychological tests (Abbiati et al., 2016) are also used. Research conducted by Doherty and Nugent (2011) acknowledged that certain personality characteristics influence both medical students' and doctors' performance and that the personality trait recognised as conscientiousness has been found to be a significant predictor of performance in medical school. However, in the same study, the authors noted that the relationship between personality and performance becomes increasingly significant as learners advance through medical training. Other personality characteristics such as sociability (i.e., extraversion, openness, self-esteem, perfectionism, and neuroticism) can impact the mental health and well-being of medical students. Povis (2015) noted that good selection of medical students is 'an unresolved challenge'.

What Is the Meaning of Mental Health and Well-Being and the Significance of the Long White Coat?

The pilgrimage to obtain admission to and graduate from a medical programme is exceptionally competitive, and it is not surprising that the stress associated with undertaking a medical degree poses a significant problem for some students (Adsett, 1968; Dyrbye & Shanafelt, 2011; Hutchins, 1964; Lancet, 1980; McGuire, 1966; Strecker, Palmer, & Braceland, 1936). Furthermore, as recently as December 6, 2016, a major research study on medical students' mental health released in the *Journal of the American Medical Association* confirmed information about medical students' mental health and well-being known to the medical profession, but it was a shock to many worldwide. Specifically, the study pooled data from more than 195 individual studies of medical student depression and suicide totalling 129,000 medical students from 43 countries and found that 27% of medical students were depressed or had depressive symptoms, while 11% reported thoughts of suicide, and 15% had sought psychiatric care (Rotenstein, 2016). According to this study, the results support the contention that more research efforts are necessary to improve the mental health and well-being of medical students. Specifically, the report stated, 'The overall prevalence of depressive symptoms among medical students in this study was higher than that reported in the general population, which underscores the need for effective preventive efforts and increased access to care for medical students.'

While some studies report the high incidence of medical student and physician suicide, others highlight the deterioration in mental health of medical students over time and attribute its cause to the outcome of stress related to poorer academic performance, substance abuse, eating disorders, decline in personal self-care, and loss of self-confidence in addition to myriad distress symptoms and behaviours such as competitiveness, preparing for examinations, and hidden curriculum issues (Doja et al., 2016; Williams, 2016).

These findings from evidence-based reports on documented medical student distress to the point of decline in this population's ability to embody humanistic qualities and empathy (Schwenk et al., 2010) is at odds with the primary goal of medical education to prepare and graduate knowledgeable, skilled, and professional physicians (Mayo Clinic, 2005). Similarly, other researchers suggested that, on a personal level, some aspects of medical education may have unintended consequences that negatively influence medical students' mental health and well-being (Association of American Medical Colleges, 2016; LCME, 2003; Noori et al., 2016).

In addition to the known stresses associated with medical training, an added pressure is assumed by many students because of the purported prestige and power family, friends, and society believe will be bestowed upon the medical student after graduation. To understand how the perception of wearing a long white coat is viewed in society in contrast to what it means in the health professions is helpful in conceptualising how its attainment may present another unintended negative stressor in the lives of medical students.

The Long White Coat

For centuries, a white coat has symbolised the medical doctor. The long white coat today demonstrates that a medical student has successfully navigated the pilgrimage from student to intern, to resident, and finally, to attending physician. All over the world, students don short white coats to symbolise the beginning of a career that embodies professionalism, caring, and trust. In the United States, a white-coat ceremony is intended to create a 'psychological, intellectual, and ethical contract for the profession and promotes empathy in the practice of medicine from the inception of a student medical education' (Columbia School of Physicians and Surgeons, 2017).

Furthermore, the tradition of wearing a white coat began in the early twentieth century, as doctors previously wore black, formal attire. It is considered that the white coat was adopted to enhance the credibility and image of doctors as learned scientists. At Columbia School of Physicians and Surgeons, the tradition of the white-coat ceremony began in 1993 and is practised at more than 130 schools of osteopathy and medicine in America and at four medical schools in Israel and other countries. Today, a long white coat is still a symbol of status in the medical field and communities around the globe. Studies revealed that getting through medical school is challenging in a variety of ways, and the effects of the stress on the mental health and well-being of medical students has been documented (Dyrbye et al., 2005; Rotenstein et al., 2016; Slavin, 2016; Wasson et al., 2016).

MENTAL HEALTH

The beginning of a student's medical training is the best point at which medical schools should explain that mental health conditions are common and that there are students who had mental health issues in the past who went on to successful residencies and practices. Additionally, medical schools ought to clearly explain why it is critical for admissions officers to know about students' health conditions prior to the start of the programme. Open and honest discussions between students and the medical school is necessary so that proactive plans can be implemented on a student-by-student basis as opposed to the reactive measures most medical programmes offer in response to medical student distress. A powerful teaching point for medical schools is to clearly explain what sound mental health and well-being look like as a benchmark for students to understand how to manage their own self-care, and later, their patients' care. The consequences of these disorders in terms of lost health are tremendous. A sound state of mental health and well-being are fundamental to our collective and individual ability as humans to think, interact with one another, earn a living, and enjoy life. On this basis, the promotion, protection, and restoration of mental health can be regarded as a vital concern of individuals, communities, and societies throughout the world.

The implications, then, for medical educators, medical students, their families, and society at large are imperative in understanding what is considered good mental health and well-being.

The constitution of the World Health Organisation ([WHO], 1969) notes, 'Health is a state of complete physical, mental and social well-being and not merely the absence of disease or infirmity'. WHO (2016) defines mental health as a 'state of well-being in which an individual realises his or her own abilities, can cope with the normal stresses of life, can work productively and is able to make a contribution to his or her community'. The WHO (2016) definition clarifies an understanding of what constitutes positive mental health, and these traits can serve as benchmarks in recognizing the following:

- Mental health is more than the absence of mental disorders.
- Mental health is an integral part of health; indeed, there is no health without mental health.
- A range of socio-economic, biological, and environmental factors determines mental health.

According to WHO (2016), some factors to better understand the construct of mental health, as well as some related determinants of mental health, include the following:

- Multiple social, psychological, and biological factors determine a person's level of mental health at any point in time. For example, persistent socio-economic pressures are recognised risks to mental health for individuals and communities. The clearest evidence is associated with indicators of poverty, including low levels of education.
- Poor mental health is also associated with rapid social change, stressful work conditions, gender discrimination, social exclusion, unhealthy lifestyle, risk of violence, physical ill health, and human rights violations.
- Specific psychological and personality factors also make people vulnerable to mental disorders.
- Lastly, there are some biological causes of mental disorders, including genetic factors, that contribute to imbalances in chemicals in the brain.

Another report released by WHO (2017) indicated that the number of people living with depression increased by more than 18% between 2005 and 2015. These statistics are also found in a study completed by Global Burden of Disease (2015). A study by Baxter (2013) supports the findings that reveal an overall growth trend of the global population mental health deterioration as well as a proportionate increase in the age groups at which depression is more prevalent. Syntheses of the available epidemiological literature on the prevalence of depression and other common mental disorders have been undertaken as part of earlier iterations of the Global Burden of Disease study and are available through WHO (2015). Globally, the total number of people with depression was estimated to exceed 300 million in 2015. Nearly that number again suffers from a range of anxiety disorders. Since many people experience both depression and anxiety disorders simultaneously (comorbidity), it is inappropriate to simply add these two figures together to arrive at a total for common mental disorders.

Sound mental health is comprised of the emotional resilience that allows us to enjoy life; survive pain, disappointments, and sadness; and contribute to and engage productively in our communities and society. There is a personal sense of self-worth as well as the same in others.

WELL-BEING

There are many documented definitions and models of well-being. In order for administrators, faculty, staff, medical professionals, families, and medical students to embrace the idea of a multidisciplinary approach to proactive care for distressed students, it is necessary to establish a common ground for understanding what well-being entails. In the 2017 book, *Attending: Medicine, Mindfulness, and Humanity*, Ronald Epstein addresses the meaning of well-being by considering the question: 'What is well-being, anyway?'

There is no universal consensus on what constitutes well-being. The foundations of human well-being may be discussed in terms of sustainability of the environment and human spirit. Yet there is no universally accepted definition of sustainability. Despite this lack, maintaining and fortifying the human foundations of well-being is an everyday challenge. The foundations of human well-being are freedom, self-determination, intimacy with another, a social community, protection from the elements, food, water, health, entertainment, accumulation of things of value to promote human well-being, knowledge and opportunity to prosper, and opportunity to use one's talents. These foundations generally are linked to the culture of a community—a tribe or government (Vachon, 2012).

Epstein (2017) noted that when people have a deep sense of meaning and fulfilment, attainment of superficial achievements tends to be less important and may actually serve as distractions. On the other hand, people with a 'sense of purpose, satisfaction, joy and meaning' experience an intrinsic sense of fulfilment, and it is this deeper kind of 'well-being' worth pursuing (Epstein, 2017, p. 168). Another definition of well-being is based upon the 12 pillars of well-being created by Rick Hanson and used in the Foundations of Well-Being Program by applying what Hanson refers to as the four sources of well-being—recognising, resourcing, programme, and relating—to three fundamental needs of safety, satisfaction, and connection. The model provides a comprehensive strategy for understanding and applying self-care techniques to improve the quality of life. Other important definitions of well-being are offered by organisations such as the Association of American Medical Colleges (2016), who, in response to the crisis of mental health concerns amongst its professionals and students, launched a new Web site on well-being in academic medicine.

A recent study by the Public Research Bureau (2015) defined well-being as:

[H]aving an objective dimension—by determining whether an individual's basic needs for food, shelter, economic security, social relationships, and health care are being met.

Most researchers have examined two main aspects of subjective well-being as a dimension of well-being and found that because these two measures capture different aspects of well-being, using them together can provide a rich picture of life satisfaction and quality. A third type of subjective well-being, known as *eudaimonic* well-being, measures an individual's sense that his or her life has meaning and purpose (Deci & Ryan, 2008). Although aspects of this measure overlap with the other two, it is distinct in that it is based upon an understanding that people are motivated by factors beyond their own personal happiness or satisfaction (National Research Council, 2013).

A Centres for Disease Control and Prevention (2016) concept paper offers this definition of well-being: 'Wellbeing as judging life positively and feeling good'. From this perspective, the ideal of well-being integrates mental health (mind) and physical health (body), resulting in a more holistic approach to health promotion and disease prevention (Dunn, 1973). Some researchers using experimental, longitudinal, and cross-sectional studies found that well-being is associated with factors in the social and physical environment, with numerous health-, job-, family-, and economically related benefits, such as social connectedness, mental and physical illness, longevity, self-perceived health, healthy behaviours, and productivity (Lyubomirsky et al., 2005). Higher levels of well-being are associated with decreased risk of disease, illness, and injury; better immune functioning; speedier recovery; and increased longevity. Some researchers purport the view that positive emotions—central components of well-being—are not merely the opposite of negative emotions but are independent dimensions of mental health that can and should be fostered (Bradburn, 1969; Dunn, 1973).

Other research has noted that a substantial proportion of the variance in well-being can be attributed to heritable factors (Barry, 2007; Lykken & Tellegen, 1996) and that environmental factors play an equally, if not more, important role (Diener et al., 2006; Frey & Stutzer, 2002). The bottom line in considering well-being is the idea that a good state of mental well-being is possible, although an individual might be diagnosed with mental illness. Another way of thinking about mental health and well-being is to examine how it relates to the concept of wellness. The founder of the National Wellness Institute (NWI), Bill Hetter (1996), developed a six-dimension wellness model that has proven to be effective in the helping professions. This holistic model focuses on the following six aspects of life related to wellness:

- **Occupational Health:** At least two different focus areas contribute to occupational wellness. The first is creating a healthy work environment that can help to reduce stress, such as staying hydrated at work and staying active in the office. The second area focuses on feeling fulfilled. This means the self-recognition of the importance of work in which one is engaged as well as holding the perception that one's career is fulfilling.
- **Emotional Health:** The ability to balance the different priorities in life contributes to emotional health. Examples include balancing work, volunteering, family, and downtime. Being emotionally healthy means being in control of one's emotions and a general feeling of good well-being.
- **Intellectual Health:** Learning new job skills, vocabulary, life skills, games, or fun habits are all ways to enhance intellectual health. The opportunity to learn new things is an important factor in intellectual health.
- **Social Health:** This involves creating and maintaining healthy relationships. These relationships can help build a strong support system. In today's society, social health can also encompass cultural health—another common wellness dimension.
- **Physical Health:** This includes everything from physical activity and nutrition to hydration and even illness. How a person's body physically functions entails physical health.
- **Spiritual Health:** This can be closely associated with emotional health. Some medical schools attempt to address emotional well-being through activities such as meditation, yoga, and mindfulness training. Spiritual health is generally associated with a range of connectedness, which in turn provides benefits for one's well-being.

According the National Wellness Institute (1996). 'Wellness is an active process through which people become aware of, and make choices toward, a more successful existence'. The following three questions were devised by the National Wellness Institute to help individuals and organisations assess the degree to which wellness is incorporated into a particular approach or programme:

- Does this help people achieve their full potential?
- Does this recognise and address the whole person (multidimensional approach)?
- Does this affirm and mobilise peoples' positive qualities and strengths?

Supporting Hetter's (1996) wellness model, the Centres for Diseases Control and Prevention (2016) suggest that 'Wellness focuses on improving how one's body works rather than meditating or reflecting on a current state of being'. This definition of wellness places the focus on progress. This type of thinking can be useful in helping medical students create and maintain small healthy habits that amount to a complete wellness.

Well-Being and Wellness: Alike or Different?

Well-being and wellness are related concepts. Well-being is associated with numerous health, job, family, and economically related benefits. For example, higher levels of well-being are associated with decreased risk of disease, illness, and injury; better immune functioning; speedier recovery; and increased longevity (Pressman, 2005). Individuals with high levels of well-being are more productive at work and are more likely to contribute to their communities (Frey, 2002; Tov, 2008).

Well-being is a holistic state of being. It is an overall positive existence that includes being emotionally, spiritually, socially, and mentally grounded. A positive state of well-being is characterised by overall contentment and balance in one's life. To ensure a holistic approach to helping medical students cope with the pressures of medical education, concepts of mental health, well-being, and wellness are useful constructs from which the question becomes less about what the problem is and more about promoting high levels of mental health, something research has proven is associated with productivity, increased learning, prosocial behaviour, and positive social connections (Diener, 2009; Herrman, 2005).

Ultimately, the author contends that mental health is complex. Having a common ground from which an understanding of what is meant by mental health, well-being, and wellness will go a long way in helping everyone concerned about the deteriorating mental health and well-being of medical students to contribute to the prevention of mental health conditions in an open and honest environment. Students will have different needs and variance in their experience of mental health problems, including how they choose to think about their issues and whether they want to share their difficulties. Therefore, keeping in mind that mental illness or mental health difficulties can beset students at any point in the academic career is essential. All mental health problems are not directly related to the stressors and pressures of medical education. Slavin (2016) called for medical education professionals to recognise that the 'responsibility for student well-being should not be limited to one office and one administrator; student wellness must be everyone's concern'.

ISSUES, CONTROVERSIES, AND PROBLEMS

Globally, What Pressures Contribute to College Students' Mental Health Crises?

University and related organisations worldwide are grappling with many of the same pressures to manage the growing crisis of college students' mental health and well-being. A global scan of the literature in higher education associated with mental health problems and mental illnesses reveals a problem of great magnitude.

Kadison and Digeronimo (2004) noted that the mental health of university students in the United States has suggested that there is a crisis in mental healthcare in colleges. Research conducted by the National Alliance on Mental Illness (2017) on mental health on college campuses shows that the top five mental health issues facing students included depression, anxiety, suicide, eating disorders, and addiction. Other statistics noted from the same study showed the following:

- One in four college students has a diagnoseable illness.
- Forty per cent of college students do not seek help.
- Eighty per cent of college students feel overwhelmed by their responsibilities.
- Fifty per cent of college students have been so anxious they struggled in school.

Mascaskill (2012) found that the rates of mental illness in students equalled those of the general population, but only 5.1% were currently receiving treatment. Second-year students reported the most significant increases in psychiatric symptoms (Maunder et al., 2010). In their work on mental health problems and help-seeking behaviour among college students, Hunt and Eisenberg (2010) summarised much of the current literature on the prevalence of mental health problems in college-age students. The key findings when compared to the mental health state of nonattending college peers include the following:

- A lower prevalence of drug use disorders and nicotine use,
- A higher prevalence of alcohol use disorders,
- Approximately the same overall 12-month prevalence of mental disorders.

A summary of the scope and prevalence of data examined from the Centre for Collegiate Mental Health Report (2010) confirms that 'There is a general consensus amongst colleges and university counselling centres that the prevalence and severity of college student mental health is on the rise' (p. 16). Canada, the United Kingdom, and Australia were amongst the leading countries noted as having a strong interest in the mental health of youth, including college and university students. Adlaf et al. (2004) cited results from the Canadian Campus Survey that described the prevalence of mental health problems among Canadian undergraduate students. Four key findings from the survey indicated that students seeking higher education were found to present mental health issues, hazardous and harmful drinking, alcohol and other drug use, and gambling.

In the United Kingdom, an increased awareness of the importance of mental health and well-being at the government level is evident in the 2011 publication, *No Health Without Mental Health: A Cross-Governmental Health Outcomes Strategy for People of All Ages*, which sets forth a framework for its mental health system to focus on individuals by combining efforts with the community at large to improve mental health and well-being and to promote mental well-being for all citizens. Similarly, Scotland's (2012) mental health strategy was created to integrate system-wide quality for people with mental health issues. Wales's 10-year plan, *Together for Mental Health: A Strategy for Mental Health and Wellbeing in Wales* (Wales, 2010), demonstrates the international commitment to improving the mental health and well-being of citizens at large.

Factors contributing to the increase in students presenting with mental health issues are linked to the findings in the literature on mental health generally. For discussion purposes in this chapter, these findings are organised into three broad areas: general societal pressures, pressures associated with higher education settings, and pre-existing mental health issues.

General Societal Pressures

Support for the contention that anxiety and depression are a possible source of the mental health distress seen around the world in higher education settings is based upon recent statistics from WHO (2017), indicating that more than 350 million people in the world suffer from depression and related disorders. It can be said that today's students are living in an age of anxiety, and depression reports similar to WHO's statistics indicate clear trends in the increase of depression. Depression is a common mental disorder—it is one of the main causes of disability worldwide—and more women are affected than men. Specifically, in the WHO European region, statistics show that if anxiety and depression were combined, then 4 out of 15 people are affected by these mental health and related disorders.

Studies show that the rates of depression in America have risen dramatically in the past 50 years. Anxiety disorders are the most common mental illnesses in the United States, affecting 40 million adults age 18 and older, or 18% of the population

(National Institute of Mental Health). Nearly half of those diagnosed with depression are also diagnosed with an anxiety disorder. It is not uncommon for a person with an anxiety disorder to also suffer from depression or vice versa (Anxiety and Depression Association of America, 2016).

A possible explanation from the data regarding the college student mental health crisis is the fact that mental health and well-being distress are a global phenomenon. Underlying this assumption, questions about what is causing the deterioration of mental health in society at large should be considered. The causes are speculative in nature, but some scholars in the area of mental health and well-being suggest that the current mental health crisis has been influenced by rapid social and academic changes over the past few decades. Some examples of critical areas of change have been observed in areas such as the following:

- Psychopharmacology and the increase of the disease-pill model of mental illness has skyrocketed over the past few decades, reflecting the use of medication to manage psychological symptoms (America's State of Mind, 2011). It is worrisome that an entire report is an inventory of pill usage for the treatment of psychological and behavioural problems.
- Disintegration of the traditional family structure has been viewed as a source of contention globally, as research documented many problems that stem from the unstable environment and lack of structure needed for children to build a secure base. Instances of divorce, 'modern families', and confusion of roles have been cited as an enigma to providing what some scholars consider necessary so that children get what they need the most: predictable family structures and stable, loving, and supportive homes.
- Loss of moral compass and purpose, according to Barry Schwartz in his book *Battle for Human Nature: Science, Morality, and Modern Life* (1987). His work offers a fascinating sociological explanation for the impact the emergence of science has had on society, both positively and negatively. In particular, Schwartz describes how religion has been de-emphasised and replaced by a focus on materialism and hedonism, both associated with lower levels of well-being. Furthermore, Schwartz contends that the displacement of religion in society opens a door for people to construct their own lives based upon their own moral decisions. As a result, people are fundamentally uncertain of what they believe and why. They lack a philosophy of life.
- Along the same lines, another insightful book that presents a view on the inability of today's young adults to ground their actions from a moral perspective is *Lost in Transition: The Dark Side of Emerging Adulthood* by Christian Smith, Kari Christoffersen, Hilary Davidson, and Patricia Snell

Herzog (2011). One characteristic described is the confused state of purpose from which deep-seated problems may be created, such as depression, anxiety, and other mental illnesses. Students appear to be pursuing higher education to ensure long-term financial gain as opposed to developing a meaningful philosophy of life.

These examples must be viewed from a context of the larger societal values. It is important to bear in mind that the terminology *emerging adulthood* was coined in 2000 by Jeffrey Arnett to describe a whole additional period of development in the lifespan (18–37 years of age). It is attributed to the rise of the modern society and its complexities, thus requiring a longer period of development before functioning independently. This development is worth considering in respect to its impact on mental health and well-being.

Another possible issue impacting mental health and well-being is the fact that the economic upheaval worldwide in 2008 continues to wreak havoc for many people. The fallout of the economic depression is relevant to college-seeking youth, as more of them have to work to pay for college, fight the rising costs of attending an institution of choice, and live with the uncertainty of job prospects at the end of college. Mounting personal debt at the beginning of adulthood is overwhelming and discouraging, as unemployment or underemployment still pervades (FRB, 2003).

Pressures Associated With Higher Education Settings

College was traditionally reserved for society's elite until several decades ago. Major strides have made higher education more accessible to a diverse population. As a result, through legal changes, accommodations and support for students with mental health difficulties are available as part of most campus services. However, the transition is extremely stressful, in particular for those students in the traditional age range. In a time of 'helicopter' and 'snowplough' parenting, some students are totally unprepared for the stressful environment and competitiveness encountered.

The significant social upheaval experienced by students seeking higher education is a concern because a major risk factor for affective mood disorders can result from a lack of social support, especially when coupled with major stressors (Kashani et al., 1994). The stress associated with the transition to university life adds additional risk factors (e.g., Bryde & Milburn, 1990; Chemers et al. 2001; Gall, 2000; Montgomery & Côté, 2003). This frequently involves living away from home for the first time, having to make new friends, handling finances, adjusting to new learning regimes, and creating a new identity as a student (Scanlon, Rowling, & Weber, 2010).

Academic expectation and performance factors are often a surprise for students. In particular, those in the traditional age group who have been accustomed to getting top grades in high school may be unprepared when faced with college-level academic performance. Consequently, a vicious cycle of stress associated with poor academic skills and unpreparedness for the rigours of the higher education environment can result in some students' failure in the face of greater pressure to succeed.

Other sources of major distress for students are associated with the spiralling cost of higher education, especially in the United States, where the rise in college fees and tuitions has outpaced the rate of inflation while funding for higher education has continued to be reduced. The financial burden experienced as a result of policy decisions directly impacts students' abilities to attend college without working. In many instances, students work beyond the recommended part-time 10–20 hours; instead, some are forced to work full time, thus resulting in delayed graduation. Other noteworthy areas of problems and issues that have increased include drug and alcohol abuse, sexual assault, gender problems, family and relationship problems, and grief.

Previous Mental Health Issues

Mental illness is more publicised today than it was in the past; yet, in many circles, stigma still follows the people with the problem and is avoided by those around them. The attitude towards mental illness remains a dynamic that requires massive education, awareness, access to care, and a system that fosters well-being rather than avoiding these problems. Mackean (2011) confirmed that students experience mental health challenges right at the period of development in which they are entering the higher education system:

- The years between 15 and 25 are a natural age for the onset of mental disorders, an age where young people are pursuing higher education.
- Pre-existing mental health issues are more prevalent amongst students pursuing higher education.
- The prevailing stigma toward mental illness forces students and families not to disclose pre-existing conditions due to the fear and shame attached to these struggles.

The literature suggests that the failure of students and their families to disclose information about existing mental health difficulties during the recruitment and admission process creates another barrier at the onset of higher education pursuits. In addition to students' omission of mental health problems, a worrisome trend on many campuses is the inability of counselling departments to keep up with the demands for service from those who do seek help in a timely fashion.

There is a growing recognition that students with clinically recognised levels of mental difficulties are studying in larger numbers. It is important to note that some level of stress does not necessarily have to have a negative impact and can be stimulating. For all students, engaging in higher education can also make a positive contribution to mental well-being in that it contributes to the following:

- Provides a purposeful environment.
- Provides opportunities for personal and academic achievement that can lead to a fuller life, creating a sense of identity and increased self-esteem.
- Offers opportunities to build confidence, as new experiences provide the chance to manage a variety of demands.
- Extends through more diverse student bodies the chance to build new relationships.
- Provides an opportunity to make a contribution to a community while learning how to take care of oneself.

The evidence suggests that, with young people, early intervention can play a crucial role in outcome (Kosky & Hardy, 1992), so the task for universities is to make it easier for students to access specialist treatment by ensuring they provide adequately resourced services. Additionally, institutions need to help students capitalise on the positive mental health benefits of higher education while identifying and providing appropriate support to those who are more vulnerable to its pressures. Research on what causes pressures in students pursuing higher education holds many implications for medical education to benefit from the lessons learnt around the world in a variety of university and college settings.

Models of wellness to support students suffering with mental health issues require higher education institutions to promote self-agency, resilience, and independence in an academic environment that is not based upon a deficit model where only students who reach crisis points are offered support. Higher education institutions are not only seeking to improve the environment for students, faculty and staff, for the sake of students. By its nature, much of the core business of higher education means that student, faculty, and staff concerns are interrelated and interdependent.

The Healthy Universities Initiative (Healthy Universities Network, 2010) is a model for how higher education institutions can create holistic healthy settings for the support and management of mental health issues and problems. Healthy settings are physical and social settings, such as schools, workplaces, hospitals, and communities, that serve as supportive environments for health protection and health promotion activities (Yusoff et al., 2013)

Other lessons from higher education include the awareness that the response to mental ill health is the job of everyone in the institution. But it is imperative to remember that students often prefer to get help from those they know and trust—for example, family and friends. For mental well-being-related information to be effective, dissemination routes should encompass the whole institutional population.

Research on what causes pressures in higher education students holds many implications for medical education to benefit from the lessons learnt around the world in a variety of university and college settings. A conclusion drawn from research by Douce and Keeling (p. 6. 2014) reminds us that 'not all students who could benefit from mental or behavioural health services will come to the counselling centre today, or any day. Students may not recognise the need for or recognise the availability of services'.

The purpose of this literature scan was to explore the extent to which the crisis has been documented globally and why this crisis holds implications for medical education. The scan does not purport to be a depth-and-breadth review of the literature on this subject matter. Providing a connected culture of care will maximise learning and produce resilient and healthy world citizens.

What Is Medical Student Life Like, and What Pressures Encountered During Medical Education Negatively Impact Mental Health and Well-Being?

The lived experience of medical students involves a range of activities, pressures, and outcomes. In general, students perceive the medical profession as one that brings power and status. As early as the beginning of medical education, medical students experience feelings of omnipotence reflecting the role of physicians in society. However, at the same time, they face situations of pain, suffering, death, and social realities different from their own. Some students may experience an ambivalence of feeling satisfied coupled with the fears, demands, pressures, and insecurities of the medical profession. They consider that a medical school demands exclusive dedication, and indeed, they devote a large part of their time to it, to the detriment of other areas of their lives. When they compare themselves to other young people from other programmes, they feel that more is demanded from them. They also feel more stressed, more responsible, and less capable of managing their personal and financial lives. Considering these ambivalent experiences, students must learn to leave this 'mesh' and differentiate good from bad experiences in academic life. Thus, in the midst of this mix of sacrifice and renouncement, they also recognise rewards and satisfaction, leading to a sense of personal pride.

The fact that stress is cited as the single greatest impediment to academic achievement by both genders, with depression and anxiety ranked as the top reasons for the crisis in college student mental health distress, is significant. Similarly, issues of depression, stress, anxiety, and related tensions are common pressures experienced by some medical students during the years of medical education. To support this well-known situation, researchers from Singapore analysed 77 studies, examining nearly 63,000 medical students across the globe (Puthran et al., 2016). The results from this meta-analysis found that 28% of medical students are depressed and that 5.8% have considered suicide.

Distress in medical students is not just a first-world problem. The percentage of students with depression or depressive symptoms ranged from 20% in Europe to 31.8% in the Middle East. Medical students in North America had the second highest prevalence at 30.3%. Still, there were no statistically significant differences in depression by region, sex, or even between medical students and nonmedical students (Yusoff et al., 2013). Yusoff et al.'s study supports views that medical training is not an optimal environment for the psychological health of medical students.

It is important to note that the following discussion is a general overview of pressures associated with medical training and the fact that suicide, depression, anxiety, and related tensions appear to be the most prevalent problems experienced by medical students globally and that awareness of the cultural impact on students in different countries will vary. For example, in China, acceptance to medical school is not necessarily as prestigious as it is in the United States. Students with the highest scores pursue careers in computer science; for those whose examination scores are not high enough, medicine is the second career choice

To understand the range of pressures medical students are exposed to, the author attempted to synthesise from a scan of the literature how these problems manifest into issues, problems, and even controversy during the pursuit of medical education. The discussion is organised into the following three broad categories: academic pressures, social and personal pressures, and medical school debt on medical students' mental health and well-being (American Medical Association, 2015; Claassen et al., 2016; Edwards & Zimet, 1976; Tempski et al. 2012).

Academic Pressures

- **Formal Curriculum Stressors:**

The academic pressures associated with obtaining a medical education exemplify a culture of high achievement, commitment, connection, and focus. However, the configuration of many medical education curricula into three distinct learning and teaching segments as denoted by a formal, informal, and hidden curriculum provides a systematic method of thinking about the particular types of stresses experienced by medical students.

The formal curriculum includes what is to be taught, while the informal curriculum may be defined by how teachers teach and how students and teachers interact. The most controversial area of a medical school culture is known as the hidden curriculum. Hafferty (1998) proposed that a set of influences that function at the organisational structure and culture of a medical school is deemed the hidden curriculum. However, characteristics of the hidden curriculum, such as a commonly held understanding of how to behave, what is really expected of students, and what issues or problems should not be taken on, is implicit in student interactions with administration, staff, and faculty. The controversial nature of the hidden curriculum still needs to be studied in respect to its impact on medical student distress.

Most medical students will admit to becoming stressed out or panicked about life in medical school on a fairly regular basis. The programme of study varies across medical schools around the world in the scope, sequence, and length of preparation. What is common, however, is the transitions that students experience as they progress from one stage of training to another—for example, first year versus third year, then internships followed by residencies requires adaption to new a transition.

Noteworthy pressures experienced by medical students may include some of the following stressors closely related to the formal and informal curriculum.

- **Colossal Information Overload:**

Students are shocked by the extraordinary amount of medical information to be memorised and applied at some point in the near future. For many students, the realization that it is impossible to remember every detail from the extensive medical information, as well as master it, can forge feelings of stress. The vast amount of information in medical school is overwhelming, and during the first half of the programme, many students drop out (Karpf, Perman, & Higdon, 2006; Lazin & Nuemann, 1991; Lorgren et al., 2006).

- **Fear of Failing:**

The author informally discussed this topic with a third-year medical student who summed up just how distressing the underlying fear of failure can be for students beyond passing the medical school formal curriculum, boards, and other forms of evaluation along the pilgrimage towards becoming a physician: 'Just graduating is fine, but it does not matter if you do not match for residency'.

- **Peer Competition:**

Competitiveness among peers has been reported due to concerns related to continuing education in highly requested residency programmes (usually those with specialisation in areas of potentially better income). For many students, medical school is the first time they encounter equally smart, or perceived smarter, people. They deem them as threats, and this in turn might impact academic performance (Supe, 1998).

- **Mastering Medical Knowledge:**

The ability to not only learn a massive amount of information but also to attempt to master the material at a rapid pace can be a source of distress. This challenge is amplified for students with learning disabilities (Stewart et al., 1999). Additionally, students are faced with learning in an unstructured environment to prepare for the continuous high-stakes examinations at the end of each course and between transition years, such as the USMELE 1 or COMLEX 1, which determine academic advancement. The distress that may result from constant evaluation is also heightened because, as students rotate through clinical training, medical knowledge becomes more specialised, and rather than highlighting students' progress, deficiencies are amplified.

- **Bad Role Models:**

Unfortunately, it has been documented that medical school training is characterised by a decline in humanitarianism and empathy (Crandall et al., 1993; Woloschuk Harasym, 2004). & These traits are highly valued in the helping professions; yet, the apparent cynicism towards students by medical academic faculty, staff, and administrators appears for some to be a normal strategy for interacting with students. Statements such as 'Medical school is extremely rigorous', 'If students are not strong enough to handle the stress, then another career should be pursued', or just the dismay expressed towards students when additional help is needed can negatively impact students (Hafferty, 1998).

In a qualitative research study, Tempski et al. (2009) noted an insensitivity to students' needs and students' perceptions by insensitive faculty: 'Bad teachers and coordinators, and classes without a didactic approach worsen quality of life'. Much of medical student training involves performing in front of colleagues and peers. Students report extreme distress when faced with the negativity commonly observed during routine medical teaching and learning situations. Most medical students have a memory of a negative incident whereby, for example, 'pimping' resulted in a wrong response, and the resident insulted the student. The pain and distress associated with this teaching method—teaching by intimidation—has been reported as adversely affecting the mental health of students. The extent to which this type of teaching strategy is used in medical training is described in the book *How Doctors Think* by (Groopman, 2007), in which he explains that physicians are trained to always entertain the worst-case scenarios first in order not to miss important diagnoses. Instructors rely on the dynamic known as negativity bias and use it as a technique for pushing students to think critically. Unfortunately, negative experiences seem to have more influence than positive experiences. This is the thinking behind the continued use of the pimping teaching strategy, to the emotional demise of students (Vaish et al., 2008).

Personal and Social Pressures

- **Hidden and Informal Curriculum:** The pressures associated with the adjustment to the medical school environment extend beyond the stressors related to academic expectations and academic performance. Other sources of distress for many students, such as a deficit in hours of sleep, physical activity, lack of social interactions, and adapting to the myriad behaviours inherent in the informal and hidden curriculum of medical education, are problematic as well as controversial (Lempe, 2004; Parkernson et al., 1990; Tempski et al., 2009).

Students reported a variety of difficulties and crises during medical school (Tempski et al., 2012) that affected them personally and socially. According to Goldman, Shah, and Bernstein (2015), 'Medical training involves numerous risk factors for mental illness, such as role transition, decreased sleep, relocation resulting in fewer available support systems, and feelings of isolation'. Issues associated with the hidden and informal curriculum add to the personal burdens and internal struggles for students that include an inability to handle problems related to the bureaucratised medical school culture.

- **Bureaucratised Medical School Culture:** The organisational structure of many medical programmes is a source of contention for students, and in some instances, for staff and faculty. Specifically, the academic side of the medical programme is operated independently of the student affairs division, as each has its own responsibilities and budgets. Historically, the integration and collaboration between these two divisions remained separated. While this model seems effective, the resources allocated to each has a direct impact on the ability of the medical institution to provide a plethora of services that might be needed to support the mental health of students. For example, most dedicated funds are allocated to the academic side of the institution to support faculty salaries, research, and continuous improvements to the academic environment. The student affairs division that handles the counselling, learning support, and advising of students in academic, personal, and extracurricular activities is usually unable to meet student demands for help in a timely fashion. Additionally, students resist using many of the services offered by the student affairs division for fear that confidentiality might be compromised, thereby forcing a student to go outside the institution for help. Overall, the lack of coordination in meeting student needs between these two divisions is likely to be a barrier to students receiving timely support.

- **Informal Curriculum:** The messages students pick up from interactions with faculty, administrators, other students, and eventually, from residents and physicians appear to negatively influence and impact them. Medical students report being at the bottom of the medical system hierarchy, where they are often disrespected and subjected to abuse by allied health professionals and unsatisfied physicians, are unlikely to take proactive actions in self-defence. Adding to these stressors is the student's need to ensure strong evaluations and recommendations to advance to the next stage of medical training by making good impressions on supervisors.
- **No Time to Be Sick:** Some students' mental and physical health is compromised because they have not engaged with a personal physician. Others ascribe to the 'hidden' messages collected in the hallways of medical schools, hospitals, and related environments. For example, some students reported a lack of care associated with their own health and well-being according to the harmful habits observed and adopted by teachers (Thislethwaite et al., 2010).

When it comes to mental health and well-being, students afraid of stigma resort to self-care and suffer silently. The hypocrisy endemic in the medical school culture, although being addressed, is far from a reactive disease approach rather than a preventive model. Such a model would advocate first for the health of students and doctors before giving them the responsibility of ensuring the health of society at large. Many reasons are reported for student lack of self-care in addition to problematic scheduling to allow for personal well checks and follow ups with a primary doctor. Finally, studies have shown that doctors self-manage, self-treat, and enter into hallway conversations about their own health needs (Cohen & Rhydderch, 2013). Where issues of ill health are minimised and resilience expected, medical students learn coping methods from the informal and hidden curriculum. Furthermore, students learn to self-manage illness early in the process of medical education, which increases during training, where access to drugs becomes more available.

- **Student Abuse:** Amongst medical students, the perception of being taken advantage of or abused is common and most noted during the clinical years. However, institutional abuse, such as racial discrimination and unfair grades, has been attributed to prolonged stress and anxiety, hostility, low self-esteem, and increased use of alcohol by students who were affected by abuse (Silver & Glicken, 1990). Verbal abuse is the most common stressor within this category of abuse and includes cases of pimping, which involves being humiliated in front of peers, residents, and staff and produces high levels of pressure. The severity of verbal abuse is not reported due to student perceptions of potential reprisals or repercussions on performance evaluations (Elnicki et al., 2002).

- **Gender and Race:** The syndrome known as the invisible white coat describes the behaviour of patients who assume that the student is a nurse even though a white coat is being worn. This issue is a double-edged sword for women of colour (Russo et al.2006; Swift, 2017). used data from a documented study to analyse gender differences in perceived pressures and distress in medical students. Their findings revealed that female students appeared to be at a higher risk for anxiety than male students. Related to the higher level of anxiety found in female students was peer competition compared to male students who reported more anxiety in regards to the long hours. The stress associated with gender and race adds a significant burden to medical students who have to deal with an additional source of stress.
- **General Personal Life Events:** Personal life events such as marriage have proven to have a positive impact on students' stress levels, although having children has proven more stressful for females while in medical school (Katz et al., 2000). Personal illness and death of a family member adds to distress. Greater study into the impact of family member deaths and the illness of peers on medical students is needed.
- **Forming Professional Identity:** Due to the variations in medical school structures, curriculum, missions, and values, many important facets of forming a professional identity are left to incidents and information gathered by medical students' observations, perceptions, and exposures during formal training. Sources of distress related to managing the transition, especially in the third year of medical education when students go from classroom and laboratory settings to rotations where decisions and first-time experiences in dealing with patients, presenting cases, dealing with death and suffering, or being present at an unexpected death causes students enormous distress, as most have had very limited training, if any, on how to handle these aspects of the profession. Student training is deficient in this area of the curriculum. The informal curriculum conveys powerful messages about professional norms, values, and character. The unfortunate models of cynicism and unethical behaviour witnessed by students in the clinical setting is often shocking and contradicts the lessons taught in medical school (formal/structured curriculum) versus those learnt in practice. Students are left with conflicted emotions and an ethical conflict between doing what is right or following the examples

of seasoned practitioners to whom they rely upon for recommendations to advance. As one third-year medical student noted, finding a balance between being assertive and being an annoying 'gunner' is difficult.

- **Social Pressures:** Educational and clinical demands leave little time for the health and social activities that promote well-being. Many medical schools have buddy schemes and a wide range of societies to help combat isolation; yet, studying medicine can still seem exceedingly lonely. Medical students' schedules are different, which can be a barrier to establishing or maintaining relationships. Some students may not reach the typical milestones of same-aged peers because instead of thinking about buying a house or starting a family, the focus is on studying and working towards the next phase of the pilgrimage towards obtaining a long white coat.

There are varying attributes of social pressures experienced or perceived by medical students, and although not a mental disorder, the issue of the 'imposter syndrome' may cause distress. The imposter syndrome is characterised by chronic feelings of self-doubt and fear of being discovered as an intellectual fraud. The personal expectation set by students once they announce a medical school career to family and friends may compound the problem of pressures. It behoves medical educators to reconsider facets of medical education (i.e., shame-based learning and overall teaching style) and to optimise the medical learning environment (Villwock et al., 2016).

- **Medical School Debt:** Financial debt is a key determinant that predisposes students to depression, as noted by Jenkins et al., (2008) who established a clear link between financial debt and poor mental health. The impact of debt on the mental health of medical students has not been studied to a great extent. However, in the first study of its kind, Walsemann et al. (2015) posed two important questions: 'What is the association between the amounts that students accrue during studies and their wellbeing post-graduation when they are between the ages of 25–31?' and 'What is the association between annual loan student borrowing and the mental wellbeing of currently enrolled students?' This is the first nationally known study in the United States that attempted to examine the effects of student loans on health. According to Walsemann et al., the possible impact of these high debts could influence other life decisions, such as occupational choices. This finding is already evident in the medical profession, where a study by Phillips et al. (2014) indicated that medical students are staying away from family medicine practice because the income and rate of debts owed are not panning out, thus a significant shortage in primary healthcare providers by 2025 is anticipated and will be a be a major issue for healthcare. While medical student debt is increasing, the effect of debt on student well-being and performance remains unclear (Morra et al., 2016).

Having surveyed the types of pressures associated with the challenges and barriers confronting medical students, what lessons have been learnt, and what ought to be done to prevent medical student distress? The solutions and recommendations offered next result from the considerations of lessons students with similar challenges to mental health and wellbeing: college students, graduate and doctoral level learners.

SOLUTIONS AND RECOMMENDATIONS

How Can the Culture of Medicine and Medical Education Create Policy, Planning, and Administrative and Curricular Innovations to Improve the Mental Health and Well-Being of Future Physicians?

Currently, many of the proposed solutions to address student mental distress are externally designed and managed through changes in the resource allocation of the medical school, institutional policies, and evaluation activities that do not bear on the internal or intrinsic needs of future physicians. Although the hidden curriculum may hold convoluted messages of self-sacrifice that stop students from seeking help, there are solutions aimed at the prevention of common pressures associated with medical training at each major transition point in medical education designed to promote sound mental health and well-being. The following solutions and recommendations are general ideas that warrant further exploration and research:

1. A global network of curricular benchmarks and best practices to help students adapt to entry into medical education, thus preparing them for the huge academic requirements and fostering critical thinking and a realistic understanding of how to take care of themselves.
2. Specific strategies aimed at solutions for subpopulations of medical students who experienced other pressures within the medical school structure. Women, students with disabilities, and students from ethnically and culturally diverse backgrounds in many cases require more support in managing medical school challenges. All struggling students require opportunities for individualised support.
3. Train the trainers programmes designed to teach medical educators how to organise the massive amount of information deemed necessary for students to

traverse the medical school system. Pedagogical training in teaching methods will provide a structure within the curriculum to avoid both faculty and student burnout. Research is needed to determine how medical faculty are deciding what, how much, and the rate which medical knowledge should be imparted to students. Collaborative teaching strategies, where two teachers are actually in a classroom at the same time as opposed to the singular approach used to deliver high volumes of information, are more appealing to students. The dynamics of co-teaching have been proven successful in other teaching institutions. Furthermore, the overemphasis on rote learning has been proven ineffective for long-term memorisation and understanding. Bloom's Taxonomy (Bloom 1956) exists as proof that teaching scientific concepts, critical thinking, and higher-order learning techniques whereby subject matter is interrelated contributes to long-term learning.

4. The focus on students' internal motivation when entering medical training where traits such as strong work ethic, altruism, and intrinsic motivation provide a basis for reducing the stress associated with the overreliance on GPA rankings. The success of future doctors as caring, compassionate, and competent physicians has to be based upon something other than GPA and high ratings on the board examinations as the strongest indicators for future success.
5. Stakeholders at the national, regional, and institutional levels must collaborate on how funding is to be implemented within the medical education structure to provide prevention education in the systems associated with training physicians. Funding is necessary to train the trainers and to increase staff in the student development and counselling areas so that students receive treatment immediately for problems encountered.
6. Common ground training for recruiters of prospective medical students beginning at the middle-school levels and into college.
7. Common ground information for families, spouses, and professionals close to medical students in layman's terms. Topics should include how to recognise change within the student and how to provide support for and information about what is generally being experienced by the student. The awareness that students have to learn a lot of information does not describe student daily lived experiences of attending lectures and learning massive amounts of material in addition to earlier immersion in hospital settings where they encounter life-and-death situations, sometimes before being academically prepared.
8. Common and realistic pre-entry training for medical school students that includes basic testing for pre-existing mental health problems, learning problems, and issues related to becoming ready to matriculate into the academic rigours associated with medical training. Similar processes are deemed necessary to

prepare students to transition between classroom training, labs, early entrance into hospitals, and working with patients to managing the internship and residency experiences. Sharing known literature and best practices based upon practical knowledge of seasoned doctors can help students learn in advance how to prepare for transitions, thus preventing trial-and-error experiences.

9. Revamp the structure of medical education. Theories of how adults learn and lessons learnt from medical schools with best practices should be embraced. The culture of medicine warrants changes in the components of the formal, informal, and hidden curriculum; institutional policies; and culture of medical schools from academically driven agendas to development of physicians as complete people.

FUTURE RESEARCH DIRECTIONS

While new and innovative strategies designed to assist medical students with mental health issues include changing grading systems from letter grades to pass/fail, voluntary classes in mindfulness, and creation of wellness initiatives in many more medical educational institutions, future research is imminent. The following questions remain to be addressed:

- What is the best structure for medical education?
- How do medical students learn best?
- What is the best type of curriculum change requisite to ensure that medical education prepares students on a spectrum of well-being and wellness areas to extend into social, personal, financial, emotional, and physical well-being?
- How can medical schools educate the public, prospective students, and their families about the rigours associated with medical training?
- How can students seek help without the stigma associated with mental illness impacting future internships, residencies, and job placements?
- How can the dollars and human resources in medical education be allocated beyond the academic side of the programmes to include proactive well-being student support services?

Finally, more research is needed from the perspective of the medical student on the pressures associated with medical school at each stage of training. Outside of medical student blogs, there is insufficient literature from the student perspective.

CONCLUSION

Medical school is supposed to be a time of personal and professional development. There is enough data to show that medical training leads to mental ill health in medical students and residents. The moment to re-engineer medical education is present, and all our lives depend upon drastic measures designed to help medical students navigate medical education with sound mental health and well-being.

REFERENCES

Abbiati, M., Baroffio, A., & Gerbase, M. W. (2016). Personal profile of medical students selected through a knowledge-based exam only: Are we missing suitable students. *Med Educ Online, 21*(29705). doi:.v21.2970510.3402/meo

Adlaf, E. M., Begin, P., & Sawka, E. (2005). *Canadian Addiction Survey (CAS): A national survey of Canadians' use of alcohol and other drugs: Prevalence of use and related harms: Detailed report.* Ottawa, Canada: Canadian Centre on Substance Abuse.

Adsett, C. A. (1968). Psychological health of medical students in relation to the medical education process. *Journal of Medical Education, 43*(6).

Age of Anxiety. (n.d.). In *The Concise Oxford Dictionary of Music.* Retrieved March 02, 2017 from Encyclopedia.com: http://www.encyclopedia.com/arts/dictionaries-thesauruses-pictures-and-press-releases/age-anxiety

AlFaris, E., Irfan, F., Qureshi, R., Naeem, N., Alshomrani, A., Ponnamperuma, G., … van der Vleuten, C. (2016). Health professions' students have an alarming prevalence of depressive symptoms: exploration of the associated factors. BMC Medical Education, 16(279).

American Association of Medical Colleges. (1984). *Physicians for the Twenty-First Century.* The GPEP Report: Report of the Panel on the General Professional Education of the Physician and College Preparation for Medicine. ERIC Number: ED252102.

American Association of Medical Colleges. (2016). *Creating a Culture of Wellbeing and Resilience in Academic Medicine.* AAMC's Leadership Forum, Washington, DC. Retrieved 27 February http://www. aamc.org.AAMCacrnml

American Medical Association (AMA). (2014). *Education.* Retrieved from http://www.ama-assn.org/ama

Anxiety and Depression Association of America (ADAA). (2016). *Master's Level Videos*. Retrieved from http://www.adaa.org

Arnett, J. (2000). Emerging Adulthood: A theory of development from the late teens to the late twenties. *The American Psychologist*, *55*(5), 469–480. doi:10.1037/0003-066X.55.5.469 PMID:10842426

Association of American Medical Colleges (AAMC). (1984). *Physicians for the Twenty-First Century*. AAMC.

Barry, M. M., & Jenkins, R. (2007). *Implementing Mental Health Promotion*. Oxford, UK: Churchill Livingstone, Elsevier.

Baxter, A. (2013). Global prevalence of anxiety disorders: A systematic review and meta-regression. *Psychological*, *43*, 897–910.

Bloom, B. S. (Ed.). (1956). Taxonomy of Educational Objectives. In Handbook I: The Cognitive Domain. New York: David McKay Co Inc.

Bradburn, N. M. (1969). *The structure of psychological well-being*. Chicago: Aldine.

Bryde, J. F., & Milburn, C. M. (1990). Helping to make the transition from school to college. In R. L. Emans (Ed.), *Understanding undergraduate education* (pp. 203–213). Vermillion, SD: University of South Dakota Press.

Carter, R., Golant, S. K., & Cade, K. E. (2010). Within Our Reach: Ending the Mental Health Crisis. Rodale Press, Inc.

Center for Collegiate Mental Health. (2015, January). *2010 Annual Report* (Publication No. STA 15-30). Author.

Chemers, M. M., Hu, L., & Garcia, B. F. (2001). Academic self-efficacy and first-year college student performance and adjustment. *Journal of Educational Psychology*, *93*(1), 55–64. doi:10.1037/0022-0663.93.1.55

Cohen, D., & Rhydderch, M. (2013). *Support for tomorrow's doctors: getting it right, meeting their needs*. Retrieved from occmed.oxfordjournals.org/content/63/1/2.full

Columbia School of Physicians and Surgeons (CSPS). (2017). *The white coat ceremony*. Retrieved from http://psclub.columbia.edu/orientation/whitecoatceremony

Crandall, J. S., Volk, R. J., & Loemker, V. (1993). Medical Students Attitudes Toward Providing Care for the Underserved: Are We Training Socially Responsible Physicians? *JAMA*, *269*(19), 2519–2523. doi:10.1001/jama.1993.03500190063036 PMID:8487415

Deci, E.L., & Ryan, R.M. (2008). Hedonia, Eudaimonia, and wellbeing. *Journal of Happiness Studies, 9*(1). doi:10.1007/s10902-006-9018-1

Department of Experimental and Clinical Medicine. (n.d.). *Frontiers in Psychology* [2016, 7:1682]. Retrieved from www.europepmc.org.mg alt="Cover image" src="http://ars.els-cdn.com/content/image/1-s2.0-S0272735813X00078-cov150h.gif"class="toprightlogo

Diener, E. (2009). Assessing well-being: the collected works of Ed Diener. New York: Springer.

Diener, E., Lucas, R. E., & Scollon, C. N. (2006). Beyond the hedonic treadmill: Revising the adaptation theory of well-being. *The American Psychologist, 61*(4), 305–314. doi:10.1037/0003-066X.61.4.305 PMID:16719675

Doherty, E. M., & Nugent, E. (2011). Personality factors and medical training: A review of the literature. *Med Educ., 45*(2), 132-40. doi: . 20.10.1111/j.1365-2923

Doja, A., Bould, M. D., Clarkin, C., Eady, K., Sutherland, S., & Writer, H. (2016). The hidden and informal curriculum across the continuum of training: A cross-sectional qualitative study. *Medical Teacher, 38*(4), 410–418. doi:10.3109/0142159X.2015.1073241

Douce, L. A., & Keeling, R. P. (2014). *A strategic primer on college student mental health. American Council on Education (ACE).*

Dunn, H. L. (1961). *High-level wellness*. Arlington, VA: Beatty Press.

Dunn, H. L. (1973). *High level wellness*. Arlington, VA: R.W. Beatty, Ltd.

Dyrbye, L. N., & Shanafelt, T. D. (2011). Commentary: medical student distress: a call to action. Academic medicine. *Journal of the Association of American Medical Colleges, 86*(7), 801–803. doi:10.1097/ACM.0b013e31821da481

Dyrbye, L.N., Thomas, M.R., & Shanafelt, T.D. (2005). Medical student distress: Causes, consequences, and proposed solutions. *Mayo Clinic Proc., 80*(12), 1613-1622.

Edwards, M. T., & Zimet, C. N. (1976). Problems and concerns among medical students. *Journal of Medical Education, 51*(8).

Elnicki, D. M., Curry, R. H., Fagan, M., Friedman, E., Jacobson, E., Loftus, T., & Linger, B. et al. (2002). Medical students' perspectives on and responses to abuse during the internal medicine clerkship. *Teaching and Learning in Medicine, 14*(2), 92–97. doi:10.1207/S15328015TLM1402_05 PMID:12058552

Enns, S. C., Perotta, B., Paro, H.B., Gannam, S., Peleias, M., Mayer, F. B., … Zen, T. P. (2016). Medical Students Perception of Their Educational Environment and Quality of Life: Is There a Positive Association?. Academic Medicine, 91(3), 409-417.

Epstein, R. (2017). *Attending: Medicine, Mindfulness, and Humanity.* Scribner.

Federal Reserve Bank of San Francisco (FRB). (2003). *What effects do recessions have on college students?*. FRB.

Fenlkenstein, C., Brownstein, A., Scott, C., & Lan, Y. (2007). Anxiety and stress reduction in medical education: An intervention. *Medical Education, 41*(3), 258–264. doi:10.1111/j.1365-2929.2007.02685.x PMID:17316210

Firth, J. (1986). Levels and sources of stress in medical students. *British Medical Journal (Clinical Research Ed.), 292*(6529), 1177–1180. doi:10.1136/bmj.292.6529.1177 PMID:3085772

Frey, B. S., & Stutzer, A. (2002). *Happiness and economics*. Princeton, NJ: Princeton University Press.

Gall, T. L., Evans, D. R., & Bellerose, S. (2000). Transition to first-year university: Patterns of change in adjustment scores across life domains and time. *Journal of Social and Clinical Psychology, 19*(4), 44–67. doi:10.1521/jscp.2000.19.4.544

General Medical Council (GMC). (2009). *Tomorrow's Doctors. Outcomes and standards for undergraduate medical education.* Available from: http://www.gmc-uk.org/Tomorrow_s_Doctors_1214.pdf_48905759.pdf

Glasser, W. (1999). *Choice Theory: A New Psychology of Personal Freedom*. New York, NY: Harper Perennial.

Global Burden of Disease (GBD). (2015). Disease and injury incidence and Prevalence Collaborators, and others. Global, regional, and national incidence, prevalence, and years lived with disability for 310 diseases and injuries, 1990–2015: A systematic analysis for the Global Burden of Disease Study 2015. *Lancet, 388*, 10053.

Global Knowledge Exchange Network (GKEN). (2009). *An overview of educators and training requirements for global healthcare professionals-Physicians, Workforce and Training Task Force*. Author.

GMC. (2013). *Medical students: professional values and fitness to practice*. Available at www.gmc-uk.org/education/undergraduate/professional behaviour.asp

Groopman, J. (2007). *How doctors think*. Houghton Mifflin Harcourt.

Gunderman, R. (2006a). *Medical Student depression and our health system*. Academic Press.

Gunderman, R. (2016b). *What Do High Rates of Medical Student Depression Say About Health System?* Retrieved from www.realclearhealth.com/.../2016/.../what_do_high_rates_of_medical_student_depres

Hafferty, F. W. (1998). Beyond curriculum reform: Confronting medicines hidden curriculum. *Academic Medicine*, *73*(4), 403–407. doi:10.1097/00001888-199804000-00013 PMID:9580717

Haight, S. J., Chibnall, J. T., Schindler, D. L., & Slavin, S. J. (2012, April). Associations of medical student personality and health/wellness characteristics with their medical school performance across the curriculum. *Academic Medicine*, *87*(4), 476–485. doi:10.1097/ACM.0b013e318248e9d0 PMID:22361792

Hanson, R. (2017). *The 12 Pillars of the Path of Well-Being*. Retrieved from https://fwb.rickhanson.net/affiliate/4474

Healthy Universities. (2010). Retrieved at http://www.healthyuniversities.ac.uk/index.php?s=1

Herrman, H. S., Saxena, S., & Moodie, R. (2005). Promoting Mental Health: Concepts, Emerging Evidence, Practice. A WHO Report in collaboration with the Victoria health Promotion Foundation and the University of Melbourne. Geneva: World Health Organization; Retrieved from http://www.who.int/mental_health/evidence/MH_Promotion_Book.pdf

Hetter, H. M. G. (2011). *No health without mental health: A cross-governmental mental health outcomes strategy for all ages*. 10.1016/j.socscimed.2014.11.027

Hunt, J., & Eisenberg, D. (2010). Mental health problems and help-seeking behaviour among college students. *The Journal of Adolescent Health*, *46*(1), 3–10. doi:10.1016/j.jadohealth.2009.08.008 PMID:20123251

Hutchins, E. B. (1964). The AAMC longitudinal study: Implications for medical education. *Journal of Medical Education*, *39*, 265–267. PMID:14130655

Jenkins, R., Bhugra, D., Bebbington, P., Brugha, T., Farrell, M., Coid, J., & Meltzer, H. et al. (2008). Debt, income, and mental disorder in the general population. *Psychological Medicine*, *38*(10), 1485–1493. doi:10.1017/S0033291707002516 PMID:18184442

Kadison, R., & Digeronimo, T. F. (2004). *College of the overwhelmed: The campus mental health crisis and what to do about it*. San Francisco, CA: Jossey-Bass.

Kashani, J. H., Canfield, L. A., Borduin, C. M., Soltys, S. M., & Reid, J. C. (1994). Perceived family and social support: Impact on children. *Journal of the American Academy of Child and Adolescent Psychiatry*, *33*, 819-823. PMID:8083138

Kavan, M. G., & Brumback, R. A. (2009). The White Coat Ceremony: A tribute to the humanism of Arnold P. *Gold. Journal of Child Neurology*, *24*(8), 1051–1052. doi:10.1177/0883073809336133 PMID:19448139

Koenig, T.W., Parrish, S.K., Terregino, C.A., Williams, J.P., Dunleavy, D.M., & Volsch, J.M. (2013). Core personal competencies important to entering students' success in medical school: what are they and how could they be assessed early in the admission process?. *Acad Med*, *88*(5), 603-13. doi: 10.1097/ACM.0b013e31828b3389

Kosky, R., & Hardy, J. (1992). Mental health: Is early intervention the key? *The Medical Journal of Australia*, *3*, 47–58. PMID:1545713

Lazin, R., & Nuemann, L. (1991). Student Characteristics as predicators of drop-out from medical school: Admissions to Beer-Sheva over a decade. *Med Educ.*, *25*(5), 396-404.

LCME. (2003). *The Changing Face of Medical Education Accreditation*. Retrieved from www.flbog.edu/documents_meetings/0017_0088_0736_9.pdf

LCME. (2016). *Functions and Structure of a Medical School Standards for Accreditation of Medical Education Programs Leading to the MD Degree*. Accessed http://med.virginia.edu/ume-curriculum/wp-content/uploads/sits/216/2016/2017-18_Functions-and-Structure_2016-03-24.pdf

Legassie, J., Zibrowski, E. M., & Goldszmidt, M. A. (2008, July). Measuring Resident Well-Being: Impostorism and Burnout Syndrome in Residency. *Journal of General Internal Medicine*, *23*(7), 1090–1094. doi:10.1007/s11606-008-0536-x PMID:18612750

Lempe, H., & Seale, C. (2004). The hidden curriculum in undergraduate medical education: Qualitative study of medical students perceptions of teaching. *British Medical Journal*, *329*(7469), 770–773. doi:10.1136/bmj.329.7469.770 PMID:15459051

Lievens, F., Coetsier, P., De Fruyt, F., & De Maeseneer, J. (2002). Medical students personality characteristics and academic performance: A five-factor model perspective. *Medical Education*, *36*(11), 1050–1056. doi:10.1046/j.1365-2923.2002.01328.x PMID:12406265

Lippman, J. (2016). *What does a doctor's white coat really mean?*. Retrieved from www.kevinmd.com/blog/2016/12/doctors-white-coat-really-mean.html

Lorgren, R., Karpf, M., Perman, J., & Higdon, C. M. (2006). The U.S. health care system is in crisis: Implications for academic medical centers and their missions. *Academic Medicine, 81*(8), 713–720. doi:10.1097/00001888-200608000-00007 PMID:16868424

Lykken, D., & Tellegen, A. (1996). Happiness is a stochastic phenomenon. *Psychological Science, 7*(3), 186–189. doi:10.1111/j.1467-9280.1996.tb00355.x

Lyubomirsky, S., King, L., & Diener, E. (2005). The benefits of frequent positive affect: Does happiness lead to success? *Psychological Bulletin, 131*(6), 803–855. doi:10.1037/0033-2909.131.6.803 PMID:16351326

Mackean, G. (2011). *Mental health and well-being in post-secondary education settings: A literature and environmental scan to support planning and action in Canada. Canadian Association of College and University Student Services*. CACUSS.

Maher, B. M., Sweeney, C., Khashan, A. S., ORouke, M., Doran, K., Harris, A., & OFlynn, S. (2013). Medical School Attrition-Beyond the Statistics A Ten Year Retrospective Study. *BMC Medical Education, 13*(1), 13. doi:10.1186/1472-6920-13-13 PMID:23363547

Mahon, K.E, Henderson, M.K., & Kirch, D.G. (2013). Selecting tomorrow's physicians: the key to the future health care workforce. *Acad Med, 88*, 1806.

Mascaskill, A. (2012). *University student mental health in crisis: A United Kingdom perspective*. Retrieved from https://pdfs.semanticscholar.org/1f78/2c0eb86b7f3d32bc067bfdf8fcbc3b276ae0.pdf

Maunder, R. E., Gingham, J., & Rogers, J. (2010). Transition in higher education: Exploring the experiences of first and second year psychology undergraduate students. *Psychology of Education Review, 34*(1), 50–54.

Mayer, F. B., Itamar, S. S., Paulo, S. P., Silveira, M. H., Itaqui, L., Souza, A. R., & Tempski, P. et al. (2016). Factors associated to depression and anxiety in medical students: A multicentre study. *BMC Medical Education, 16*, 1. PMID:26727954

Mayo Clinic. (2005). *Medical Student distress: Causes, consequences and proposed solutions*. Mayo Clinic proceedings.com

McGuire, F. L. (1966). Psycho-social studies of medical students: A critical review. *Journal of Medical Education, 41*, 728–734. PMID:5328333

McManus, I., Woolf, K., Dacre, J., Paice, E., & Dewberry, C. (2009). The academic backbone: Longitudinal continuities in educational achievement from secondary school and medical school to MRCP(UK) and the specialist register in UK medical students and doctors. *BMC Med., 11*(242).

McManus, S., Meltzer, H., Brugha, T., Bebbington, P., & Jenkins, R. (2009). Adult psychiatric morbidity in England, 2007: Results of a household survey. London: National Centre for Social Research.

Miller, G. D., Kemmelmeier, M., & Dupey, P. (2013). Gender differences in worry during medical school. *Medical Education, 47*(9), 932.

Monroe, A., Quinn, E., Samuelson, W., Dunleavy, D. M., & Dowd, K. W. (2013). An overview of the medical school admission process and use of applicant data in decision making: What has changed since the 1980s?. *Acad Med, 88*, 672-81.

Montgomery, M. M., & Côté, J. E. (2003). College as a transition to adulthood. In G. R. Adams & M. D. Berzonsky (Eds.), *Blackwell handbook of adolescence* (pp. 149–172). New York: Blackwell Publishing.

Morra, D. J., Regehr, G., & Ginsburg, S. (2009). Anticipated debt and financial stress in medical. *Medical Education, 41*(2), 105.

Mousa, O. Y., Dhamoon, M. S., Lander, S., & Dhamoon, A. S. (2016). The MD blues: Under-recognised depression and anxiety in medical trainees. *Plos*. Retrieved from nim.nih.gov

Mucci, N., Giorgi, G., De Pasquale, C. S., Fiz-Perez, J., Mucci, F., & Arcangeli, G. (2016). Anxiety, Stress-Related Factors, and Blood Pressure in Young Adults. Academic Press.

National Alliance on Mental Illness (NAMI). (2017). *Fact sheets*. Retrieved from http:// www.nami.org

National Institute of Health. (2017). *Transforming the understanding and treatment of mental illnesses*. Author.

National Research Council. (2013). *Subjective Well-Being: Measuring Happiness, Suffering, and Other Dimensions of Experience* (A. Stone & C. Mackie, Eds.). Washington, DC: National Academies Press.

No health without mental health: A cross-governmental health outcomes strategy for people of all ages: The mental health strategy for England-GOV.UK. (2011). Retrieved from https://www.gov.uk/government/publications/the-mental-health-strategy-for-england

Noori, S., Blood, A., Meleca, J., Kennedy, V., & Sengupta, D. (n.d.). *Current directions in medical student wellbeing: A primer for students.* Retrieved February 2017 from https://www.aamc.org/download/450164/data/medstudentwellbeing.pdf

O'Connor, M. C., & Paunonen, S. V. (2007). Big five personality predictors of post-secondary academic performance. *Pers Indiv Diff., 43*, 313-315. 10.1080/01421590801953000

Parkernson, G. R., Broadhead, W. E., & Tse, C. J. (1990). The Health Status and Life Satisfaction of First-year Medical Students. *Academic Medicine, 65*(9), 586–587. doi:10.1097/00001888-199009000-00009 PMID:2400477

Phillips, J. P., Petterson, S. M., Bazemore, A. W., & Phillips, R. L. (2014). A Retrospective Analysis of the Relationship Between Medical Student Debt and Primary Care Practice in the United States. *Annals of Family Medicine, 12*(6), 542–549. doi:10.1370/afm.1697 PMID:25384816

Population Reference Bureau (PBR). (2015). *Research on Health and Well-Being Aims to Improve Quality of Life in Later Years.* Accessed: http://www.prb.orf

Povis, D. (2015). Selecting medical students: An unresolved challenge. *Medical Teacher, 37*(3), 252–260. doi:10.3109/0142159X.2014.993600 PMID:25532428

Pressman, S. D., & Cohen, S. (2005). Does positive affect influence health? *Psychological Bulletin, 131*(6), 925–971. doi:10.1037/0033-2909.131.6.925 PMID:16351329

Pscyho, R. C. (2011). *Mental Health of Students in Higher Education.* Retrieved at http://www.rcpsych.ac.uk/files/pdfversion/cr166.pdf

Puthran, R., Zhang, M. W. B., Tam, W. W., & Ho, R. C. (2016). Prevalence of depression amongst medical students: A meta-analysis. *Medical Education, 50*(4), 456–468. doi:10.1111/medu.12962 PMID:26995484

Richardson, M., Abraham, C., & Bond, R. (2012). Psychological correlates of university students' academic performance: A systematic review and meta-analysis. *Psychol Bull, 138*(353), 87.

Richardson, T., Elliott, P., & Roberts, R. (2013). The relationship between personal unsecured debt and mental and physical health: A systematic review and meta-analysis. *Clinical Psychology Review, 33*(8), 1148–1162. doi:10.1016/j.cpr.2013.08.009 PMID:24121465

Rosenthal, O. (2005). White Coat Mood indigo: Depression in Medical school. *NEJM.*

Ross, S., Cleland, J., & Macleod, M. J. (2006). Stress, debt and undergraduate medical student performance. *Med Educ, 40*(6), 584–589.

Rotenstein, L. S., Ramos, M. A., Torre, M., Segal, J. B., Peluso, M. J., Guille, C., & Mata, D. A. et al. (2016). Prevalence of Depression, Depressive Symptoms, and Suicidal Ideation Among Medical Students: A Systematic Review and Meta-Analysis. *Journal of the American Medical Association, 316*(21), 2214. doi:10.1001/jama.2016.17324 PMID:27923088

Russo, N. F., & Pirlott, A. (2006). Gender-Based violence: Concepts, methods and findings. *Annals of the New York Academy of Sciences, 1077*(1), 178–205. doi:10.1196/annals.1385.024 PMID:17189506

Rutter, M. (2012). Resilience as a dynamic concept. *Development and Psychopathology, 24*(2), 335–344. doi:10.1017/S0954579412000028 PMID:22559117

Scanlon, L., Rowling, L., & Weber, Z. (2010). You don't have an identity... you are just lost in a crowd: Forming a student identity in the first-year transition to university. *Journal of Youth Studies, 10*(2), 223–241. doi:10.1080/13676260600983684

Schwartz, B. (1987). The Battle for Human Nature: Science, Morality and Modern Life Paperback. W.W. Norton & Company.

Schwenk, T. L., Davis, L., & Wimsatt, L. A. (2010). Depression, stigma, and suicide ideation in medical students. *Journal of the American Medical Association, 304*(11), 1181–1190. doi:10.1001/jama.2010.1300 PMID:20841531

Silver, H. K., & Glicken, A. D. (1990). Medical student abuse. Incidence, severity, and significance. *JAMA, 264*(13), 1657-60.

Slavin, S. J., & Chibnall, J. T. (2016). Finding the why, changing the how, improving the mental health of medical students, residents, and physicians. *Academic Medicine, 91*(9), 1194–1196. doi:10.1097/ACM.0000000000001226 PMID:27166866

Smajdor, H. A., & Stöckl, A. (2012). Towards an understanding of resilience and its relevance to medical training. *Med Educ., 46*, 349-356.

Smith, C., Christoffersen, K., Davidson, H., & Herzog, P. (2011). Lost in Transition: The Dark Side of Emerging Adulthood. Oxford University Press, Inc.

Sobral, D. T. (2004). What kind of motivation drives medical students learning quests?. *Medical Education, 38*(9), 950–957. doi:10.1111/j.1365-2929.2004.01913.x PMID:15327676

Strecker, E. A., Appel, K. E., Palmer, H. D., & Braceland, F. J. (1936). Psychiatric studies in medical education: Neurotic trends in senior medical students. *The American Journal of Psychiatry, 92*(4), 937–957. doi:10.1176/ajp.92.4.937

Swift, D. (2017). *The 'Invisible White Coat': Black Women in Medicine*. Medscape Medical News.

Tempski, P., Bellodi, P. L., Paro, H., Enns, S. C., Martins, M. A., & Schraiber, B. (2012). What do medical students think about their quality of life? A qualitative study. *BMC Medical Education, 12*(1), 106. doi:10.1186/1472-6920-12-106 PMID:23126332

Tempski, P., Martins, M. A., & Paro, H. B. (2012). Teaching and learning resilience: a new agenda in medical education. *Med Educ., 46*(4), 345-6. doi: 10.1111/j.1365-2923.2011.04207.x

Tempski, P., Perotta, B., Pose, R. A., & Vieira, J. E. (2009). A questionnaire on the quality of life of medical students. *Medical Education, 43*(11), 1107–1108. doi:10.1111/j.1365-2923.2009.03476.x PMID:19874519

The Gypsy Nesters. (2007-2017). *Boomer Travel, Food, Laugher*. Gypsynester.com.

The Lancet. (1980). Stress in medical students. *Lancet, 1*, 129-130.

Thistlethwaite, J. E., Quirk, F., & Evans, R. (2010). Medical students seeking medical help: A qualitative study. *Medical Teacher, 32*(2), 164–166. doi:10.3109/01421590903434177 PMID:20163234

Together for Mental Health: A strategy for mental health and wellbeing in 2010. (n.d.). Retrieved from gov.wales/topics/health/nhswales/mental-health-services/policy/strategy/?lang=en

Tov, W., & Diener, E. (2008). The well-being of nations: Linking together trust, cooperation, and democracy. In B. A. Sullivan, M. Snyder, & J. L. Sullivan (Eds.), *Cooperation: The psychology of effective human interaction* (pp. 323–342). Malden, MA: Blackwell Publishing.

UNESCO. (2011). *International standard classification of education*. Montréal: UNESCO Institute for Statistics.

University of South Carolina. (2015, January 22). How are student loans affecting the well-being of young adults?. *Science Daily*. Retrieved March 4, 2017 from www.sciencedaily.com/releases/2015/01/150122114430.htm

U.S.A. Centres for Disease Control Prevention (CDC) Concept Paper. (n.d.). *Wellbeing*. Retrieved 1 March, 2017 www.cdc.gov/hrqol/wellbeing.htm

Vachon, R. (2012). *Foundations of human wellbeing: Social, environmental, economic*. Retrieved from http://www.sustainabledevelopment.un.org

Vaish, A., Grossmann, T., & Woodward, A. (2008). Not all emotions are created equal:the negativity bias in social-emotional development. *Psychological Bulletin*, *134*(3), 383–403. doi:10.1037/0033-2909.134.3.383 PMID:18444702

Vansteenkiste, M., Lens, W., & Deci, E. L. (2006). Intrinsic versus extrinsic goal contents in self-determination theory: Another look at the quality of academic motivation. *Educ Psychol.*, *41*(1), 19–31. doi:10.1207/s15326985ep4101_4

Villablanca, , Li, Beckett, & Howell. (2017, February). Evaluating a Medical School's Climate for Women's Success: Outcomes for Faculty Recruitment, Retention, and Promotion. *Journal of Women's Health*. PMID:28170291

Villwock, J. A., Sobin, L. B., Koester, L. A., & Harris, T. (2016). *Impostor syndrome and burnout among American medical students: A pilot study*. Academic Press.

Walsemann, K. M., Gee, G. C., & Gentile, D. (2014). Sick of our loans: Student borrowing and the mental health of young adults in the United States. *Social Science & Medicine*, 124.

Wasson, L. T. Cusmano, A., Meli, L., Louh, I., Falzon, L., Hampsey, M., … Davidson, K. W. (2016). Association between learning environment interventions and medical student wellbeing: A systematic review. *Journal of the American Medical Association*. doi:10.1001/jama.2016.17573

Watch. (n.d.). *Treating Anxiety Disorders*. Retrieved from https://www.adaa.org/resources-professionals/practice-guidelines-tools

WHO Constitution. (n.d.). Retrieved February 2017 http://www.who.int/about/en/

Williams, D. (2016). Cracking the code on the "hidden curriculum" in medical education pipeline and its contribution to attrition. *Journal of Unschooling & Alternative Learning*, *10*(19), 82–99.

Wolf, T. (1994). M: Stress, coping and health: enhancing well-being during medical school. *Medical Education*, *28*(1), 8–17. doi:10.1111/j.1365-2923.1994.tb02679.x PMID:8208174

Woloschuk, W., & Harasym, P. H. (2004). *Attitude change during medical school: A cohort study*. Retrieved from onlinelibrary.wiley.com/doi/10.1046/j.1365-2929.2004.01820.x/pdf

World Health Organisation. (2011). *America's State of Mind Report*. Retrieved from http://apps.who.int/medicinedocs/en/d/Js19032en/

World Health Organisation (WHO). (2016/2017). *Mental Disorders Fact sheet*. Retrieved from http://www.who.int

World Health Organisation (WHO). (2015). Retrieved from http://www.who.int/healthinfo/global_burden_disease/estimates

World Health Organization (WHO) & World Federation for Medical Education (WFME). (2005). *WHO/WFME Guidelines for Accreditation of Basic Medical Education*. Available from: http://wfme.org/accreditation/whowfme-policy/28-2-who-wfme-guidelines-for-accreditation-of-basic-medical-education-english/file. www.gken.org

Yusoff, M. S. B., Rahim, A. F. A., Baha, A. A., Ismail, S. B., & Pa, M. N. (2013). The impact of medical education on psychological health of students: A cohort study. *Journal of Psychology. Health & Medicine*, *18*(4), 420–430. doi:10.1080/13548506.2012.740162

KEY TERMS AND DEFINITIONS

Graduate Medical Education (GME): The period after graduation from a medical education programme. Recognised by entry into an internship and residency period ranging from 3 or more years, depending upon the speciality area of study.

Healthy Universities: Institutions with initiatives designed to create holistic settings that incorporate many interrelated factors in the academic environment. These factors include academic, social, economic, and environmental areas that may impact the mental health of students.

Higher Education: Education provided by a college or university.

Medical Education: Education related to the training of being a medical doctor or physician. The process of obtaining a medical education generally begins after the completion of higher education at the bachelor and/or master's degree level. Across the world, training varies in academic requirements and programme lengths. Generally, medical education programmes include 4 years or more of undergraduate medical training. This programme of study is followed by what is known as graduate medical education and encompasses an internship, residency, and fellowship training. The residency and fellowship training periods vary according to specialities. Graduate medical education leads to licensure. Some countries, such as the United States, the United Kingdom, Canada, and Australia, have specific continuing medical education activities designed to help physicians increase the knowledge, skills, and professional performance necessary to stay current.

Medical School: The educational organisation providing a basic (undergraduate) programme in medicine. It is synonymous with medical faculty, medical college, medical academy, or medical university.

Mental Health Promotion: Improving the capacity of everyone to take control of their lives and to improve their mental health. At the community level, it involves public policy to enhance the personal skills and services necessary for achieving optimal mental health.

Mental Ill Health: A mental health problem can feel just as bad, or worse, than any other physical illness, only you cannot see it.

Section 2

Problems, Issues, and Controversies

Chapter 2
Medical Students' Perceived Stigma in Seeking Care:
A Cultural Perspective

Virginia Joseph
Spartan Health Science University, Saint Lucia

Jozelle M Miller
Milton Cato Memorial Hospital, Saint Vincent and the Grenadines

ABSTRACT

This chapter discusses the stigma and the barriers, which hinder medical students from seeking help for both physical and mental health conditions. Stigma will also be explored from a cultural perspective; the authors will demonstrate how it is embedded in help seeking behaviour. The authors will explore the existing literature to highlight these issues, and demonstrate how negative help seeking behaviour contributes to the poor academic performance of the students, as well produces chronic mental and physical health conditions. Solutions and interventions to address this perceived stigma will also be discussed. The authors will emphasise the importance of educators and staff of medical schools taking a more proactive role, in providing the necessary environment to facilitate such change in behaviour, by implementing some of these interventions.

INTRODUCTION

According to a Mayo Clinic study in 2006,

Students enter medical school with mental health profiles similar to their peers from college. But they begin to show higher rates of mental distress as they progress

DOI: 10.4018/978-1-5225-2811-1.ch002

through medical school. The same study found that the most depressed students often are the least likely to reach out for help because of stigma related to mental illness. (Rapporteur, 2016, p. 47)

Many studies have shown that medical students experience high levels of mental and physical health issues, such as depression and anxiety (Amarasuriya, Jorm, & Reavley, 2015; Roh, Jeon, Kim, Han, & Hahm, 2010; Tjia, Givens, & Shea, 2005). It might be associated with the stress they experience due to their academic courses and the university experiences. Furthermore, medical students suffering from such mental health problems are shown to be at the risk of facing academic difficulties and potential drop-out from the medical school (Roh et al., 2010); and they also suffer from mental health problems later, in their careers as future doctors (Pullen, Lonie, Lyle, Cam, & Doughty, 1995). Therefore, it is important for medical students affected by such problems, to receive necessary assistance.

It is expected that medical students have a greater opportunity of receiving exposure to mental and physical health information, as compared to non-medical students; Hence, it would be expected that they have higher levels of mental health knowledge, i.e., information relevant to recognition, treatment and prevention of mental disorders (Amarasuriya, Jorm, & Reavley, 2015). Other researchers such as Dahlin and Runeson (2007) showed that being a medical student and the amount of years spent in training are linked to more advanced mental health knowledge.

However, as a professor of behavioural science, the author(s) have observed that the students that are exposed to literacy on mental health, the ones taking Doctoring 1 and Doctoring 11 (Behavioural Science course in medicine), tend to show increased signs of mental illness. This might be due to exposure to information that trigger or re-traumatise past experiences. From observation, these students start the course displaying no signs or complaints of mental health issues. However, the authors found no supporting literature to support this theory after a thorough search, which highlight the need for this theory to be further researched to explore the relationship between mental health literacy and the increase in mental health issues. Nonetheless, Jorm et al. (1997) introduced the term 'mental health literacy' and defined it as 'knowledge and beliefs about mental disorders which aid their recognition, management or prevention'. They believe that mental health literacy plays an important part in seeking help. In light of this conclusion, it would also be anticipated that medical students who experience mental health problems would seek the necessary professional assistance to treat mental health issues. However, studies show a different outcome to this expectation; that a small percentage of these students seek help. The study also shows medical students who seek help turn to informal sources, such as family and friends (Amarasuriya, Jorm, & Reavley, 2015). Most common reasons medical students mention for unwillingness to seek help for mental health issues, is the fear of the impact on academic records, confidentiality, stigma and fear of discrimination by others (Amarasuriya, Jorm, & Reavley, 2015; Givens & Tjia, 2002).

Stigma is understood as a negative stereotype and prejudice, ascribed to a person or action that falls outside the conventional expectation of the popular group (Corrigan, 2004). Stigma can be real or perceived. Stigmatised persons may internalize perceived prejudices to the extent of affecting their behaviour. In this chapter, the authors will seek to look at the perceived stigma experienced by medical students, as they access help for both medical and psychological conditions.

Stigma has been identified as an important barrier to seeking help for mental health issues, for college students as stated by Eisenberg et al. (2009). In this chapter, the authors will discuss how these stigmas are embedded in the culture of medical students. Understanding help seeking barriers such as, stigma towards mental health, student's culture, religion, spirituality and confidentiality has particular significance in medical student populaces for several reasons; as it contributes to poor academic performance and well-being. The authors will explore and discuss effective interventions and recommendations, to reduce such barriers and improve medical students' well-being.

BACKGROUND OF RESEARCH

Understanding Stigma

The concept of 'stigma' has its roots in the work of sociologist Erving Goffman (2009), who cited stigma as being a process based on the social construction of identity. To be stigmatised is a mark of disgrace that sets a person apart; It involves assigning labels and stereotypical classifications by others in an undesirable and less acceptable way. Goffman made it clear that stigmatisation was an interactive social process, but some interpreted his work as indicating that the blame lay with the person carrying the stigma. More recently, the term stigma has been used in a wider sense to refer to the reaction of other people, or even to include the attitude and behaviour of both the victim and the perpetrator.

For proper communication, it is important to define which concept of stigma we are working with. For the purpose of this discussion, the authors are using Scambler's (1998) definition of the terms, which he developed during his work on epilepsy. He coined the terms: felt stigma and enacted stigma. Felt stigma (internal stigma or self-stigmatisation) refers to the shame and expectation of discrimination that prevents people from talking about their experiences and stops them from seeking help. Enacted stigma (external stigma, discrimination) refers to the experience of unfair treatment by others. Felt stigma can be as damaging as enacted stigma, since it leads to withdrawal and restriction of social support.

In this chapter, the authors will examine the stigma experienced by medical students, as it relates to seeking medical care. Research shows that medical students experience higher stress levels, depression and anxiety than people in the general population. While stigma does exist, there have also been instances where people experienced stigma purely within their minds and not in actuality. The idea of felt stigma versus enacted stigma deserves a worthwhile consideration, in contextualizing a medical student's feelings and reactions to the stigma they feel has been meted out to them (Gray, 2002).

Culture and Its Impact on Help Seeking Behaviour

Belonging to the black ethnic minority, and serving as educators in medical universities, and ones who provide psychological services; the authors believe it is imperative to understand the role that one's ethnicity and culture plays in the understanding and perception of mental health and well-being.

According to the Oxford Dictionary (1990), ethnicity is defined as, 'a group of mankind having common national or cultural tradition'. This definition of ethnicity implies common values, rituals and traditions and it is a widely-accepted view. Stuart Hall (1992) states 'the term ethnicity acknowledges the place of history, language and culture in the construction of the subjectivity and identity, as well as the fact that all discourse is placed, positioned, situated, and all knowledge is contextual' (p. 257). Having a sense of belonging, historical continuity and identity with one's own people is a basic psychological need. Ethnicity, the concept of a group's 'peoplehood' refers to a group's commonality of ancestry and history, through which people have evolved their shared values and customs over the centuries. Based on a combination of race, religion, and cultural history; ethnicity is retained, whether or not members realise their commonalities with one another. Its values are transmitted over generations by the family structure, and reinforced by the surrounding community (Modood, et al., 1997).

Culture has been described by William (1993, p.87) as, 'one of the two or three most complicated words in English language'. The complexity arises from the variety of meanings associated with the concept of culture such as 'race', 'is dynamic in nature' and 'defies simple definitions'. Kirmayer (2006) defines 'culture' as a 'system of knowledge and practise that provide individuals with conceptual tools for self-understanding and rhetorical possibilities for self-preservation and social positioning'.

Christopher (2001) argues that life is not conceivable without culture, because it provides common understandings that allow people to make sense of the social and physical preservation and social positioning (p.163). He implies that 'culture' is located in and emanates from the real lives of real people. It comes out of the struggles and connections with one another; and from the wishes and dreams of ordinary people against a background of heritage, or what we inherit culturally. Culture provides shared meanings that function as a background set of assumptions and values that structure existence and orient people to life.

Culture profoundly affects behaviour, ways of seeing and thinking about the world, understanding relationships between people, things and events, preferences and the established world. Culture permeates social functioning, and gives meaning and coherence to daily life in a way that is not innately available to us as infants. Kagawa-Singer and Chung (2002) also describe, 'Culture provides the lens through which its members view reality and, for mental well-being, shapes the expectations of cure and the management of emotional distress. The structural content of beliefs, values, and practises form the cognitive map that creates the refraction through which its members see the world' (p. 55). Without these definitions and conceptualizations of what culture and ethnicity is, it would be difficult to understand how they can be a barrier to seeking professional help.

Goldston et al. (2008) indicated that there are many cultural factors such as acculturation, enculturation, family, collectivism and individualism, stigma, cultural mistrust, religion and spirituality, which can influence the manifestation and interpretation of psychological distress; And as a result hinder help seeking behaviour for individuals, specifically in ethnic minorities. Leong and Lau (2001) discussed four categories that act as barriers to seeking help across culture. They identified them as: cognitive, affective, value orientation, and physical.

Leong and Lau (2001) believe the cognitive barriers are one's conceptions of the nature, causes, and cures of mental illnesses which are culturally influenced. This behaviour is seen predominantly in Asian and African culture where psychological distress or symptoms are expressed physically, through aches, pains, low mood or depression, instead of as a psychological symptom. Individuals from these cultural backgrounds understand the mind and body as one, in comparison to dominant western conceptualisation that views the mind and body as separate units (Allen, 1988; Gopaul-McNicol & Brice-Baker, 1997). For effective barriers, they expressed it as one's perception of seeking help. For some cultures, specifically Asian ones, they may become more concerned about the social image and as a result may decide to protect their family reputation by not seeking help. Ethnic minority medical students may acknowledge having psychological issues; however, their desire to report psychological problems may be hindered by their perceptions of stigma and shame.

Leong and Lau (2001) discussed value orientation barriers, as cultural values that govern norms regarding how one manages and communicates about their emotions. African and Asian cultures perceive that disclosure of personal problems may bring shame to family members and the community. This is also supported by Leong, Wagner, and Kim (1995), who emphasise that Asian Americans and African Americans might be unwilling to discuss personal issues with strangers, such as psychologists, outside of their accepted social support network of family, friends, and community advisers. They argued that the value placed on these beliefs creates a hostile reaction to traditional Western psychotherapy orientations, which place a high value on open communication. Lastly, they describe physical barriers as a lack of awareness about available services and their inability to access these services, due to economic and geographic realities.

One of the authors, in her many years of experience as a faculty member in a multicultural medical school, noticed that most ethnic minorities, such as the African, West Indians and Asian students stay very committed to their cultural values and beliefs, even when they are in a host country with different culture. Acculturation and enculturation have both been factors that influence individuals help seeking behaviour. Acculturation is described as a process by which members of a minority group (immigrants or ethnic minorities) change their behaviours and attitudes to resemble those of the host or majority group (Pasupuleti, 2013). Many researchers have showed that the individuals, who have low levels of acculturation, may perceive a more negative attitude towards seeking help. Likewise, enculturation refers to the extent to which ethnic minority individuals retain and are socialised to the norms of their indigenous culture. Therefore, it is evident that a medical student that practises enculturation in their cultural values might allow that value system to impede in the professional help seeking behaviour. This was supported by Kim (2007) who stated that an Asian American who has strong cultural values would view seeking professional help, as the shame of personal failure and weaknesses.

Spirituality has been embedded in many cultures, cultural identity, and personal well-being (Schulte, Skinner, & Claibom, 2002). It is claimed that Asian Indians use a religious framework to explain psychological distress and certain disorders. This belief was also supported by Ramisetty-Mikler (1993), who indicated that this cultural group believes physical and mental illness to be a consequence of God's Will or past Karma, which can result in a non-caring attitude, which deters help-seeking behaviour. Here, one can understand that medical students, who are from such cultures and hold strong spiritual values can view their mental issues as God's will or a punishment. This is also supported by Whitley, Kirmayer, and Groleau (2006), who did a study on West Indians' attitude to seeking help, and found a reluctance to use mental health services because of their belief in the curative power of non-medical interventions, notably God, and, traditional folk medicine; and found that they have similar spiritual values and belief. Previously, the authors discussed that black ethnic minority would prefer to seek guidance and support from religious persons, instead of visiting a counsellor; Here, one would understand that this behaviour is stemming from their strong spiritual values that is embedded in their culture. However, it is also stated that those seeking support from clergy's or spiritual persons are not for psychological distress but for spiritual guidance (Utsey, Adams, & Bolden, 2000).

The belief of Obeah or witchcraft is a deep- seated cultural belief. This is one of African rites that has survived slavery, and has been passed on through the generations (Gopaul-McNicol, 2006). Therefore, medical students from such cultures; African Americans or West Indians would resort to this method for help. These practitioners of the craft, Obeahmen, are consulted for a variety of reasons: to cure illness, predict the future, interpret dreams, allay fears, exact revenge or grant favour (Neki, et al., 1986). Many of these reasons are similar to the reasons why people seek psychotherapy (Brice-Baker, 1994). Gopaul-McNicol also noted that Africans as well as West Indians rarely evoke psychological explanation for their mental illness. Their mental illness is most often attributed to demon or spirit possession by a vengeful spirit. Consequently, consultation with a powerful witchdoctor or an Obeahman, is one way of attempting to alleviate the symptoms, which an individual may be experiencing. The Obeahman may offer help in the form of (1) medicine (herbal preparations), (2) insight into the spiritual force, both seen and unseen, that may be at the root of the individual's anxiety, and (3) working spells on the person or what the person's views as the source of stress (Gopaul-McNicol and Brice-Baker, 1997).

Here, it can be observed that medical students' ethnicity can be a strong barrier to seeking help for mental health issues, due to strong stigma embedded within their culture.

CONTROVERSIES AND ISSUES

Medical students through their journey in school are faced with many mental health issues, such as anxiety around exams, parents' expectations, fear of not good enough to make it as a professional, the demands of the curriculum and depression. Several studies show that the prevalence of stress, depression and anxiety among medical students is greater than the general population (Amarasuriya, Jorm, & Reavley, 2015; Schwenk, Davis, & Wimsatt, 2010). These reports also highlight deterioration in mental health over time as they progress through their training. Yet it has shown that medical students have a perceived stigma, which hinders them in seeking help for mental illnesses.

A study done by Givens and Tjia (2002) on 1st and 2nd year medical students showed that depressed medical students were reluctant to use mental health counselling services. They showed that the most frequently cited barriers to using these were stigma allied with using mental health services which form (30%), lack of confidentiality (37%), and fear of documentation on academic record (24%) among others. From this research, it is highlighted that stigma towards seeking help for mental health issues contributed to 30% of these students. Stigma, as discussed earlier in this chapter can be either, felt stigma (internal stigma or self-stigmatization) and enacted stigma (external stigma, discrimination). Felt stigma is where a person feels shame and expects others to discriminate against them; hence, preventing that individual from talking about their experiences and stops them seeking help. Enacted stigma on the other hand refers to the experience of actual unfair treatment by others.

Medical students struggle with internal stigma or self-stigmatisation. This is where the student will internalise how they will be seen in the eyes of others, when they seek help. Through their own self-stigmatisation, they might believe others see them as weak and incompetent to be in medical school (Kim, 2007). This internal stigma can be part of who these students are, and stem from their culture. As discussed earlier in this chapter, one's culture plays an important role in their help seeking behaviour through enculturation. This is where their cultural values might allow value system to impede in professional help seeking behaviour.

This is also supported by Givens and Tjia (2002), who stated medical students do not seek help for mental health issues, because they perceive that others will hold prejudicial and discriminating behaviour towards them. There is an assumption that if one is seeking psychological help or 'going to therapy', they are seen as 'crazy or they are mental'. Wahl (1999) support this through a study that showed public stereotypes and prejudices about a mental illness have a deleterious impact on obtaining and keeping good jobs, that people see one with mental health issues as 'dangerous and therefore people become afraid of them'. There is also the perception that they should be locked up or isolated from society. Hence, one could understand a student who holds such stigma will suffer in silence for fear of these treatments, as well as demonstrate a denial of their illness due to such stereotypical perceptions.

Other Barriers to Help Seeking Behaviour

Many medical students have the notion that their problem does not necessitate help or intervention. Eisenberg, Hunt, and Speer (2012) reviewed the epidemiological data of stigma in medical school as it relates to mental health treatment, especially in the United States; They noted that medical students do not often seek treatment, due to the perception that their problem does not require help or intervention. They also implied that there is a strong relationship between perceiving a need for help, and intention to seek help. The most common reasons which was highlighted for not seeking help was, 'their' problem will get better by itself; stress is normal in college or graduate school; they question how serious their problem is; they prefer to handle their problems on their own; and they do not have time to seek treatment'. Theories around help-seeking imply that help-seeking beliefs and intentions is a common concept within the help-seeking process, both considered important indicators of help-seeking behaviours (Celluci, Krogh, & Vik, 2006; Eisenberg, Hunt, Speer, & Zivin, 2011).

In a research done by Amarasuriya et al. (2015) on medical students in Sri Lanka found that even if medical students had positive help seeking beliefs, it did not result in their intentions; These students did not act on their belief and get help. However, the study also indicated that those who had intentions to seek help resorted to family and friends for support, instead of health professionals. This behaviour can be a result of issues of confidentially, as well as internal stigma 'that they do not discuss their problems with a stranger, their problems stays at home'. This is also supported by Leong, Wagner, and Kim (1995), who implied that Asian Americans as well as Africans are reluctant to discuss personal issues with strangers, such as psychologists. As a result, students may seek help from family and friends. Sue and Sue (1999) found that people of colour have a tendency to seek help from more informal sources, including family members, friends, the clergy and indigenous healers.

Confidentiality and trust also seem to be major barriers to seeking help by medical students. Goyal, Kohli, Kishore, and Jiloha (2013) conducted a study on depressed medical students, and found most common reasons for not seeking help was they believed they would not be understood by others, and their fear of lack of confidential treatment. A study by Chew, Rogers and Yassin (2003) found that medical students dread seeking help as they perceived it might be seen as a sign of weakness and might have negative impact on their future career, as their mental illness would be on their records, as well as issues of confidentiality. The issue of trust has been noted, as a major hindrance for medical students. A study by Jackman et al. (2016) of medical students on barriers towards help seeking behaviour found that trust was an important factor in choosing a support service. The study also revealed that students would prefer to get support from someone they know and had regular contact with, rather than going to a mental health support service. This is also supported by Berk (2010), who argued that a personal and individual bond between a student and a mentor is critical in the success, and satisfaction of the relationship, and is strongly associated with attendance and positive outcome.

Culture differences in relation to the language barrier can also be a hindrance to seeking help. Students might feel that the counsellor will not be able to understand them. Chang and Berk (2009) found that misunderstandings that emerge from cultural differences in communication may lead to alienation and/or an inability to develop trust and rapport, which in turn may lead to early termination of treatment.

Stigma Associated With Medical Students Seeking Medical Treatment

It is important that the issue of self-treatment is addressed in medical schools; as such attitudes are already present among many junior doctors. Strategies aimed at doctors' self-treatment should focus on challenging the culture of doctors' self-reliance, and their unwillingness or inability to show their vulnerability or need in relation to seeking treatment when sick.

The intimate reflections of some doctors who experienced major illness in the past suggested that the 'pull yourself together and just get on with it' mentality is a significant barrier to seeking appropriate treatment (Armstrong, 1997). In a South Wales study, Pullen, Lonie, Lyle, Cam, and Doughty (1995) found that 26% of doctors experienced a condition warranting medical consultation, but felt inhibited about consulting a doctor. It was further noted that when doctors do seek external care, evidence suggests they receive a lesser quality of care than lay patients. Self-treatment for doctors includes diagnosing and treating one's own illness, and prescribing for oneself. It also includes undertaking informal, or 'corridor', consultations and self-referring to a specialist.

In a study conducted by Vaz et al. (2012) in Goa Medical College, they examined the health seeking behaviour among medical students. Data collection was done with the help of a structured pretested questionnaire. Various aspects of health seeking behaviour were studied. Data was analysed using SPSS statistical software package. A total of 281 students were studied across three semesters/clinical years. Some form of illness in the preceding twelve months was reported by 80.4% of the student population. Students reported an average of 2.2 doctor visits over twelve months' period. It was found that 31.3% had self-investigated and 66.3% had taken self-treatment. Around 38.4% of the students felt that it was alright to self-investigate, while 35.9% felt it was alright to take self-treatment. There is a need to have a formal health programme for medical students, set guidelines for students to follow if they fall ill, and for provision of medicines. Students needed to be made aware of the dangers of self-treatment and investigation.

It is important that an in-depth exploration be conducted of a doctor's perception on the acceptable limits to self-treatment; and to identify the barriers for doctors seeking appropriate healthcare services. According to Chambers (1993), when doctors experience ill health, they disregard the advice they give their patients; And the medical community has over the years developed a culture in which working through illness and self-treating became the norm (McKevitt, Morgan, Dundas, & Holland, 1997; Thompson, Cupples, Sibbett, Skan, & Bradley, 2001).

SOLUTIONS AND RECOMMENDATIONS

What can be done to assist with effectively eradicating the de-stigmatising attitudes and behaviours as it relates to medical students seeking help in the health care system; be it for medical or mental health related issues? Below will be a discussion on past research highlighting the necessary measures and effective interventions, to de-stigmatise attitude and behaviour of seeking help amongst medical students.

Mental Health Literacy for Medical Students and Educators

The stigma of mental illness among medical students is a prevalent concern that has far reaching negative consequences. Attempts to combat this stigma through educational initiatives have had mixed results. These results suggest that it is possible to create an environment in which medical student attitudes towards mental illness can be shifted in a positive direction.

In a study by Papish et al. (2013) looking at reducing the stigma of mental illness in the undergraduate medical education; it was noted that 'the results supported previous findings which show that medical students do carry a stigma towards mental illness' (Chew-Graham, Rogers, & Yassin, 2003; Schwenk, Davis, & Wimsatt, 2010). The results also provided support to the notion that comprehensive medical education can be effective in reducing the stigma of mental illness and can increase medical students' confidence in working with people who have mental illness. Furthermore, it was suggested that it is possible to create an environment in which medical student attitudes towards mental illness can be shifted in a positive direction. However, despite the improvement in attitudes, the stigma towards mental illness remained greater than that for a stigmatised physical illness (Hooper, 1981), such as a diagnosis of type 2 diabetes mellitus.

Another plausible solution may be that medical students required additional knowledge, throughout their course of study; but specifically, in their first year of training at medical school, to help tackle the stigma of mental illness. Providing accurate knowledge can help correct misinformation, reduce ignorance and improve mental health literacy, especially when combined with contact strategies (Thornicroft, Brohan, Kassam, & Lewis-Holmes, 2008). It must also be noted that specific types of knowledge might not be helpful in reducing the stigma of mental illness. There has been emerging evidence that education about the biological nature of mental illness; framing it as a neurological brain disease may perpetuate the stigma even deeper by suggesting to some that it is irreversible and creating wider social divisions. The understanding should be that while some mental illnesses may not be curative, with treatment people can function optimally and lead fulfilling lives (Rosenberg, 2014).

A number of studies have examined the effects of providing educational programmes to health care providers who are still in training e.g., pharmacy, medical, occupational therapy students (Beltran, Scanlan, Hancock, & Luckett, 2006: Mino, Yasuda, Tsuda, & Shimodera, 2001: O'Reilly, Bell, Kelly, & Chen, 2011). The findings of these studies revealed that health care providers in training can exhibit positive changes in attitudes several weeks after exposure to educational interventions (Beltran et al., 2007; Altindag, Yanik, Ucok, Alptekin, & Ozkan, 2006). Bahora et al. (2008) also reiterated evidence of the beneficial nature of education in eradicating stigma; 'They pointed out that an extensive 40- hour crisis intervention training for police officers has resulted in officers feeling increased self-efficacy regarding working with people in crisis, increased knowledge and more positive attitudes toward people with mental illness (Compton et al., 2006), and less stigma toward people in crisis' (Bahora et al., 2008; Compton et al., 2006). Added to that, these trainings may also have reduced the use of force and unnecessary arrests, and increased referrals to psychiatric facilities (Bowler and Pettit, 2001; Steadman, Deane, Borum, & Morrissey, 2000).

In a research conducted by Pinfold et al. (2003) with young people at a secondary school which was aimed at increasing mental health literacy and challenging negative stereotypes associated with severe mental illness; the researchers found that a school-based programme combining education and social contact with people with mental illness was associated with improvements in stigmatising attitudes among adolescents six months later. The programme included having a health professional speaker to discuss personal experiences of living with depression or schizophrenia and also showed that students who know someone with mental health problems learned more from the sessions than those who did not associate the subject area with a personal contact. From this research, it can be noted that if medical students are exposed or are in close contact, whether it is having a family member or friend with mental illness, this can result in reducing the stigma attached to mental health problems. Medical universities can engage more school campaigns as a way to educate the students about mental illnesses. This can reduce both internal and enacted stigma held by them.

Supporting Pinfold et al. (2003), one of the authors at Spartan Health Science University School of Medicine based in the Caribbean has started a programme, where second year medical students are taken on a field trip to a mental hospital which is part of their curriculum. The students are exposed to individuals with mental illness. The authors believe that learning about mental illness at medical school and being in close contact with someone with mental illness has a greater impact on the students. What the author has observed that after the field trip, most students would enrol as a member in a group which the author has formed at the university, which aims to bring about mental health awareness to the students and the community. The group project is a charitable trust which assists patients at the mental hospital and in the community. Students who are members of this programme also go out to secondary schools where they educate students on different mental health issues, such as 'peer pressure, bullying, drug abuse, physical abuse, teenage pregnancy, anxiety etc.'. It has been observed that students who joined this group became more aware of mental illness and showed more compassion and empathy towards mentally ill persons than before joining.

Pinfold et al. (2003) also found in their research that students reported after the workshop less- stigmatising descriptions for a person with mental health issues; the attention was more on feelings, such as sad, dazed, lonely, scared, and normal than the label. The authors plan to use this on-going programme at Spartan Health Science University school of Medicine to investigate these observations on the effectiveness of changing students held stigma towards mental health and seeking behaviour, and also how it affects their academic performance. Here, the authors believe if medical universities introduce school programmes or community outreach programmes where students are actively involved in assisting persons with mental health issues or taking part in educating others about mental illness, it will reduce this stigma towards mental illness.

Research by Bond, Jorm, Kitchener, and Reavley (2015) on medical and nursing students in Australia showed that providing these students with mental health first aid course was effective in decreasing their stigmatising attitudes about their mentally ill peers, as well increased health knowledge and confidence in assisting someone who is experiencing mental illness. The mental health first aid course is a 12-hour training course, which teaches individuals how to respond to a person who is developing mental illness or experiencing a mental health crisis. Other studies have shown that this course is very effective in improving the attitude to mental health treatment, decreasing stigma towards those with mental health problems and also increasing confidence in providing support to people experiencing mental health problems. It has also shown to be effective with high school teachers and pharmacy students (O'Reilly et al., 2011).

The authors believed if Mental Health First Aid (MHFA) training is provided in medical schools to students, as well as the faculty and the staff; this might reduce student's stigmatised behaviour towards mental health improving help seeking behaviour. Also, through this training students being mental health first aiders, will be more proactive in assisting fellow colleagues who face mental illness and also easily notice early signs of mental health issues in friends and peers, as well as in themselves. Faculties with such training will be more aware when students are displaying early signs of mental health issues, and therefore will be more knowledgeable as how to assist with early interventions. Kutcher, Wei, McLuckie, and Bullock (2013)) found in their research that there is potential value of mental health literacy training, as it improves the mental health knowledge and attitudes of the educators. They noted that this may be necessary in order for schools to provide effective mental health promotion and prevention programming.

It is being suggested that the medical colleges take the initiative to be the focal points in the dissemination of accurate information, as it relates to mental illness and more so, mental wellness. This initiative should undoubtedly form a part of the curriculum with an understanding that medical students are usually quite predisposed to mental challenges, due to the intense work load. As such, it is imperative that they learn to show empathy and due care, as they may be the recipients of the same at some point in their lives.

Social Norms-Based Interventions

Social norms-based interventions aim to alter individual health-related attitudes and behaviours by correcting misperceptions about peers' behaviours and attitudes, and have been widely used in campus health promotion campaigns (Wechsler, Nelson, Lee, & Keeling, 2003). According to Frauenfelder (2001), the social norms approach is an environmental strategy gaining ground in health campaigns. The social norms approach is founded upon the concept of pluralistic ignorance, which is a set of assumptions that individuals incorrectly perceive, about the attitudes or behaviours of others that may be different from their own, when in reality they are similar. It is largely because individuals assume the most memorable and salient, often extreme, behaviour is representative of the behaviour of the majority. This may lead individuals to adjust their behaviour to that of the presumed majority, by adhering to the pseudo-norms created through observing such memorable behaviour.

Social norms interventions have been found to be effective in changing the behaviour of the moderate or the occasional-drinking majority (pluralistic ignorance), as well as confronting and changing the behaviour of the heavy drinking minority. The authors suggest that such interventions can also be applicable to the population of medical students, who may adhere to the misconceived thought that medical students should not readily seek medical help for their illnesses, but instead attempt to treat themselves.

To avoid having medical students conducting self- examinations and treating themselves, a senior practitioner should be assigned to conduct consultations specifically for students who can provide the required guidance in diagnosis and treatment. They can also allow students to be an active part of the process, therefore facilitating learning in the process. Many students would express a desire for a formal health programme for medical students within their colleges; which outlines the guidelines for seeing specific doctors or medical/mental health related issues; also at a cost affordable to students place needed sanctions against the idea of self-medicating. Drugs should not be readily dispensed to medical students without the proper prescription written up by a registered physician.

Another effective intervention in social norms is group mentoring. In an article on US News and world report issued that New Medical School Programs Help Students Battle Burnout. Wellness and social programmes are aimed at helping medical students achieve work-life balance. Hobson (2013) stated that Johns Hopkins University and the University of Virginia, among others, have moved from fail to pass grades in the first two years, as a result of implementing a mentoring programme where students meet in mentoring groups with faculty members for an hour every month to discuss such topics, as managing stress and conflict and dealing with mistakes. This can be another method of medical student dealing with mental health issues, similar to being in therapy; can share their issues in the group. This can help reduce both self-stigmatisation and enacted stigma for students. Also, students become aware that they are not the only ones with mental health issues, eliminating issues around the fear of confidentiality.

Culturally Competent Counsellors

Having counsellors that are multi-culturally competent foster to a more positive perception and relationship. Many health professionals noted that racial or ethnic factors may act as impediments to counselling (Alladin, 2002; Diamond, 2005). They also implied that misunderstanding that arises from cultural variations in communication may lead to alienation and/or an inability for the clients to develop trust and rapport. Medical universities need to employ multicultural and linguistically competent university staff and faculty, and train them properly. It is important for student affairs practitioners including counsellors to be more sensitive to cultural differences related to their comfort to seeking help and maintaining awareness of the impact of therapy, when there is a language barrier depending where the students come from geographically.

Furthermore, Yakunina and Weigold (2011) stated that practitioners could frame counselling, as a positive way to promote academic and career success; as this could lessen their stigma toward and fear around confidentiality. Medical universities can also consider renaming mental health counsellors differently, such as advisor for well-being. This might help students feel less stigmatized.

Screening and Referral

Since students have issues around confidentially seeking help, it might be beneficial for medical schools to have a screening system, where students are screened for mental health issues instead of relying on self-referrals. This method was proven effective for the American Foundation for Suicide Prevention's Interactive Screening Program, where they used a web-based screen to identify students with higher risk for suicides. Additionally, in an effort to cause medical students to feel comfortable about asking for help for mental health conditions, it would be important that they understand the extent to which the services they are accessing are confidential. Students should have access to or know about the support service confidentiality policy.

FUTURE RESEARCH DIRECTIONS

Areas of further research can be explored for both medical students as well focus on training for medical school educators and staff. Another critical area of further research in regards to medical students can be around culture, as well as multicultural training. Through this chapter, what was highlighted as a major barrier to seeking help was the stigma embedded within a student's culture. It was supported by research that black ethnic minority medical students were less likely to seek help. Since, this has been a main focus, it would be important to explore what are the variables within their culture 'black culture', that impact such negative behaviour. Variables, such as, experience, up-bringing, racism, and prejudice can be explored. This research could share more light in changing cultural stigma.

Also, the authors mentioned a programme 'Spartan Mental Health Awareness Trust (SMHAT)' which is currently used at a medical university, where it has been observed to have a positive impact in changing student's stigma towards mental health. It would be beneficial, if a study is conducted on that programme to measure its effectiveness to changing stigma; as it can be a model used in other medical universities.

Most of these recommendation and interventions will not be effective, if educators and staff of medicals school do not have mental health literacy. This is important, as it will improve of awareness of students displaying symptoms, as well as providing the necessary intervention. The authors believe that this area of research requires further exploration to highlight effectiveness.

CONCLUSION

Research has shown that there is a major problem facing medical students in their help seeking behaviour, for both mental and medical health issues; which impact both their well-being and academic performance. Here, the authors have highlighted stigma and discussed some of the major barriers that might be factors for students not seeking help. Importantly, recommendations and solutions are also presented in this chapter, as it aims to assist in changing medical students' attitudes towards seeking help. Emphasis must be placed on the importance of educators and staff of medical schools, to take a more proactive role in providing the necessary environment to facilitate such change in behaviour, by implementing some of these interventions. Research has indicated that stigmatising attitudes vary significantly across subgroups within medical school populations, which suggests that stigma-reduction efforts may be more effective, if strategies are tailored accordingly. The authors hope that this chapter would not only shed light on an important phenomenon, but it would allow for behaviour change and tolerance as it relates to a patient's (be it medical student, or not) human right to seek out the needed care in an environment which is safe, confidential and well-equipped.

REFERENCES

Alladin, W. J. (2002). Ethnic Matching in Counselling: How Important is it to Ethnically Match Clients and Counsellors? In S. Palmer (Ed.), *Multicultural Counselling: A Reader*. New York: SAGE.

Allen, A. A. (1988). West Indians. In *Clinical Guidelines in Cross-cultural Mental Health*. Oxford, UK: John Wiley & Sons.

Altindag, A., Yanik, M., Ucok, A., Alptekin, K., & Ozkan, M. (2006). Effects of an Antistigma Programme on Medical Students Attitudes Towards People with Schizophrenia. *Psychiatry and Clinical Neurosciences*, *60*(3), 283–288. doi:10.1111/j.1440-1819.2006.01503.x PMID:16732743

Amarasuriya, S., Jorm, A., & Reavley, N. (2015). Perceptions and intentions relating to seeking help for depression among medical undergraduates in Sri Lanka: A cross-sectional comparison with non-medical undergraduates. *BMC Medical Education*, *15*(1), 162. doi:10.1186/s12909-015-0453-8 PMID:26419827

Amarasuriya, S. J. A., & Reavley, N. (2015). Perceptions and intentions relating to seeking help for depression among medical undergraduates in Sri Lanka: A cross-sectional comparison with non-medical undergraduates. *BMC Medical Education*, *15*(1), 162. doi:10.1186/s12909-015-0453-8 PMID:26419827

Arboleda-Flórez, J., & Stuart, H. (2012). From Sin to Science: Fighting the Stigmatisation of Mental Illnesses. *Canadian Journal of Psychiatry*, *57*(8), 457–463. doi:10.1177/070674371205700803 PMID:22854027

Armstrong, E. (1997). Rehabilitating troubled doctors. *BMJ (Clinical Research Ed.)*, 7095.

Ayalon, L., & Young, M. (2005). Racial Group Differences in Help-Seeking Behaviours. *The Journal of Social Psychology*, *145*(4), 391–403. doi:10.3200/SOCP.145.4.391-404 PMID:16050338

Bahora, M., Hanafi, S., Chien, V. H., & Compton, M. T. (2008). Preliminary Evidence of Effects of Crisis Intervention Team Training on Self-Efficacy and Social Distance. *Administration and Policy in Mental Health*, *35*(3), 159–167. doi:10.1007/s10488-007-0153-8 PMID:18040771

Beltran, R. O., Scanlan, J. N., Hancock, N., & Luckett, T. (2006). The Effect of First Year Mental Health Fieldwork on Attitudes of Occupational Therapy Students Towards People with Mental Illness. *Australian Occupational Therapy Journal*, 42–48.

Berk, R. A. (2010). Where's the Chemistry in Mentor-Mentee Academic Relationships? Try Speed Mentoring!. *The International Journal of Mentoring and Coaching*, 85-92.

Bond, K. S., Jorm, A. F., Kitchener, B. A., & Reavley, N. J. (2015). *Mental health first aid training for Australian medical and nursing students: An evaluation study. BMC Psychology.*

Bowler, D. L., & Pettit, W. G. (2001). The Albuquerque Police Department's Crisis Intervention Team: A Report Card. *FBI Law Enforcement Bulletin*, 1-6.

Brice-Baker, J. (1994). West Indian Women: The Jamaican Woman. In *Women of Colour: Integrating Ethnic and Gender Identities in Psychotherapy* (pp. 139–160). New York: Gilford Press.

Celluci, T., Krogh, J., & Vik, P. (2006). Help seeking for alcohol problems in a college population. *The Journal of General Psychology*, *133*(4), 421–433. doi:10.3200/GENP.133.4.421-433 PMID:17128960

Chambers, R. (1993). What should doctors do if they become sick? *Family Practice*, *10*(4), 416–423. doi:10.1093/fampra/10.4.416 PMID:8168678

Chang, D., & Berk, A. (2009). Making cross-racial therapy work: A phenomenological study of clients experiences of cross-racial therapy. *Journal of Counseling Psychology*, *56*(4), 521–536. doi:10.1037/a0016905 PMID:20414342

Chew-Graham, C., Rogers, A., & Yassin, N. (2003). I wouldn't want it on my CV or their records: Medical students experiences of help-seeking for mental health problems. *Medical Education*, *37*(10), 873–880. doi:10.1046/j.1365-2923.2003.01627.x PMID:12974841

Christopher, J. C. (2001). Culture and Psychotherapy: Towards a Hermeneutic Approach. *Psychotherapy (Chicago, Ill.)*, *38*(2), 115–128. doi:10.1037/0033-3204.38.2.115

Compton, M., Esterberg, M., McGee, R., Kotwicki, R., & Oliva, J. (2006). Brief Reports: Crisis Intervention Team Training: Changes in Knowledge, Attitudes, and Stigma Related to Schizophrenia. *Psychiatric Services (Washington, D.C.)*, *57*(8), 1199–1202. doi:10.1176/ps.2006.57.8.1199 PMID:16870973

Corrigan, P. W. (2004). How stigma interferes with mental health care. *The American Psychologist*, *59*(7), 614–625. doi:10.1037/0003-066X.59.7.614 PMID:15491256

Dahlin, M., & Runeson, B. (2007). Burnout and psychiatric morbidity among medical students entering clinical training: A three year prospective questionnaire and interview-based study. *BMC Medical Education*, *7*(1), 6. doi:10.1186/1472-6920-7-6 PMID:17430583

Diamond, G. M. (2005). Counseling and Therapy with Minority Group Counselors /Therapists. In D. W. Sue & D. Sue (Eds.), *Counseling the Culturally Diverse: Theory and Practice* (pp. 317–344). Hoboken, NJ: Wiley.

Eisenberg, D., Hunt, J., & Speer, N. (2012). Help Seeking for Mental Health on College Campuses: Review of Evidence and Next Steps for Research and Practice. *Harvard Review of Psychiatry*, *20*(4), 222–232. doi:10.3109/10673229.2012.712839 PMID:22894731

Eisenberg, D., Hunt, J., Speer, N., & Zivin, K. (2011). Mental health service utilisation among college students in the United States. *The Journal of Nervous and Menal Disease*, 301-308.

Frauenfelder, M. (2001, December 9). The Year in Ideas: A to Z.; Social-Norms Marketing. *The New York Times Magazine*.

Givens, J., & Tjia, J. (2002). Depressed Medical Students Use of Mental Health Services and Barriers to Use. *Academic Medicine. Journal. Association of American Medical Colleges*, 918–921. doi:10.1097/00001888-200209000-00024

Goffman, E. (2009). *Stigma: Notes on the Management of Spoiled Identity*. New York: Simon and Schuster.

Goldston, D. B., Molock, S. D., Whitbeck, L. B., Murakami, J. L., Zayas, L. H., & Hall, G. C. (2008). Cultural considerations in adolescent suicide prevention and psychosocial treatment. *The American Psychologist*, *63*(1), 14–31. doi:10.1037/0003-066X.63.1.14 PMID:18193978

Gopaul-McNicol. (2006). Non-Western Approach to Helping. In C. Lago (Ed.), *Race, Culture and Conselling*. Maidenhead, UK: Open University Press.

Gopaul-McNicol, S., & Brice-Baker, J. (1997). Caribbean Americans. In S. Friedman (Ed.), *Cultural Issues in the Treatment of Anxiety* (pp. 65–68). New York: Guilford Press.

Goyal, M., Kohli, C., Kishore, J., & Jiloha, R. C. (2013). Effect of an Educational Booklet on Knowledge and Attitude Regarding Major Depressive Disorder in Medical Students in Delhi. *International Journal of Medical Students*, 16-23.

Gray, A. J. (2002). Stigma in Psychiatry. *Journal of the Royal Society of Medicine*, *95*(2), 72–76. doi:10.1258/jrsm.95.2.72 PMID:11823548

Hall, S. (1992). New Ethnicities. In J. Donald & A. Rattansi (Eds.), *Race, culture and Difference* (pp. 441–449). London: SAGE.

Hobson, K. (2013, March 21). New Medical School Programmes Help Students Battle Burnout. *US News*.

Hopper, S. (1981). Diabetes as a Stigmatised Condition: The Case of Low-Income Clinic Patients in the United States. *Social Science and Medicine. Medical Anthropology*, *15*(1), 11–19. doi:10.1016/0160-7987(81)90004-1 PMID:7209601

Hunt, J., & Eisenberg, D. (2010). Mental Health Problems and Help-Seeking Behaviour Among College Students. *The Journal of Adolescent Health*, *46*(1), 3–10. doi:10.1016/j.jadohealth.2009.08.008 PMID:20123251

Jackman, S., Ellis, J., Quince, T., Wilkinson, P., Davies, R., & Thiemann, P. (2016). *Improving barriers to medical student mental health help-seeking*. University of Cambridge.

Jorm, A. F., Korten, A. E., Jacomb, P. A., Christensen, H., Rodgers, B., & Pollitt, P. (1997). "Mental health literacy": A survey of the public's ability to recognise mental disorders and their beliefs about the effectiveness of treatment. *The Medical Journal of Australia*, 182–186. PMID:9066546

Kagawa-Singer, M., & R. C. Y., C. (2002). Towards a new paradigm: A cultural systems approach. In K. Kurasaki, S. Okazaki, & S. Sue (Eds.), *Asian American Mental Health* (pp. 47-66). New York: Kluwer Academic.

Kim, B. S. (2007). Adherence to Asian and European American Cultural Values and Attitudes Toward Seeking Professional Psychological Help Among Asian American College Students. *Journal of Counseling Psychology*, *54*(4), 474–480. doi:10.1037/0022-0167.54.4.474

Kirmayer, L. J. (2006). Beyond the New Cross-cultural Psychiatry: Cultural Biology, Discursive Psychology and the Ironies of Globalization. *Transcultural Psychiatry*, *43*(1), 126–144. doi:10.1177/1363461506061761 PMID:16671396

Kutcher, S., Wei, Y., McLuckie, A., & Bullock, L. (2013). Educator Mental Health Literacy: A Programme Evaluation of the Teacher Training Education on the Mental Health & High School Curriculum Guide. *Advances in School Mental Health Promotion*, 83-93.

Leong, F. T., & Lau, A. S. (2001). Barriers to Providing Effective Mental Health Services to Asian Americans. *Mental Health Services Research*, *3*(4), 201–214. doi:10.1023/A:1013177014788 PMID:11859966

Leong, F. T., Wagner, N. S., & Kim, H. H. (1995). Group counseling expectations among Asian American students: The role of culture-specific factors. *Journal of Counseling Psychology*, *42*(2), 217–222. doi:10.1037/0022-0167.42.2.217

McKevitt, C., Morgan, M., Dundas, R., & Holland, W. (1997). Sickness absence and working through illness: A comparison of two professional groups. *Journal of Public Health*, *19*(3), 295–300. doi:10.1093/oxfordjournals.pubmed.a024633

Mino, Y., Yasuda, N., Tsuda, T., & Shimodera, S. (2001). Effects of a One-Hour Educational Programme on Medical Students Attitudes to Mental Illness. *Psychiatry and Clinical Neurosciences*, *55*(5), 501–507. doi:10.1046/j.1440-1819.2001.00896.x PMID:11555346

Miville, M. L., & Constantine, M. G. (2007). Cultural Values, Counselling Stigma, and Intentions to Seek Counseling Among Asian American College Women. *Counseling and Values*, *52*(1), 2–11. doi:10.1002/j.2161-007X.2007.tb00083.x

Modood, T., Berthoud, R., Lakey, J., Nazroo, J., Smith, P., Virdee, S., & Beishon, S. (1997). *The Fourth National Survey of Ethnic Minorities: Ethnic Minorities in Britain*. London: Policy Studies Institute.

Mojtabai, R., Olfson, M., Sampson, N. A., Jin, R., Druss, B., Wang, P. S., & Kessler, R. C. (2011). Barriers to mental health treatment: Results from the National Comorbidity Survey Replication. *Psychological Medicine*, *41*(08), 1751–1761. doi:10.1017/S0033291710002291 PMID:21134315

Neki, J., Joinet, B., Ndose, N., Kilonzo, G. J. H., & Duvinage, G. (1986). Witchcraft and Psychotherapy. *British Journal of Psychotherapy*, 145–155. PMID:3535977

OReilly, C. L., Bell, J. S., Kelly, P. J., & Chen, T. F. (2011). Impact of Mental Health First aid Training on Pharmacy Students Knowledge, Attitudes and Self-Reported Behaviour: A Controlled Trial. *The Australian and New Zealand Journal of Psychiatry*, *45*(7), 549–557. doi:10.3109/00048674.2011.585454 PMID:21718124

Papish, A., Kassam, A., Modgill, G., Vaz, G., Zanussi, L., & Patten, S. (2013). Reducing the stigma of mental illness in undergraduate medical education: A randomised controlled trial. *BMC Medical Education*, 1–10. PMID:24156397

Pasupuleti, R. V. (2013). *Cultural Factors, Stigma, Stress, and Help-seeking Attitudes Among College Students*. University of Rhode Island.

Pinfold, V., Huxley, P., Thornicroft, G., Farmer, P., Toulmin, H., & Graham, T. (2003). Reducing psychiatric stigma and discrimination - Evaluating an educational intervention with the police force in England. *Social Psychiatry and Psychiatric Epidemiology*, *38*(6), 337–344. doi:10.1007/s00127-003-0641-4 PMID:12799785

Pullen, D., Lonie, C., Lyle, D., Cam, D., & Doughty, M. (1995). Medical care of doctors. *The Medical Journal of Australia*, 481–484. PMID:7746206

Ramisetty-Mikler, S. (1993). Asian Indian immigrants in America and sociocultural issues in counseling. *Journal of Multicultural Counseling and Development*, *21*(1), 36–49. doi:10.1002/j.2161-1912.1993.tb00581.x

Rapporteur, P. (2016). *Envisioning the Future of Health Professional Education: Workshop Summary*. The National Academic Press. https://doi.org/10.17226/21796

Roh, M., Jeon, H., Kim, H., Han, S., & Hahm, B. (2010). The prevalence and impact of depression among medical students: A nationwide cross-sectional study in South Korea. *Academic Medicine*, *85*(8), 1384–1390. doi:10.1097/ACM.0b013e3181df5e43 PMID:20453812

Rosenberg, D. (2014, October 28). *The Secret Dual Lives of People Living With Mental Illness*. Retrieved from Slate Blog: http://www.slate.com/blogs/behold/2014/10/28/liz_obert_dualities_looks_at_the_hidden_and_visible_worlds_of_people_living.html

Scambler, G. (1998). Stigma and disease: Changing paradigms. *Lancet*, *352*(9133), 1054–1055. doi:10.1016/S0140-6736(98)08068-4 PMID:9759769

Schulte, D. L., Skinner, T. A., & Claibom, C. D. (2002). Religious and spiritual issues in counseling psychology training. *The Counseling Psychologist*, *30*(1), 118–134. doi:10.1177/0011000002301009

Schwenk, T., Davis, L., & Wimsatt, L. (2010). Depression, stigma, and suicidal ideation in medical students. *Journal of the American Medical Association*, *304*(11), 1181–1190. doi:10.1001/jama.2010.1300 PMID:20841531

Steadman, H. J., Deane, M. W., Borum, R., & Morrissey, J. P. (2000). Comparing Outcomes of Major Models of Police Responses to Mental Health Emergencies. *Psychiatric Services (Washington, D.C.)*, *51*(5), 645–649. doi:10.1176/appi.ps.51.5.645 PMID:10783184

Sue, D., & Sue, D. W. (1999). *Counselling the culturally different*. New York: Wiley.

Thompson, W. T., Cupples, M. E., Sibbett, C. H., Skan, D. I., & Bradley, T. (2001). Challenge of culture, conscience, and contract to general practitioners' care of their own health: Qualitative study. *BMJ (Clinical Research Ed.)*, *323*(7315), 728–731. doi:10.1136/bmj.323.7315.728 PMID:11576981

Thornicroft, G., Brohan, E., Kassam, A., & Lewis-Holmes, E. (2008). Reducing stigma and discrimination: Candidate interventions. *International Journal of Mental Health Systems*, 3-10.

Tjia, J., Givens, J., & Shea, J. (2005). Factors associated with undertreatment of medical student depression. *Journal of American College Help*, 219-224.

Utsey, S., Adams, E., & Bolden, M. (2000). Development and initial validation of the Africultural Coping Systems Inventory. *The Journal of Black Psychology*, *26*(2), 194–215. doi:10.1177/0095798400026002005

Vaz, F. S., Ferreira, A., Kulkarni, M., Perni, S., Dsouza, D., & Dsouza, L. (2012). Study of health seeking behavior among medical students in Goa, India. *Asian Journal of Medical and Clinical Sciences*, 140-141.

Wahl, O. (1999). Mental health consumers experience of stigma. *Schizophrenia Bulletin*, *25*(3), 467–478. doi:10.1093/oxfordjournals.schbul.a033394 PMID:10478782

Wechsler, H., Nelson, T. F., Lee, J. E., Seibring, M., Lewis, C., & Keeling, R. P. (2003). Perception and reality: A national evaluation of social norms marketing interventions to reduce college students heavy alcohol use. *Journal of Studies on Alcohol*, *64*(4), 484–495. doi:10.15288/jsa.2003.64.484 PMID:12921190

Whitley, R., Kirmayer, L. J., & Groleau, D. (2006). Understanding immigrants'reluctance to use mental health services: A qualitative study from Montreal. *Canadian Journal of Psychiatry*, 205–209. PMID:16629344

William, R. (2005). Towards understanding culture. In C. Lago (Ed.), *Race, Culture and Counseling* (pp. 40–49). Maidenhead, UK: Open University Press.

Yakunina, E. S., & Weigold, I. K. (2011). Asian International students' intentions to seek counseling: Integrating cognitive and cultural predictors. *Asian American Journal of Psychology*, *2*(3), 219–224. doi:10.1037/a0024821

KEY TERMS AND DEFINITIONS

Ethnicity: People who share a common culture or nationality.

Medical School Culture: Customs, rules, and ethics which medical schools place on the management of the institution, being on structure or student's well-being.

Mental Health Literacy: The understanding of mental health in regards to awareness, presenting symptoms, and how to seek help.

Obeah: A form of folk magic and belief among black culture, especially African and West Indian. It is used to ward off misfortune or to cause harm and also prescribed herbal medicine.

Religious Beliefs: Behaviours that are attached to one's religion.

Spirituality: one's faith or religion.

Western Psychotherapy: The different theoretical approaches to counselling based on taking cure, which focus on psychological symptoms.

Witchcraft: The act of magic, sorcery or supernatural powers' use to protect from harm or cause harm and embedded in the African and West Indian cultures.

Chapter 3
Perfectionism:
Addressing Lofty Expectations in Medical School

Samantha Ilia Smith
West Virginia School of Osteopathic Medicine, USA

Mitchell Dandignac
West Virginia School of Osteopathic Medicine, USA

ABSTRACT

Perfectionism is the refusal to accept any standard short of perfect. Perfectionist students might strive for 'faultless performance, meticulous attention to detail and high levels of competency' (Humphris & Kaney, 1998). In a field as complex and advanced as medicine, faultless performance is unrealistically expected. This chapter will discuss how the rigours of medical school promote perfectionistic behaviours in students. What is perfectionism? How does perfectionism in medical school affect students? How can educators and administrators identify perfectionism, provide psychoeducation, or address maladaptive perfectionism? How can students address perfectionism? It is essential to recognise perfectionism in medical students as research has shown that maladaptive perfectionism has been correlated to physician suicide (Scutti, 2014). The chapter concludes with recommendations on how students and medical educators can employ strategies to promote sound mental health and wellbeing during medical school.

INTRODUCTION

The negative impact of medical school on students' general and mental health been made clear by research (Voltmer et al., 2010; Guthrie, 1998; Dyrbye, 2005; Doherty & Nugent, 2011). The research found that, compared to students studying

DOI: 10.4018/978-1-5225-2811-1.ch003

other subjects, or peers in the same age range, medical students face an increased risk of developing depression, anxiety, and burnout. Ahmed et al. (2012) and Prinz (2012), support the prevalence of these mental health issues. In addition to these significant mental health problems experienced after students begin medical school, other signs of distress are noticeable in the personality of some students, according to the research referenced above.

Studies documenting personality types refer to many medical students and doctors as having Type A personalities. People described as having Type A personalities may have higher rates of some health problems. For instance, Type A personality behaviour was first mentioned as a potential risk for heart disease by cardiologists Meyer Friedman and Ray Rosenman in the 1950s. Behaviours commonly viewed as being associated with the Type A temperament include excessive ambition, aggression, competitiveness, drive, impatience, need for control, focus on quantity over quality and unrealistic sense of urgency (Lipsenthal 2014). The personality type of medical students may have an important impact on both their academic performance and emotional adjustment during medical school (Turiano et al., 2012; Jerant et al., 2012; Plaisant et al., 2011; Friedman et al., 2010; Henning et al., 1998). Thus, when students who display Type A personality traits are exposed to the demands of medical school, they are more likely to develop maladaptive perfectionistic behaviours.

When examining the culture of medicine and medical education, a typical expectation is that medical students will perform at a high level and on a consistent basis (Hafferty, 1998). Striving for excellence and maintaining distinction are worthy goals. The hidden curriculum in medicine appears to shun students who do not live up to the firm beliefs that medicine is both rigorous and demanding, and that if students are not tough enough to handle these high expectations, then another career ought to be considered (Hafferty, 1998).

Medical students are expected to learn an immense amount of information, study for long hours, and pass a series of examinations designed to serve as yardsticks before being able to advance to the next course or phase of medical training. The pressures to constantly achieve may compromise the mental health of students, as well as doctors, who work to live up to high expectations from family, medical educators, the rest of the medical community and patients who all expect a high level of competence. The stress associated with trying to match or exceed these expectations often lead to the development of feelings of inadequacy (Bhatia, 2016). In the literature, feelings of inadequacy are often discussed in terms of the phenomenon known as 'imposter syndrome'. According to a study conducted by Henning et al. (1998), strong associations were found between students suffering from psychological distress, perfectionism and imposter syndrome. Imposter syndrome occurs when students deemed high achievers chronically question their abilities to succeed and live in fear of being considered by others to be intellectual frauds.

Perfectionism has been viewed by some as a positive personality trait, but it can lead to self-defeating behaviours that in turn prevent the achievement of goals (Scutti, 2014). The issue of perfectionism as a deterrent to sound mental health in medical students and doctors has been studied extensively (Egan, 2008, Hill, 2004 & Hollender, 1978). Enns et al. (2001) study on perfectionism in doctors concluded that perfectionism in medical students differs systematically from perfectionism in general arts students. Melrose (2011), in her study of nurses, revealed similar patterns of personality disorders related to perfectionism and depression. Perfectionism has been conceptualised as a personality construct that may positively or negatively impact a person's behaviour (Benson, 2003). Distinguishing adaptive and maladaptive aspects of perfectionism is important in understanding the cross-sectional and longitudinal implications of perfectionism for medical students.

The goal of this chapter is to highlight some of the evidence-base literature describing perfectionism and to offer suggestions for students, medical educators and administrators on how to recognise when students' mental health and well-being are threatened by maladaptive perfectionism. Specifically, the following questions will be discussed:

- What is perfectionism?
- How does perfectionism in medical school affect students?
- How can educators and administrators identify perfectionism, provide psychoeducation, or address maladaptive perfectionism?
- How can students address perfectionism?

The chapter concludes with a series of solutions and recommendations presented from evidenced-based literature and the personal experiences of the authors. These recommendations may provide a guideline to assist students, medical academic faculty, and others who may be tasked with recognising perfectionistic behaviours, in addition to providing appropriate interventions that promote sound mental health and well-being in medical students.

BACKGROUND

Perfectionism has been linked to stress, burnout, depression (Moate, Gnilka, West, & Bruns, 2016), and personality disorders (DiMaggio et al., 2015). Upon recognising the various stressors that affect medical students, it is no surprise that they often suffer from these mental health issues. Stressors that lead to these symptoms in medical school students range from the expected changes such as less time for socialising and extracurricular activities, to rising financial debt, information overload, and time pressure (Enns, Cox, Sareen & Freeman, 2001). Medical students typically have very high expectations imposed upon them by parents, family, the medical education community, and the general population. Furthermore, these expectations continue beyond graduation, into Graduate Medical Education (GME) and practicing years. Students accustomed to being at the top of the class, are not apt to change high standards to a lower level of accomplishment as the educational advancement progresses. However, many of these students face a difficult transition into medical school and it is statistically impossible for everyone to remain in the top 10% of the class. There is a new bell curve (SciTechDaily, 2012) and it is used in a learning environment as a means of appraising performance and as a result create doubts in the mind of students even though performance may be adequate to pass. Hypothetically, a medical student could be doing very well but still feel as though failing is imminent because their grades are lower than those achieved during undergraduate courses. The frequency of 'perceived' failure during medical training may lead to a loss of morale and further deterioration of performance (Bhatia, 2016). Feelings and thoughts of inadequacy is normal but for some students, medical school pushes those insecurities into high gear, leading to some maladaptive behaviours. In the literature, a connection between conscientiousness and perfectionism has been explored to the extent of categorisation of different types of behaviours resulting in distress as a result of a negative use of the perfectionistic trait.

What Is Perfectionism?

According to Mosby's Medical Dictionary (2009), 'perfection is a subjective state in which a person pursues an extremely high standard of performance and, in many cases demands the same standards of others. Failure to attain the goals may lead to feelings of defeat and other adverse psychological consequences'. The perfectionist aims to complete chores in the most perfect manner possible. Fletti et al. (2002) and Frost et al. (1990) noted that 'People who are perfectionists strive for flawlessness, set excessively high standards of performance, and tend to be overly critical of behaviour'. Stoeber & Yang (2010) state that perfectionism is 'the state of ongoing trial to be perfect and to fix probable flaws.

An examination of the 'multidimensional definitions' of perfectionism in the evidence-based literature reveals that a definitive definition of perfectionism is lacking. Instead, many studies have focused upon the personality types that frequently demonstrate perfectionistic behaviours (Bieling, Israeli, & Antony, 2004). Recent studies have explored the relationship between perfectionism and personality, with most focusing on the Big Five model, representing five dimensions of normal personality: neuroticism, extraversion, openness to experience, agreeableness and conscientiousness (Costa & McCrae, 1992). There have been some proposals that perfectionism is a personality trait (Zuroff, 1994); other researchers have argued that it is a process that consists of cognitive and behavioural elements (Egan et al., 2011) and that maladaptive aspects of perfectionism can be reduced through cognitive-behavioural treatment (Shafran, Egan, & Wade, 2010; Egan, Wade, Shafran, & Antony, 2014). The theory of perfectionism as a behaviour pattern, as opposed to a personality trait, offers support for the effectiveness of reduction through treatment.

Personality research suggests that tendencies toward perfectionism are a consequence of extreme conscientiousness (Hogan, 2005). Conscientiousness is the personality trait commonly associated with high job performance (Hogan & Hogan, 2001). Hogan's research suggests that environmental pressures and high work expectations play into the stress levels of people. Extreme stress causes strengths such as conscientiousness to become overtaxed and to develop into dysfunctional behaviours. Hogan (2005) points out that the interaction between environmental pressures and high work demands with personality traits 'triggers perfectionism'.

The pressures associated with medicine today demand that physicians do more work, in a more expedient manner, of higher quality, and often, with fewer resources. The intense scrutiny of the public, the media, regulatory agencies, and others in the medical community itself, can 'wreck-havoc' on the mental health of doctors (Peters & King, 2012). Such lofty expectations from every possible stakeholder connected to the medical student may cause an increase in the levels of anxiety experienced. According to Peters & King (2012), these characteristics, when they become chronic, can lead doctors to experience feelings of doubt and persistent guilt, thus resulting in flawed decision-making when dealing with co-workers and patients. The awareness of the fact that most people engage in perfectionistic behaviour in some areas of life is different from those people who are unable to carry out tasks for fear of being perceived as being incompetent.

It has been well established that perfectionism is correlated with traits of neuroticism. For example, socially prescribed perfectionism is positively correlated with neuroticism (Cruce, Pashak, Handal, Munz, & Gfeller, 2012; Dunkley, Blankstein, & Flett, 1997). Socially prescribed perfectionism is characterized by people's beliefs or perceptions that the influential people in their lives are putting unrealistic standards on them, evaluating them severely, and exerting pressures on them to be absolutely perfect (Hewitt & Flett, 1991). Moreover, a number of studies have found that higher levels of perfectionism are related to 'lower agreeableness' (Dunkley et al., 1997; Dunkley, Sanislow, Grilo, & McGlashan, 2004; Zuroff, 1994). Only one study (Stumpf & Parker, 2000) did not find any evidence linking the perception of people with perfectionistic traits as being less agreeable. Numerous studies have demonstrated that conscientiousness has a positive correlation with perfectionism (Cruce et al., 2012; Dunkley et al., 1997; Dunkley, Blankstein, Zuroff, Lecce, & Hui, 2006; Stumpf & Parker, 2000). Studies utilising the Dysfunctional Attitudes Scale (DAS; Weissman & Beck, 1978) to measure perfectionism, have found positive correlations between neuroticism and perfectionism and negative correlations between extraversion and perfectionism (Dunkley et al., 1997; Dunkley et al., 2004; Zuroff, 1994). In this section of the chapter, the definition of perfectionism is based upon the behaviours referred to in the literature as adaptive and maladaptive perfectionism (Enns, 2001, Rice & Lopez, 2004; Wei et al, 2006).

Adaptive, Maladaptive and Non-Perfectionist Perfectionism

Perfectionism can be a useful characteristic. Hollender (1978; cited in Shafran & Mansell, 2001) is one of the first researchers to explain perfectionism: this researcher defined perfectionism as 'the practice of demanding oneself or others a higher quality of performance than is required by the situation' to refer to the manner in which a person performs or aspires to perform. Burns (1980), definition of perfectionism, adds: Many perfectionistic people are characterised by all or nothing thinking describes and are people who set high, irrational standards for themselves. An understanding of the behaviours associated with perfectionism is useful in understanding the phenomenon. The following descriptions of adaptive versus maladaptive perfectionism provides insight into the role perfectionism plays in some medical students. Eagan (2008) studied perfectionism scores among students in medicine, dentistry, pharmacy, and nursing students in America and revealed that perfectionism scores were higher in medicine and pharmacy students. The mean score of perfectionism was 46.9 for the students. It also showed that female students are more likely to be perfectionists than male students. A comparative study in Canada showed that positive perfectionism in medicine students is higher as compared to art students (Choy & McInerney, 2007). Hill et al. (2004) affirmed that negative perfectionism is negatively correlated with the academic performance of medicine students.

Enns et al. (2001) noted that medical students' cognitive and emotional characteristics have a significant impact on emotional adaptation to medical education and academic performance. Perfectionism according to researchers (Humphris & Kaney, 1998) is another contributing factor to the success of medical students. Interesting findings from a study by Soltani-Kouhbanani & Khosrorad (2015) indicate that there is a significant correlation between perfectionism in male and female students.

According to research there is a three-class model of perfectionism; adaptive perfectionism, maladaptive perfectionism, and non-perfectionism (Enns et al., 2001). Non-perfectionists, as the name suggests, are different from adaptive perfectionists and maladaptive perfectionists because they possess lower standards. When referring to the standards of non-perfectionists, these are not necessarily on the opposite end of the spectrum from the extremely high and often unattainable standards of perfectionists, but are rather on a level that might be perceived as simply 'average' or more easily achievable.

Adaptive perfectionism is characterised as a normal, healthy type of perfectionism and is defined by deriving satisfaction from achievements made from intense effort but tolerating the imperfections without resorting to the harsh self-criticism that characterizes maladaptive perfectionism (Stoltz & Ashby, 2007). Adaptive perfectionists work well in environments that require cooperation. In general, adaptive perfectionists may not feel compelled to take on leadership roles, but are more likely to seek joint relationships (Stoltz & Ashby, 2007). Stoeber and Otto (2006) highlight the fact that there are some desired psychological outcomes associated with adaptive perfectionism. These outcomes are positive self-esteem, life satisfaction, positive affect, emotional regulation, exam performance and academic achievement, study behaviour, school motivation, career decision-making, self-efficacy, active coping, secure adult attachment, interpersonal adjustment, and perceived social support. Additionally, adaptive perfectionism has been associated with several beneficial outcomes, such as hopefulness (Ashby, Dickinson, Gnilka, & Noble, 2011), higher satisfaction with life (Rice & Ashby, 2007), and healthier personal relationships (DiPrima, Ashby, Gnilka, & Noble, 2011).

Maladaptive perfectionism, on the other hand, has been linked with several negative outcomes such as lower satisfaction with life (Gnilka, Ashby, & Noble, 2013; Rice & Ashby, 2007), negative coping skills (Gnilka, Ashby, & Noble, 2012), higher levels of depression (Ashby et al., 2001), and higher rates of procrastination (Rice, Richardson, & Clark, 2012). Among college students, maladaptive perfectionism is associated with higher rates of stress (Ashby et al., 2012; Rice, Leever, Christopher, & Porter, 2006) and burnout (Flett, Hewitt, & Hallett, 1995; Steober & Rennert, 2008). Furthermore, maladaptive perfectionists also claim very high personal standards, in both the personal and professional aspects of life. However, maladaptive perfectionists differ in the response to falling short of those lofty standards. Instead of simply acknowledging the inability to obtain a satisfactory level of achievement and coming to terms with the unmet goal, maladaptive perfectionists subject themselves to higher levels of self-critical behaviour and thinking (Rice & Ashby, 2007; Stoeber & Otto, 2006). This response to failure is fundamental to understanding how maladaptive perfectionism can impact students, especially in medical school where the stakes are higher and the chance for failure or perceived failure is substantially higher. What are the differences between the two groups? Adaptive perfectionists hold themselves to high personal standards, but do not engage in overly self-critical behaviours and thought patterns if it is impossible to meet those standards unlike maladaptive perfectionist who generally have severe and prolonged distress in reaction to failure.

What Is the Prevalence of Perfectionism in Medicine?

A scientific review of the literature to answer this question is beyond the scope of this chapter. Instead, the authors chose to examine perfectionism in evidenced-based literature that reported on the phenomena of perfectionism in medical students and reported perfectionism as a root cause of suicide in some doctors. Doctors have much higher rates of suicide than other university graduates and health care professionals (Scutti, 2014). Physician and noted author, Shanafelt (October 2012) in a keynote address to the International Conference on Physician Health in Montréal, Quebec, disclosed that 'The perception from the societal view is not matching reality and in fact, an opposite reality exists in which many doctors are suffering'. Some doctors routinely claim to be working too many hours, at too chaotic a pace and under too much time pressure. These same doctors too often self-diagnose maladies, self-treat and self-prescribe.

In an article penned by Rodger Collier (2012) entitled 'The "physician personality" and other factors in physician health', made the point that not all the factors that lead to physician distress are related to their work environment. Doctors tend to be perfectionists and hard workers to a fault. Doctors with maladaptive tendencies often demand a lot of themselves and have difficulty relaxing or allocating time for themselves, and tend to have an exaggerated sense of responsibility to patients. According to Shanafelt (2012), these characteristics can also be attributed to what is called the 'physician personality'. The prevalence of the different types of perfectionism in medicine warrants more research to assist medical educators with a deeper understanding of how to recognise and help students maintain realistic study and work habits.

MAIN FOCUS OF THE CHAPTER

Issues, Controversies, and Problems

How Does Perfectionism Affect Medical Students?

Perfectionism has been conceptualised as a personality variable that underlies a variety of psychological difficulties. Recently, however, theorists and researchers have begun to distinguish between two distinct types of perfectionism, one determined to be a maladaptive form that results in emotional distress, as opposed to a second form which is relatively benign, perhaps even adaptive. Maladaptive evaluation concerns were more strongly associated with depression, anxiety, stress, and test-taking anxiety. Lipsenthal (2005) describes several fundamental aspects related to how perfectionism can be linked to the personality types often demonstrated by people drawn to a career in medicine. Lipsenthal (2005) further reveals how perfectionism manifests in medical school and the practice of medicine. The article referred to: Type A behaviour, competitiveness, safety-seeking behaviour, social isolation and emotional disassociation as personality traits that enable medical students to endure the rigours of the experience. On the other hand, those same characteristics that push students to perform can also lead to personal distress. This concept is similar to the findings of Shanafelt (2010), whereby perfectionism can be viewed as adaptive or maladaptive.

Perfectionistic Behaviours in Medical School

Perfectionism and its effects are not limited to the routine activities of the medical school curriculum, such as examinations and studying, but often extend to personal and social interactions. In this setting, it is apparent that most perfectionistic students tend to set high academic standards for themselves and work to achieve the best grade possible, which, though certainly a worthy pursuit, may also encourage a mindset that can be a hindrance while taking an examination. Co-author of this chapter, Mitchell Dandignac, who has first-hand experience as a learning specialist working with medical students, observed several consistent areas in which perfectionism may pose an obstacle for students: test-taking, studying and socialising and in the following sections outlines how the thinking of students manifests perfectionism during each of the three situations.

Test-Taking

Based on the above literature review, one can surmise that perfectionists can often struggle on examinations, especially multiple choice examinations. Doing well on an exam is as much about sound decision-making as it is about preparation. The majority of examinations in medical school are in a multiple-choice format, typically with four to five options and the expectation is that students will be able to:

- Identify the correct response as the best choice from a set of alternatives. This action requires decision-making processing and does not simply amount to choosing the 'right' answer but rather deciding on which answer is the 'best' when compared to several other answer choices for which there is a justification. With this in mind, good decision-making becomes crucial. Perfectionism can be a factor in this situation as it is common for perfectionists to strongly desire feeling 100% certain that each answer chosen is the correct one. This behaviour can be especially detrimental due to the timed natured of medical school exams; if one spends too much time going back and forth between answers, possibly reviewing and changing them multiple times, then the test-taker's pace may be thrown off, thereby risking the loss of time to thoroughly approach future questions. It is also important to note that in many cases, medical students are able to narrow down most questions to two answers. In such cases, perfectionists will likely be less than 100% certain of the best answer and may lose a considerable amount of valuable time overthinking the question and selected response. Accompanying this, a perfectionist may think 'I'm going to get this question wrong'. This negative thought process is understandable because selecting the wrong answer choice is always a possibility. However, students with adaptive perfectionism tend to consider the correct answer choice will be chosen and may think 'there's a minimum of a 50% chance I will get this question correct'. These students understand that the thought of being correct is possible and apply a more positive mindset. As a result, these students minimise stress and poor decision-making tendencies, in addition to time spent on questions.

Perfectionists tend to treat each question as a 'do or die' question, fearing that getting a single question wrong will translate to an overall poor performance on the examination (Peters & King, 2012). However, this is certainly not the case as exams are comprised of numerous questions and ample opportunities to answer questions correctly, thus allowing for a satisfactory exam grade. Medical students must remember that it is not necessary for test-takers to get every question correct in order to achieve a good score on the exam. Recognising the fact that there is always room for error is a key difference between perfectionists and non-perfectionists. A non-perfectionist, for instance, might recognise that even without being completely certain about the correct answer choice, narrowing down the options to the more probable of the multiple-choice answers and then simply guessing, provides the opportunity to get credit for the question. Poundstone (2014) supports these observations and offer a starting point when working with students struggling with test anxiety. Co-author Dandignac offers some suggestions:

- The desire to feel 100% confident in a chosen answer can lead to the time and energy-consuming process of overthinking and lead to errors in decision-making. This may further result in students making a myriad of cognitive distortions. An example of such a distortion may arise when it takes a test-taker 10 seconds to justify the correct answer and 60 seconds to justify another answer. Poor test-takers tend to pick the answer that took 60 seconds to justify because they equated effort with accuracy, even though the process of arriving at this decision was likely based on more assumptions and torturous

> reasoning to make the answer fit. When one overthinks a question, there is more potential to start prioritising the quantity of reasons for one answer over the quality of reasons for another. Subsequently, this may promote a false sense of confidence in the selected answer choice, even though quantity of purported reasons does not necessarily correlate with quality of the reasoning behind selecting another choice. Another common problem among test takers is changing one's answer based solely on subjectivity. Many students admit to changing their initial answers due to relying on subjective reasoning, especially when they are particularly uncertain about the correct choice.

It is important to note that changing answers is not always detrimental. However, the thought process that takes place when making the decision to change an answer must be examined. When students are feeling anxious during an exam, that anxiety can radically influence their decision-making process. Instead of relying on learned material, students' anxiety might negatively influence them when choosing answers, so much so that they begin to change answers because they 'feel like it' or think 'this answer might be better'. Perfectionists can become so uncomfortable with not being 100% confident that they may tell themselves 'if I'm not sure, I might as well change it'. Perfectionists may 'torment themselves into knots of second-guessing' where they change an answer choice several times, vacillating between their original selection and the other answers (Sherman, 2012). This behaviour is noted to resemble some similarity to gambling, where the player falsely determines that every option has equal odds even though this is not the case. This mindset is often indicative of 'the grass is green on the other side' thought process. Simply stated, such test-takers change an answer just because it feels better to do so, regardless of the fact that doing so may not significantly alter the likelihood of selecting the correct choice. Although there are no guarantees that the initial answer will be the correct one for that question, the student will at least have made a good decision based on the provided information, instead of falling into the trap of second-guessing themselves. It is important to remember that you do not judge a decision based on the outcome but on the thought process involved. Sometimes good decisions have bad outcomes, but if test-takers are able to make a series of good decisions, the end result is likely to be better than abiding by a more subjective reasoning process.

Maladaptive perfectionists have a tendency to not be able to move past a situation where the perception of not meeting high standards is possible and results in distress. This might occur during the course of an exam, as a perfectionist may continue to think about questions already answered as later questions are approached. This behaviour can have a debilitating effect on one's mood as it may plant seeds of doubt and lessen personal confidence, thus feeding into all of the other test-taking issues that might occur.

Studying

Perfectionism can also manifest itself throughout the course of learning and studying the vast amount of material. Perfectionism may serve as a benefit to students as they constantly strive to not get just a working understanding of the material, but a mastery understanding of the material. Constantly setting high goals can help to maintain motivation, but as discussed earlier, there is a difference in how maladaptive and adaptive perfectionists handle not always meeting those standards. Maladaptive perfectionists may not properly cope with the failures or perceived failures throughout the process of matriculating through medical school. This is especially problematic in medical school because it is likely that prior education established the expectation that one should be able to learn something the first time it is heard or read. This is often the case with the higher performing students at the undergraduate level. Unfortunately, since the material is more challenging in medical school, learning and understanding all the material the first time is highly unlikely. It is said among some medical educators and students that absorbing medical curriculum is like drinking from a firehose. So much information comes so quickly that one simply may not have the time to learn every single detail. Perfectionists, and all students, need to appreciate that learning is a process. When attending a lecture, the expectation should not be to reach 100% comprehension of the material, but rather a more realistic expectation would be about 25% or 30%. Lofty expectations to understand lectures with new information at the 100% rate makes it difficult to maintain a positive mindset because thoughts of self-perceived failure or incompetence is likely.

Similarly, when reviewing a lecture, the expectation should not be to understand everything. Working with students has revealed that maladaptive perfectionists expect grasp every concept at that point in time. The downside to this approach is that students may get stuck on details and obsess over them for far too long. Additionally, if perfectionists struggle to do something perfectly, the tendency may be to avoid the work altogether and procrastinate until enough energy is summoned and the confidence to learn returns. In medical school, it is critical to be able to keep up with all the material. One does not have to memorise every detail, contrary to what some might suggest. It is just as important to be able to gain a conceptual understanding and the big picture view of the material. How do things relate to one another? How can they be applied to a real-life scenario?

Perfectionists' project high standards onto other things as well. For example, before a perfectionist begins to study, the need to have the environment and physical state be just right is demanded. Studying may be delayed to find some background noise, or take time to clean off desks or do some chores around the house or eat a snack. An unnecessary amount of time could be spent just trying to organise study materials. It is important that perfectionists be able to push forward and thrive in environments that are less than perfect, even more so for future physicians working in a sometimes chaotic and unpredictable medical setting. While high standards can be very beneficial, it is also important to embrace the idea of 'good enough' when a task has the potential for perceived failure.

Socialising

Perfectionism can also take on a role in social interactions and thoughts about the social self. Perfectionist students may be prone to compare their performance or their actions to their fellow classmates. It is important to understand that most medical school students were very successful in the undergraduate programmes and are used to being in the top 10% of their cohort, one or two standard deviations above the average. Perfectionists are used to being a 'big fish'. However, in medical school there is a new bell curve, and it is statistically impossible for most students to be in the top 10% (Bhatia, 2016, Science Direct Daily, 2012). This can increase the likelihood of perceived failure because living in a medical school bubble can negatively distort a person's view of themselves and their level of competence. This can be exacerbated by the fact that many medical institutions keep a class rank, which can motivate some but leave those maladaptive perfectionists at a disadvantage. It is vital that medical students realise that getting C's and B's is not a horrible thing. As many in the profession are quick to repeat, 'What do you call medical students that got through medical school with a C average? We call them doctors'.

Many students will have to go through that adjustment of managing expectations for perfect grades in medical school. Maladaptive perfectionists however, have trouble making mistakes and coping with those perceived failures. The fear of making mistakes can be a huge obstacle since making mistakes is one of the best ways to learn and remember things. For example, perfectionists might be reluctant to work in a study group because of a lack of confidence, thinking that the information should be fully understood first, and the worry of being unable to contribute in front of peers. Studying in groups though, is one of the most effective ways to learn information, make effective connections between ideas, and get different perspectives on the material. Group studying works because verbalising information and teaching information is a much more in-depth cognitive process than simply reading or listening to something. Additionally, unlike independent study, one can get immediate feedback in study groups. This technique can help build confidence in knowledge-based understanding. Therefore, participating in a study group once or twice a week would be to one's benefit even if the material is not 100% understood.

Ultimately, from the observations of medical students with perfectionism, co-author of this chapter, Dandignac offers the following scenario based upon observation and work with medical students to demonstrate how the dual-sided nature of perfectionism might coexist. A fiction writer's greatest asset is creativity and the ability to weave many intricate plots and multi-faceted characters together into an enjoyable story. The key to creativity is free-flowing thoughts and escaping from rigid thinking and constant judgement. These judgements might include grammatical revisions or rechecking the consistency of the story. A fiction writer who is constantly interrupting their creative thought processes with revisions may become discouraged. Every time the writer stops, their stream of thought is interrupted. Subsequently, the effort put forth to judge the work and continuously refocus attention back to the task at hand is challenging. Every time the writer stops, there is an acknowledgement of potential flaws in the work. Over time, the writer may even develop a strong distaste for the story because so much time was spent critiquing and detecting supposed flaws, though, in actuality, no such shortcomings would be identified by the intended readers.

SOLUTIONS AND RECOMMENDATIONS

How Medical Students Can Address Perfectionism

Becoming Adaptive

Having explored perfectionism as it pertains to medical students, the next step is to offer solutions to the various pitfalls of perfectionism. While this is hardly a comprehensive list, these are a few pieces of advice that can help promote an adaptive response to falling short of high standards instead of maladaptive responses.

1. **Forgive Shortcomings:** Everybody has many strengths and many weaknesses because nobody is perfect. As it pertains to academic pursuits, remember that learning is a process, not a destination.
2. **Regularly Revisit Priorities:** In medical school, one must strive to do something well but also in a timely manner. One must find the balance between getting a perfect result and getting something done on time.
3. **Set Goals:** As stated previously, sometimes setting perfect standards can lead to procrastination when we do not think we are capable of meeting those standards. It may help to write down specific goals that compartmentalise the day and break up big goals into smaller, more manageable goals.
4. **Jump in Head First:** When there is fear of not meeting high standards, it often leads to procrastination. This is especially true the more difficult the task. It is important to just avoid hesitating, get started, and try to generate some momentum.

5. **Delay Judgement:** Like the fiction writer from the scenario described earlier, it is helpful to delay judgement of one's progress until a substantial amount of work is completed. Otherwise, one may constantly critique and impede progress.
6. **Experiment:** There is no one right way to study or take an exam. Try out different strategies and see what works.
7. **Seek out Resources:** Most medical school institutions offer a variety of services, including counsellors and learning specialists that can offer advice and feedback on how to approach the medical school curriculum and environment.
8. **Think of Yourself as a Friend:** When failing to meet high standards, engaging in maladaptive behaviour, such as excessive criticism, might occur. However, if another experienced the same failure, we would likely choose more considerate and supportive words. Talk to yourself as if talking to a friend.

Tips to Assist Educators and Administrators With Identifying Maladaptive Perfectionism

It is important for faculty and administrators working with medical students to recognise when conscientiousness has developed into maladaptive perfectionism. Instead of being proud of their accomplishments, students exhibiting perfectionism might instead constantly compare their work or grades to those of colleagues. Some indicators of perfectionism that may be recognised in students include:

- Spending over 20 minutes writing and rewriting a short e-mail.
- Believing that missing two or three points on an exam is akin to failure.
- Emotional disassociation regarding others' successes.
- Unrealistically holding accomplishments to the standards of others.
- Focusing on the final product instead of the actual learning process.
- Excessive procrastination from studying.

A consideration when addressing the problem of medical students' socially prescribed-perfectionism; it is essential to utilise methods that also enhance academic self-efficacy (Yu et al, 2016). These authors noted that 'perfectionist traits are obviously necessary for good clinical practice but it is important to remember the line between healthy and unhealthy perfectionism'. Peters and King (2012) note several common warning signs of unhealthy perfectionism in medicine:

- All or nothing thinking (no one understands how important this is).
- Failure to delegate (no one will do it as well as I can).

- Inability to forgive oneself or others for small mistakes.
- Procrastination to avoid the possibility of error.

There are numerous psychoeducation scales available to assist educators with measuring perfectionism. Such tools can provide educators, administrators, and mental health professionals with insight into the underlying sources of perfectionism. The Multidimensional Perfectionism Scale, originally proposed by Hewitt and Flett (1990) is designed to measure specific types of perfectionism. Hewitt and Flett later developed another scale, The Perfectionistic Self-Presentation Scale. This scale rates perfectionistic behaviours in self-presentation and appears to predict psychological distress as a result of perfectionistic tendencies (Hewitt & Flett, 1990).

FUTURE RESEARCH DIRECTIONS

The authors of the chapter present first hand strategies from the viewpoints of current experiences as a learning specialist and third-year medical student. Perfectionism is one of the variables that has been studied as a multi-dimensional attribute (Stoeber, 2016). Various research studies have proposed numerous definitions of perfectionism as the maladaptive aspects of the attribute (negative). Other researchers have documented the positive outcomes of perfectionism when the traits result in success. Some medical students have been recognised to exhibit the maladaptive perfectionism stemming from a fear of failure, which is a noted consequence of perfectionism. Additional research topics that warrant further research which will enhance the field of medical education and help better prepare medical students include the following:

- Does gender play a role in creating additional stress that promotes perfectionistic behaviours?
- Does race impact the development of perfectionism?
- What impact does perfectionism in academic faculty and preceptors have on reinforcing maladaptive perfectionism?
- What methods have been proven to demonstrate a measurable change in maladaptive behaviours?

CONCLUSION

This chapter is targeted towards medical students and the medical educators who work with them; and need to recognise that many students hold themselves and many of their actions to very high standards, yet struggle to pick themselves up when they fall short of those standards. As a result, perfectionism has been linked to stress, burnout, depression (Moate, Gnilka, West, & Bruns, 2016), and personality disorders (DiMaggio et al., 2015). Perfectionism can be a very advantageous characteristic that pushes one to master the material and complete tasks with an astute attention to detail. It can also be a characteristic that fosters doubt and causes one to engage in self-critical behaviour. There are several ways to help promote more adaptive behaviour and they all revolve around a similar idea; embrace the idea of 'good enough'. It is okay to make mistakes as that is how people often learn best. In the long run, to change perfectionistic behaviour, a systematic process must be employed because simply telling a person to adjust his or her standards is advice that will be ignored.

REFERENCES

Ahmed, H., Rhydderch, M., & Cohen, D. (2012). Prevalence of common mental health disorders in medical students: A systematic review and meta-analysis. *From Awareness to Action*. Retrieved from http://www.cma.ca/multimedia/PhysicianHealth/ICPH/ ICPH2012_PrelProg_EN.pdf

Bell Curve. (2012). Retrieved from www.SciTechDaily.com

Benson, E. (2003). The many faces of perfectionism. *Monitor on Psychology, 34*(10), 18.

Bhatia, T. (2016, May 24). *Use of bell curve in performance appraisals- Good or bad?* [Weblog post]. Employee Appraisals, HR Best Practices, Human Resources, Performance Management.

Bieling, P. J., Israeli, A. L., & Antony, M. M. (2004). Is perfectionism good, bad, or both? Examining models of the perfectionism construct. *Personality and Individual Differences, 36*(6), 1373–1385. doi:10.1016/S0191-8869(03)00235-6

Brown, B. (2013). *Overcoming perfectionism.* Retrieved from http://www.huffingtonpost.com/2013/06/29/brene-brown-daring-greatly-perfectionism-oprah_n_3468501.html

Burns, D. D. (1980). The perfectionist's script for self-defeat. *Psychology Today, 14*, 34–52.

Choy, G., & McInerney, V. (2007). Multi-dimensions of perfectionism and self-concept in school Aged Children. *Paper presented at Australian international education conference*, School of Psychology, Self- Research Centre, University of Western Sydney, Australia.

Chun, K. H., Park, Y. S., Lee, Y. H., & Kim, S. Y. (2014). Academic burnout and selection-optimization- compensation strategy in medical students. *Korean Journal of Medical Education*, *26*(4), 299–308. doi:10.3946/kjme.2014.26.4.299 PMID:25800237

Costa, P. T., & McCrae, R. (1992). *Revised NEO Personality Inventory (NEO-PI-R) and NEO Five Factor Model (NEO-FFI) Professional manual.* Odessa, FL: Psychological Assessment Center.

Cruce, S., Pashak, T., Handal, P., Munz, D., & Gfeller, J. (2012). Conscientious perfectionism, self-evaluative perfectionism, and the five-factor model of personality traits. *Personality and Individual Differences*, *53*(3), 268–273. doi:10.1016/j.paid.2012.03.013

DiMaggio, G., Lysaker, P. H., Calarco, T., Pedone, R., Marsigli, N., Riccardi, I., & Paviglianiti, A. et al. (2015). Perfectionism and personality disorders as predictors of symptoms and interpersonal problems. *American Journal of Psychotherapy*, *69*(3), 317–330. PMID:26414312

DiPrima, A. J., Ashby, J. S., Gnilka, P. B., & Noble, C. L. (2011). Family relationships and perfectionism in middle-school students. *Psychology in the Schools*, *48*(8), 815–827. doi:10.1002/pits.20594

Doherty, E. M., & Nugent, E. (2011). Personality factors and medical training: A review of the literature. *Medical Education*, *45*(2), 132–140. doi:10.1111/j.1365-2923.2010.03760.x PMID:21208259

Dunkley, D. M., Blankstein, K. R., & Flett, G. L. (1997). Specific cognitive-personality vulnerability styles in depression and the five-factor model of personality. *Personality and Individual Differences*, *23*(6), 1041–1053. doi:10.1016/S0191-8869(97)00079-2

Dunkley, D. M., Blankstein, K. R., Zuroff, D. C., Lecce, S., & Hui, D. (2006). Self-critical and personal standards factors of perfectionism located within the five-factor model of personality. *Personality and Individual Differences*, *40*(3), 409–420. doi:10.1016/j.paid.2005.07.020

Dunkley, D. M., Sanislow, C. A., Grilo, C. M., & McGlashan, T. H. (2009). Self-criticism versus neuroticism in predicting depression and psychosocial impairment for 4 years in a clinical sample. *Comprehensive Psychiatry, 50,* 335–346. doi:psych.2008.09.00410.1016/j.comp

Dyrbye, L. N., Thomas, M. R., & Shanafelt, T. D. (2005). Medical student distress: Causes, consequences, and proposed solutions. *Mayo Clinic Proceedings*, *80*(12), 1613–1622. doi:10.4065/80.12.1613 PMID:16342655

Dyrbye, L. N., Thomas, M. R., & Shanafelt, T. D. (2006). Systematic review of depression, anxiety, and other indicators of psychological distress among U.S. and Canadian medical students. *Academic Medicine*, *81*(4), 354–373. doi:10.1097/00001888-200604000-00009 PMID:16565188

Egan, J. S. (2008). *An investigation of Positive and Negative Perfectionism*. Retrieved from http://adt.curtin.edu.au

Egan, J. S., Wade, T. D., Shafran, R., & Antony, M. M. (2014). *Cognitive-behavioral treatment of perfectionism*. New York: Guilford Press.

Egan, S. J., Wade, T. D., & Shafran, R. (2011). Perfectionism as a trans diagnostic progress: A clinical review. *Clinical Psychology Review*, *31*(2), 203–212. doi:10.1016/j.cpr.2010.04.009 PMID:20488598

Ellis, A. (2002). The role of irrational beliefs in perfectionism. In G.I. Flett & P.L. Hewitt (Eds.), Perfectionism: Theory, Research and Treatment (pp. 217-229). Washington, DC: American Psychological Association. doi:10.1037/10458-009

Enns, M. W., & Cox, B. J. (2001). The nature and assessment of perfectionism: A critical analysis. In G. L. Flett & P. L. Hewitt (Eds.), *Perfectionism: Theory research and treatment*. American Psychological Association.

Enns, M. W., Cox, B. J., Sareen, J., & Freeman, P. (2001). Adaptive and maladaptive perfection in medical students: A longitudinal investigation. *Medical Education*, *35*(11), 1034–1042. doi:10.1046/j.1365-2923.2001.01044.x PMID:11703639

Eum, K., & Rice, K. G. (2011). Test anxiety, perfectionism, goal orientation, and academic performance. *Anxiety Stress Coping, 24*(2), 167-78. doi: 10.1080/10615806.2010.488723

Flett, G., Heisel, M., & Hewitt, P. (2014). The destructiveness of perfectionism revisited: Implications for the assessment of suicide risk and the prevention of suicide. *Review of General Psychology*, *18*(3), 156–172. doi:10.1037/gpr0000011

Friedman, H. S., Kern, M. L., & Reynolds, C. A. (2010). Personality and health, subjective well-being, and longevity. *Journal of Personality*, *78*(1), 179–216. doi:10.1111/j.1467-6494.2009.00613.x PMID:20433617

Frost, R. O., Marten, P., Lahart, C., & Rosenblat, R. (1990). The dimensions of perfectionism. *Cognitive Therapy and Research*, *14*(5), 449–468. doi:10.1007/BF01172967

Gnilka, P. B., Ashby, J. S., & Noble, C. M. (2013). Adaptive and Maladaptive Perfectionism as Mediators of Adult Attachment Styles and Depression, Hopelessness, and Life Satisfaction. *Journal of Counseling and Development*, *91*(1), 78–91. doi:10.1002/j.1556-6676.2013.00074.x

Guthrie, E., Black, D., Bagalkote, H., Shaw, C., Campbell, M., & Creed, F. (1998). Psychological stress and burnout in medical students: A five-year prospective longitudinal study. *Journal of the Royal Society of Medicine*, *91*(5), 237–243. PMID:9764076

Henning, K., Ey, S., & Shaw, D. (1998). Perfectionism, the imposter phenomenon and psychological adjustment in medical, dental, nursing and pharmacy students. *Medical Education*, *32*(5), 456–464. doi:10.1046/j.1365-2923.1998.00234.x PMID:10211285

Hewitt, P. L., & Flett, G. L. (1990). Perfectionism and depression: A multidimensional analysis. *Journal of Social Behavior and Personality*, *5*, 423–438.

Hewitt, P. L., & Flett, G. L. (1991). Perfectionism in the self and social contexts: Conceptualization, assessment, and association with psychopathology. *Journal of Personality and Social Psychology*, *60*(3), 456–470. doi:10.1037/0022-3514.60.3.456 PMID:2027080

Hill, R. W., Huelsmann, T. J., Furr, R. M., Kibler, J., Vicente, B. B., & Kennedy, C. (2004). A new measure of perfectionism: The Perfectionism Inventory. *Journal of Personality Assessment*, *82*(1), 80–91. doi:10.1207/s15327752jpa8201_13 PMID:14979837

Hogan, R. (2005). In defense of personality measurement: New wine for older whiners. *Human Performance*, *18*(4), 331–341. doi:10.1207/s15327043hup1804_1

Hogan, R., & Hogan, J. (2001). Assessing leadership: A view from the dark side. *International Journal of Selection and Assessment*, *9*(1&2), 40–51. doi:10.1111/1468-2389.00162

Hollender, M. H. (1978). Perfectionism: A neglected personality trait. *The Journal of Clinical Psychiatry*, *39*, 384. PMID:641018

Humphris, G., & Kaney, S. (1998). The encouragement of perfect health professionals. *Medical Education*, *32*(5), 452–455. doi:10.1046/j.1365-2923.1998.00304.x PMID:10211284

Jerant, A., Griffin, E., Rainwater, J., Henderson, M., Sousa, F., Bertakis, K. D., & Franks, P. et al. (2012). Does applicant personality influence multiple mini-interview performance and medical school acceptance offer? *Academic Medicine*, *87*(9), 1250–1259. doi:10.1097/ACM.0b013e31826102ad PMID:22836836

Kim, S. J., & Lee, S. Y. (2014). The relationship between socially-prescribed perfectionism and anger suppression in college students: Self-silencing as a mediator. *Korean Journal of Counseling*, *15*(2), 729–751. doi:10.15703/kjc.15.2.201404.729

Lee, H. A., & Jo, H. I. (2013). The relation among perfectionism, academic engagement and academic burnout: The mediating effects of motives and goal processes. *Korean Journal of Counseling and Psychotherapy*, *25*, 575–601.

Lee, M. H. (2001). *The positive and negative function of perfectionism: in relations, with achievement goal, stress, psychological well-being and depression* (Unpublished master's thesis). Hanyang University, Seoul, South Korea.

Lee, S. H., & Jeon, W. T. (2015). The relationship between academic self-efficacy and academic burnout in medical students. *Korean Journal of Medical Education*, *27*(1), 27–35. doi:10.3946/kjme.2015.27.1.27 PMID:25800259

Lipsenthal, L. (2005). The physician personality: Confronting our perfectionism and social isolation. *Holistic Primary Care: News for Health and Healing.*, *6*, 3.

Melrose, S. (2011). Perfectionism and depression: Vulnerabilities nurses need to understand. *Nursing Research and Practice*, *2011*, 1–7. doi:10.1155/2011/858497 PMID:21994842

Moate, R. M., Gnilka, P. B., West, E. M., & Bruns, K. L. (2016). *Stress and burnout among* counselor educators: Differences between adaptive perfectionists, maladaptive perfectionists, and nonperfectionists. *Journal of Counseling and Development*, *94*(2), 161–171. doi:10.1002/jcad.12073

Mosby's Medical Dictionary. (2009). Elsevier.

Perfectionism. (2013). Retrieved from http://www.goodtherapy.org/learn-about-therapy/issues/perfectionism

Perfectionism. (n.d.). In *University of Illinois Counseling Center.* Retrieved from http://www.counselingcenter.illinois.edu/?page_id=113

Peters, M. & King, J. (2012). Perfectionism in doctors. *British Medical Journal, 344*, e1674.

Plaisant, O., Courtois, R., Toussaint, P. J., Mendelsohn, G. A., John, O. P., Delmas, V., & Moxham, B. J. (2011). Medical students' attitudes toward the anatomy dissection room in relation to personality. *Anatomical Sciences Education*, *4*(6), 305–310. doi:10.1002/ase.251 PMID:22065473

Poundstone, W. (2014). *Rock Breaks Scissors: A Practical Guide to Outguessing & Outwitting Almost Everybody*. New York: Little, Brown and Company.

Prinz, P., Hertrich, K., Hirschfelder, U., & de Zwaan, M. (2012). Burnout, depression and depersonalization: Psychological factors and coping strategies in dental and medical students. *GMS Z Med Ausbild*, *29*, Doc10. PMID:22403595

Rice, K., & Lopez, F. (2004). Maladaptive perfectionism, adult attachment, and self-esteem in college students. *Journal of College Counseling*, *7*(2), 118–128. doi:10.1002/j.2161-1882.2004.tb00243.x

Rice, K. G., & Ashby, J. S. (2007). An efficient method for classifying perfectionists. *Journal of Counseling Psychology*, *54*(1), 72–85. doi:10.1037/0022-0167.54.1.72

Roger, C. (2012). The "physician personality" and other factors in physician health. *CMAJ, 184*(18). doi:.10.1503/cmaj.109-4329

Scutti, S. (2014). *Perfectionists Are More Likely to Commit Suicide Than The Rest of Us*. Retrieved from http://www.medicaldaily.com/perfectionists-especiallydoctors-architects-and-lawyers-are-higher-risk-suicide-305256

Shafran, R., & Mansell, W. A. (2001). Perfectionism and psychopathology: A review of research and treatment. *Clinical Psychology Review*, *21*(6), 879–906. doi:10.1016/S0272-7358(00)00072-6 PMID:11497211

Sherman, E. (2012, January 2). *Are you a perfectionist?*. Retrieved from https://www.psychologytoday.com/blog/couch-meets-world/201201/are-you-perfectionist

Soltani-Kouhbanani, S., & Khosrorad, R. I. (2015). Investigating perfectionism in medicine and architecture majors. *International Journal of Educational Investigation*, *2*(2), 128–139.

Stoeber, J. (2016). *Comparing Two Short Forms of the Hewitt-Flett Multidimensional Perfectionism Scale Assessment*. Retrieved from https://www.ncbi.nlm.nih.gov/pubmed/?term=multidimensional+of+perfectionsim1073191116659740

Stoeber, J., & Otto, K. (2006). Positive conceptions of perfectionism: Approaches, evidence, challenges. *Personality & Social Psychology*, *10*(4), 295–319. doi:10.1207/s15327957pspr1004_2 PMID:17201590

Stoeber, J., & Rennert, D. (2008). Perfectionism in school teachers: Relations with stress appraisals, coping styles, and burnout. *Anxiety, Stress, and Coping*, *21*(1), 37–53. doi:10.1080/10615800701742461 PMID:18027123

Stumpf, H., & Parker, W. D. (2000). A hierarchical structural analysis of perfectionism and its relation to other personality characteristics. *Personality and Individual Differences*, *28*(5), 837–852. doi:10.1016/S0191-8869(99)00141-5

Turiano, N. A., Pitzer, L., Armour, C., Karlamangla, A., Ryff, C. D., & Mroczek, D. K. (2012). Personality trait level and change as predictors of health outcomes: Findings from a national study of Americans (MIDUS). *The Journals of Gerontology. Series B, Psychological Sciences and Social Sciences*, *67*(1), 4–12. doi:10.1093/geronb/gbr072 PMID:21765062

Voltmer, E., Rosta, J., Aasland, O. G., & Spahn, C. (2010). Study-related health and behavior patterns of medical students: A longitudinal study. *Medical Teacher*, *32*(10), e422–e428. doi:10.3109/0142159X.2010.496008 PMID:20854148

Wei, M., Russell, D. W., Young, S., & Hewitt, P. P. (2006). Maladaptive perfectionism and ineffective copping as mediators between attachment and future depression: A prospective analysis. *Journal of Counseling Psychology*, *53*(1), 67–79. doi:10.1037/0022-0167.53.1.67

Weissman, A. N., & Beck, A. T. (1978). *Development and validation of the dysfunctional attitude scale: a preliminary investigation*. Paper presented at the 86th Annual Convention of the American Psychological Association, Toronto, Ontario, Canada.

Yu, J., Chae, S., & Chang, K. (2016). The relationship among self-efficacy, perfectionism and academic burnout in medical school students. *Korean Journal of Medical Education*, *28*(1), 49–55. doi:10.3946/kjme.2016.9 PMID:26838568

Zuroff, D. C. (1994). Depressive personality styles and the five-factor model of personality. *Journal of Personality Assessment*, *63*(3), 453–472. doi:10.1207/s15327752jpa6303_5 PMID:7844736

KEY TERMS AND DEFINITIONS

Academic Burnout: Symptoms include physical, emotional, and psychological depletion due to fatigue, frustration, distance from studies, stress, helplessness, and cynical attitude as a result of academic overload.

Academic Self-Efficacy: An overall judgement, including self-ability to manipulate and effectuate required series of academically related tasks.

Adaptive Perfectionism: Characterized as a normal, healthy type of perfectionism,wherein individuals find a positive means to adjust to not meeting high personal standards.

Competence: Belief in own self efficacy.

Conscientiousness: Degree of organisation, persistence, control, and motivation in goal directed behaviour.

Depression: Tendency to experience feelings of guilt, sadness, despondency and loneliness.

Dysfunctional Attitude Scale: A scale used to measure perfectionism.

Maladaptive Perfectionism: Characterized as an abnormal, unhealthy type of perfectionism, wherein individuals show a tendency to engage in self-critical behaviour when there is a perception of failure.

Personality Type: A collection of behaviours that usually occur together on a consistent basis and pattern.

Socially-Prescribed Perfectionism: The excessive desire to follow the rules of society and live up to the expectations of others.

Chapter 4
Medical Student Burnout:
A Social Cognitive Learning Perspective on Medical Student Mental Health and Wellness

Robert Lubin
Technion – Israel Institute of Technology, Israel

Michael D. Hamlin
Touro University Worldwide, Israel

ABSTRACT

Medical students' mental health is a topic of great interest as it has implications not only for medical students but also for the patients of these future doctors. Medical students face many academic pressures and burnout is one possible consequence of these stressors with some studies suggesting that burnout affects up to 50% of medical students. Our own study of American students in a medical programme located outside of the U.S. showed that student perceptions of the medical learning environment were linked with burnout suggesting that reducing burnout requires a pedagogical approach that addresses academically related stress factors. This chapter contends that one institutional strategy to prevent problems such as burnout is to adopt a theory-based approach to instructional design that addresses the causes of medical student stress and burnout from the instructional side.

INTRODUCTION

Burnout has been described as 'a psychological syndrome of emotional exhaustion, depersonalization, and reduced personal accomplishment that can occur among individuals who work with other people in some capacity' (Galan et al., 2011).

DOI: 10.4018/978-1-5225-2811-1.ch004

Grounded in the realities of people's experiences Maslach's Burnout Inventory, which has been recognized for more than a decade as the leading measure of burnout, defines three dimensions of burnout. The three dimensions, Emotional Exhaustion, Depersonalization and Personal Accomplishment are related to environmental variables in different ways. Exhaustion and cynicism tend to emerge from school overload and social conflict while a sense of inefficacy arises from a lack of resources within a situation (Maslach, 2003). Maslach's theory states that burnout occurs when people lose a sense of positive connectedness with others and have a loss of shared values among peers (Maslach, Schaufeli, & Leiter, 2001).

Medical student burnout can be a predictor of depression, low self-esteem, school attrition and suicidal ideations (Chang, Eddins-Folensbee, & Coverdale, 2012) and has also been associated with intention to leave medical school and unprofessional behaviour (Dyrbye, et al., 2010). In a study conducted by the Mayo Clinic, with participants from seven U.S. medical schools, 53 percent of medical students, had symptoms of burnout. In a series of studies Drybye and her colleagues (Dyrbye, et. al, 2009, 2010, 2012) showed how burnout was associated with self-reported unprofessional conduct and less altruistic professional values among other problems.

Emotional exhaustion may lead to physical neglect, which decreases empathy and can directly affect patient care. Emotional exhaustion and loss of focus may also be the reason doctors have a higher suicide rate than the general population (Dyrbye et al., 2010). Lupo and Strous (2001) showed higher levels of anxiety among medical students in the preclinical years than the clinical years. Alternately, conflicting research cited by Rosenthal and Okie (2005) showed higher levels of anxiety in the clinical years. The conflicting data can be attributed to different types of stress factors making each phase a new learning opportunity to reflect on stressors and acknowledge symptoms.

A current thread in medical education research has examined clinical empathy and its relationship with burnout (Dyrbye et al., 2010; Hojat et al., 2004). Empathy is a universal foundation of the future physician-patient relationship (Matthews, Suchman & Branch, 1993) that promotes diagnostic accuracy, patient adherence to treatment plans and physician satisfaction (Derksen, Bensing & Largo-Janssen, 2013). Research into empathy and professional burnout has demonstrated that physicians tuned into the psychosocial needs of their patients were less likely to experience burnout (Anfossi & Numico, 2004), that empathy levels are negatively correlated with burnout (Wilczek-Ruzyczka, 2011) and that burnout is a factor with significant influence on self-assessed empathy among medical students (DiLalla, Hull & Dorsey, 2004). It has also been shown that self-perceived empathy declines significantly during the course of medical school as a result of increased contact with patients in the clinical phase of training (Neumann et al., 2011).

The capacity for empathy is important for establishing interpersonal relationships, which is crucial in the medical field where clinicians need to establish both general interpersonal relationships and doctor–patient relationships (Park et al., 2006). Within an empathetic relationship, patients talk more about their symptoms enabling the physician to collect more data and determine a more accurate diagnosis (Derksen, Bensing & Largo-Janssen, 2013). By finding a common ground between doctor and patient, trust is built, the emotional experience is recognized and the patient is able to become an active participant in the treatment (Gelhaus, 2012). Empathic communication enables patients to talk more comfortably which leads to a more accurate diagnosis and an agreeable treatment plan between physician and patient (Coulehan, et al., 2001).

Cohen, Kay, Youakim and Balacius (2009) write that empathy requires attentive listening and that empathic listening within a healthcare setting involves a higher emotional burden than what a student may have previously encountered when providing assistance in another environment. Students' discomfort at the harm they and their teachers can do to patients creates a tension between their feelings of empathy and the burnout they may experience within the medical school-learning environment.

A goal of this chapter is to demonstrate that if learning environment perceptions are associated with burnout then efforts to address these factors through theory-based instructional reform can create an environment in which burnout is addressed and assessed within a pedagogical framework. Research in medical education has pointed to two major stress-related problems for medical students. One is the stress created through academic pressures and the other is associated with social aspects of medical education. This chapter will suggest theory-based pedagogical changes in the medical school-learning environment that can address these problems and hence, reduce burnout.

A Study of Burnout, Empathy, and Perception of Learning Environment

Burnout has been demonstrated among American medical students studying in the U.S. (Dyrbye, et al., 2014) and among international medical students studying in their respective countries (Muzafar, et al., 2015; Cecil, McHale, Hart & Laidlaw, 2014). As clinical empathy has been shown to be a major beneficial factor in patient care and burnout appears to be related to the reported decline of empathy among medical students, understanding the learning environment factors related to this relationship can offer possible insights into methods that might decrease burnout in medical students.

A study of students in an international medical school programme was conducted to explore the associations between student perceptions of the learning environment and burnout. In 2014, an email survey was sent to a sample of 120 men and women medical students in an international medical programme. The identical survey was sent two times during the year at the beginning and towards the end of the academic semester. Two dimensions of burnout were measured using validated single items from the Maslach Burnout Inventory. Participants responded using a 7-point Likert scale (1=daily, 7=never) about how often he or she felt 'burned out from my work' (for emotional exhaustion) or 'callous toward people' (for depersonalization).

The Dundee Ready Educational Environment Measure (DREEM) (Alshehri, Alshehri, and Erwin, 2012) provided questions related to student perceptions of several aspects of the learning environment including self-perception about learning, student self-perception of teachers, academic self-perception, perception of atmosphere and their social situation. The DREEM was developed as a universal diagnostic inventory for assessing the whole or parts of the educational environment and climate of medical schools (Roff, et al., 1997) and is the most widely used instrument for the evaluation of medical and healthcare related courses (Alshehri, Alshehri, and Erwin, 2012).

DREEM Sub-Scales

The Student Perception of Learning sub-scale helps provide insight into the learning process and focuses on the learning style of the student. Sub-scale statements ask the student to rate their perception of learning time, focus, emphasis and confidence as well as their understanding of course objectives and class participation. The perception of learning demonstrates the operating values and beliefs of the student. A stronger self-perception is linked to a more positive self-concept (Weiner, 2000), which can be linked to a more productive learning experience.

The Academic Self-Perception sub-scale indicates how students feel about their learning environment (Alshehri, Alshehri, and Erwin, 2012). Strong positive responses can be linked to student learning as a strong connection exists between an individual's efforts and their performances (Koparan, Şahin, and Kuter, 2010).

The Perception of Teachers sub-scale measures the confidence the student has in faculty teaching, style, mannerism and delivery. Examples of these sub-scale statements include: 'The teachers give clear examples', and 'The teachers are knowledgeable'. Analysing the perception a student has of teachers provides a measure of connectivity to the faculty, which can be correlated with a student's level of academic success or failure.

The medical school-learning environment integrates classroom instruction, clinical practice, and social/professional identity formation while being impacted by the personal experiences of each student. The DREEM's Social Self-Perception subscale measures the way a student perceives their learning and development.

Certain products of professional education occur through a socialization process that crystallizes into behavioural norms and culturally appropriate beliefs. This deliberate but less conscious habitus of practice shapes perception and skilled practice (Bourdieu, 1990). The social context is important to understand when analysing learning and development of medical students.

The Jefferson Scale of Empathy

Research using the Jefferson Scale of Empathy with different classes in a medical programme has been used to demonstrate the need for a comprehensive educational approach to empathy. In this study, the Jefferson Scale of Empathy –Student Version was used to measure self-reported levels of empathy. The research team that developed the Jefferson Scale of Empathy states, 'empathy is a predominantly cognitive (rather than emotional) attribute that involves an understanding (rather than feeling) of experiences, concerns and perspectives of the patients, combined with a capacity to communicate this understanding' (Hojat, 2009, p. 413).

Results

A correlation matrix was constructed using emotional exhaustion and depersonalization as criterion variables and learning environment variables as predictor variables. Consistent with previous studies, associations were found between learning environment perceptions and burnout.

As shown in Table 1, the Academic subscale had the strongest correlation with both emotional exhaustion and depersonalization. Students' academic self-perception indicates how students feel about their performance. This relationship can also be attributed to the internal attribution of the participants. Emotional exhaustion is described as being burnt-out from a demanding job. Feeling that their performance is solely based on their level of academic acumen could relate to higher levels of emotional exhaustion. Depersonalization is described as feeling callousness towards

Table 1. Correlation matrix from collected surveys

DREEM Perceptions	Burnout: Emotional Exhaustion	Burnout: Depersonalization
Learning	0.28	0.29
Teachers	0.33*	0.27
Academic	0.36*	0.35*
Atmosphere	0.26	0.25
Social	0.29	0.32*

* 0.3-0.5 is a significant correlation

others. Using internal attributes for academic success such as doing well academically because of good studying techniques could explain the strong correlation with depersonalization.

The perception of the student influences their internal self-concept (Weiner, 2000). According to Rogers (1975, p.7), 'To perceive a new aspect of oneself is the first step toward changing the concept of oneself'. The lack of a relationship between the perception of learning and burnout could demonstrate a strong internal attribution and self-image among study participants. Participants may have attributed their understanding and level of confidence with internal attributions without reflecting on feelings of burnout.

Several studies (Dyrbye et al., 2009; 2010) have examined the links between burnout, empathy and academic performance and perceptions. In this study, there was a moderate correlation between the Learning Perceptions sub-scale and empathy (Table 2). These results demonstrate the importance of the relationship between the students' perception on the development of empathy and the learning environment. As the perception of the student influenced their control over their internal self-concept (Weiner, 2000), maintaining a supportive learning environment helped maintain their level of empathy.

In this study, an insignificant relationship was found between burnout and empathy (Table 3). In another study, results were indicative of higher burnout associations with lower empathy scores (Brazeau, Schroeder, Rovi, & Boyd, 2010). In this study, the lack of evidence for a relationship between burnout and empathy

Table 2. Correlation matrix from collected surveys

DREEM Perceptions	Empathy
Learning	0.38*
Teachers	0.22
Academic	0.23
Atmosphere	0.35*
Social	0.29

* 0.3-0.5 is a significant correlation

Table 3. Correlation matrix from collected surveys

Burnout	Empathy
Burnout: Emotional Exhaustion	0.24
Burnout: Depersonalization	0.21

* 0.3-0.5 is a significant correlation

may be indicative of the differences in how self-reported burnout is experienced by international students.

Hellsten and Prescott (2004) write about the effect the learning process has on student learning in international settings. While previous research evidence suggests that empathy declines during the clinical years (Hojat et al., 2004), data from international medical programmes do not show the same results. As well, Coulter and Abney (2009) and Deosthalee (2002) reported that visiting teachers reported less burnout than their native counterparts in Canada and India. Examining international medical programmes could produce more evidence about the cultural impact of the learning environment on teaching clinical empathy and combatting burnout.

The study failed to find a relationship between burnout and empathy as in some earlier studies but there were relationships between most of the DREEM learning environment subscales and either burnout or empathy. This leads to a conclusion that changes made on learning environment variables may reduce the stressors that lead to burnout and declines in clinical empathy found in some studies.

ISSUES, CONTROVERSIES, PROBLEMS

The Medical School Learning Environment

The learning environment in medical school needs to contain a strong clinical foundation and a structured methodology to teach effective doctor patient relationships. For instance, Larson and Yao (2005) emphasize the importance the medical school-learning environment plays in the training and development of skills like clinical empathy. Additionally, students' perception of their learning environment contributes to their academic performance (Wayne, Fortner, Kitzes, Timm & Kalishman, 2013). An assessment of teaching methods by a medical programme will have long-term benefits on problems such as student burnout. Our study provides more evidence of the relationship academic perception has on burnout.

Many medical school educational innovations are instituted to address a specific problem or gap in the curriculum but are not designed or implemented in a systematic way or with much empirical foundation. And, as Slavin and his colleagues (2014) have pointed out, efforts to address burnout often rely on additional courses or programmes designed to address the symptoms of a stressful learning environment rather than addressing the root cause which is the learning environment itself. From their perspective, rather than accepting the fact that the medical school-learning environment produces stress in students and creating programmes to address the effects of the learning environment, they chose to respond with larger scale curricular changes designed to reduce the stressful nature of learning in medical school.

From our perspective, educational innovations in the medical curriculum need to be evidenced based and should be derived from work in the learning sciences. Educators who wish to address issues with curricular and instructional change need to become aware of recent educational research, which demonstrates how learning and thinking are primarily context-oriented and involve a set of interlocking cognitive, metacognitive and affective abilities and processes. By incorporating this research, medical education can be designed with a stronger theoretical basis that can create improved learning environments and less stressful learning.

The Need to Assess the Medical Education Learning Environment

The Liaison Committee on Medical Education (LCME) emphasizes the importance of the learning environment in its accreditation standards (www.lcme.org/standard, 2014):

A medical education programme must ensure that its learning environment promotes the development of explicit and appropriate professional attributes in its medical students ...[and should] regularly evaluate the learning environment to identify positive and negative influences on the maintenance of professional standards and conduct and develop appropriate strategies to enhance the positive and mitigate the negative influences.

Hewson and Little (1998) write about the importance of creating a supportive learning environment to develop a safe place for learners to excel (Ramani and Krackov, 2012). This includes the importance of the mentoring and learning relationship established between the faculty member and the student. Research in other health care education fields has also stressed the need for a more supportive learning environment. For examples, Henderson et al., (2010) write about the benefits of a supportive learning environment for undergraduate nursing students. The study cites the importance of the educator as a learning guide and a critical factor for student achievements.

Assessing the perception of the student on their learning environment, it was found that the presence of a skilled and knowledgeable educator effectively assisted the transfer of learning. Deep learning was accomplished through effective teaching and role modeling behaviour. The relationship built between the mentor and student is instrumental in the learning process. The formal and informal support was documented as facilitating the learning process and promoting learning.

While learning can happen in every environment, the environment of the learner becomes the natural habitat for discovery. The academic learning environment is responsible for providing practical and tactical knowledge so students can develop transferable abilities. Collins, Brown and Newman (1987) state the learning environment is responsible to provide students with problem solving strategies and 'tricks of the trade' (p.14). A learning environment must be a supportive setting for students to engage, discover, explore and develop. The ideal medical school-learning environment provides academic instruction within a supportive environment.

Humanistic medical care and teaching humanism is seen as an instrumental component of medical education (Gracey, et al., 2005). Gracey, et al. (2005) defines humanism in medicine as attitudes and actions that demonstrate interest and respect for a patient and related to issues of psychological, social and spiritual concerns. Medical students should be taught to demonstrate warmth, professionalism and to validate the concerns of patients. Learning these attributes produces warm and reassuring mannerisms and more effective practitioners (Blasi, Harkness, Ernst, Georgiou & Kleijnen, 2001). Teaching, learning and living the human dimensions of care become integral in the instructional focus of a medical school. Besides the strong foundation in basic anatomy, a medical school is responsible to teach its students through formal and informal methods about humanity, empathy and effective communication.

Besides the basic science model that is taught in medical school there is a strong perspective that the social environment of the medical school has a tremendous impact on the identity development and future skills acquisition of the medical student (Suchman et al., 2004). Medical students across the world develop the 'habitus' of practice to develop professionally (Benner and Sutphen, 2007). The habitus of empathy is developed from inner experiences, patient feedback and observations and is universal in the professional experience.

Education for the Reflective Practitioner

Benbasset (2014) has stressed the role of critical reflection in reducing student anxiety and other stress-related problems such as burnout. He has also pointed out that improving positive personal perceptions such as self-awareness and awareness of others, which have been associated with increased levels of interpersonal competence, can also lead to more anxiety if students are not provided with the tools to become critical thinkers.

Critical reflection involves a critique of the presuppositions on which our beliefs have been built which transforms learning into a new experience (Mezirow, 2003). Reflection has been defined as intellectual and affective activities in which individuals engage to explore their experiences in order to lead to new understandings and appreciation (Mezirow, 2003). Educational institutions have a responsibility to provide learning environments that foster intellectual advancement while producing reflective practices.

The importance of a medical school-learning environment has been shown to be directly related to student learning and emotional development (Gracey, et al., 2005). The learning environment must train students in self-directed learning and provide guidance so each student develops their own insights and knowledge awareness (Carr and Johnson, 2013). Murinson, et al., (2010) found that student emotional development progress from first year to graduating medical student is a mark of a successful learning environment.

In relation to burnout, Maslach (2003) has pointed out that exhaustion and cynicism tend to emerge from school overload and social conflict while a sense of inefficacy arises from a lack of resources within a situation (Maslach, 2003). In our study, the majority of learning environment domains were associated with burnout which suggests that reducing burnout requires a holistic approach that may emphasize methods to improve the academic environment (Table 1). Dyrbye, et al., (2009) researched specific learning environment characteristics and burnout and found that the influences having an effect on burnout levels are variable and differ at different places in the medical curriculum. Dyrbye, et al., (2010) demonstrated that a supportive learning environment has a significant impact on student burnout and they have suggested that a supportive learning environment is important for optimal learning, facilitates the development of professionalism, and has a profound impact on student burnout.

The research and literature on burnout in medical school education has produced a number of findings about causative factors of burnout and implications for learning. Table 4 summarizes findings from two studies (Dyrbye, et al., 2010; Muzafar, et al., 2015) that identify important learning environment factors in burnout.

Table 5 shows the elements of the learning environment that were associated with burnout and student perceptions of their clinical empathy in the study presented in this chapter.

Summarizing from a number of studies that looked at the medical school-learning environment then, it can be shown that there are two main areas that should be

Table 4. Causative factors of burnout

Causative Factors of Burnout		
(Dyrbye, et al., 2010)		**(Muzafar, et al., 2015)**
Workload		Too much study with little balance
Increased student autonomy		Lack of supportive relationships
Stressed relationship with others		Lack of time for recreation
Stress of patient care		Lack of belief in what you do

Table 5. Elements of learning environment associated with burnout and empathy

	Burnout Dimensions		Empathy
	Emotional Exhaustion	Depersonalization	
Teachers	X	X	
Academic	X	X	
Social		X	
Learning			X
Atmosphere			X

addressed in efforts to create curricular changes to combat stress-related problems such as burnout. One is the stress that is created through academic pressures. The other relates to pressures associated with social aspects of medical education.

Maslach's theory of burnout states that burnout occurs when people lose a sense of positive connectedness with others and have a loss of shared values among peers (Maslach, Schaufeli, and Leiter, 2001). In medical education, Dyrbye (2010) found that strong social relationships were associated with resilience to burnout. According to McKenna, Hashimoto, Maguire and Bynum (2016) in proposing that medical education programmes need to stress the need for connection stated, 'we should prioritize connecting with one another and with our patients to build a sense of belonging within our teams, programmes, hospitals, and profession' (p. 1199).

SOLUTIONS AND RECOMMENDATIONS

This chapter argues that a culture shift is needed among medical school educators to change the conversation from segregated attempts to address burnout to a more theory-based, instructional approach (Eckleberry-Hunt, Van Dyke, Lick, & Tucciarone, 2009). As such, medical instruction and curriculum design should be evidence based and have a more humanistic, educational perspective focused on producing a more reflective and mindful practitioner. Instructional paradigms and pedagogies should be grounded in learning science and designed to produce reflective, integrative and professional medical students, which should go a long way to reduce stress and stress-related problems such as burnout, imposed by current medical curricula.

The Science of Learning

Understanding that the source of distress could stem from the learning environment, curriculum reform can be effective at improving student stress and wellbeing (Slavin, Schindler, & Chibnall, 2014). But medical educators who wish to address the need for a more supportive medical environment need to become aware of recent educational research that demonstrates how learning and thinking are primarily social activities, context-oriented and involve a set of interlocking cognitive, metacognitive and affective abilities and processes that need to be cultivated and addressed in instruction. By incorporating this research, medical education learning environments can be designed with a stronger theoretical basis about learning that can help produce practitioners who know how to assess and manage care needs, using contextualized and integrative thinking with decision making. But as this chapter will argue, education for the professions and medical education more specifically requires a new perspective and approach.

Various authors have pointed out that the unique nature of educating for practice demands an integrative pedagogy that presents knowledge, technical skills and ethical, patient-centred practices in ways that help students become reflective practitioners. Benner and Sutphen (2007) and Benner, Sutphen, Leonard, and Day (2010), for instance have called for health care education that focuses on the following:

- Contextualization

Teaching knowledge and skills separately or in a decontextualized manner produces fragmented educational experiences. Students should be taught in an environment where knowledge and thinking are situated and linked to action applied in a particular context. Faculty members must provide connections between the professional knowledge and the use of that knowledge in the practice setting.

- Authentic Learning Experiences

Teaching situations often involve impoverished settings that do not approximate the dynamic clinical setting and many assessments focus in on fine-grained or elementary competencies. Students need instruction and assessment in clinical settings encompassing a diverse set of patient care situations.

- Multiple Ways to Think

A singular focus on teaching scientific and critical thinking skills often results in a cynicism and a habitual critique of methods being taught. Scientific and critical thinking need to be augmented with other ways of thinking such as the ability to reason through the trajectory of a patient's developing situation and that integrate patient needs and the student's own life experience.

- Formation of professional identity

Health educators should transition from a focus on socialization and role taking to an emphasis on the formation of a professional identity, which supports reflective practice.

As a number of health educators such as Benner (1984), Noone (2007) and Berragan (2013) have pointed out, health professions require education for practice. Curricula and instruction must be designed to deliver education in a contextualised fashion that links knowledge, skills and ethical and reflective practice behaviour.

Situative Learning Theory in Medical Education

In the last two decades, many learning scientists have shifted their studies from a focus on the individual's cognitive processes and learning to a broader conception of thinking and learning as social activities. Learning scientists with this sociocultural perspective focus on the social nature of learning and thinking and many make the claim that all learning and thinking is situated in and tied to social contexts. Rather than focusing on the learning processes of individuals, learning scientists with this sociocultural perspective focus on communities of practice and investigate learners' interactions and patterns of participation in the activities of the group.

According to situated learning theory or what some (Greeno, 1997) have called the situative perspective, learning and cognition are thought to be the products of activity occurring in situations or communities of practice and knowledge, learning and thinking are distributed among the members and components of these communities rather than the strictly unique product of individuals (Greeno & van de Sande, 2007). The situative perspective looks at learning, cognition, motivation and achievement as social activities (Turner & Nolen, 2015) and applies the sociocultural view to research into classroom learning.

Greeno and van de Sonde (2007) have outlined the main issues in situated learning as it applies to education. Their main points include:

- Knowledge and cognition are distributed among individuals who interact within a social system
- Knowledge and cognition function as a capability for participating in activity systems

Seen from this perspective learning is a change in participation and positive learning is a change in the direction of more full, active participation. Using the situative approach to developing more effective and supportive medical learning education we would want to take into account how students coordinate interactions with each other, the learning resources and the elements of the learning environment and try to determine which learning environment elements afford positive student progress and which constrain this progress

To address the relevant pedagogical concepts from situative learning in medical education one needs to design instructional environments that incorporate notions of the social nature of thinking and learning, important aspects of discourse and guidance for the development of an appropriate professional identity. The situative perspective can inform medical education by providing guidance on how to address relevant learning affordances and the abilities and intentions to find and use them. A number of researchers (Greeno, 1992; Greeno & van de Sande, 2007; Gresalfi & Cobb, 2011) have described aspects of situative learning derived from research in the learning sciences that are relevant to medical education. Three that are particularly relevant include the social nature of cognition and learning, affordances and constraints in discourse, and an activity-based concept of identity development.

Learning in Context

One of the lines of research that stimulated the idea of learning as a social activity situated in communities of practice comes from Lave (1988) and later Lave and Wegner (1991) who studied traditional apprenticeship learning and training in authentic settings. Their work established a set of principles for learning in authentic contexts that laid the theoretical groundwork for studying cognition in practice or what has been called situated cognition.

According to Lave and Wenger, the apprentice learns and carries out tasks in a real-world context e.g. a tailor shop, a classroom or an academic medical centre, where experts and novices of varying abilities are working together. This creates a learning culture where beginners have access to expert performance and guidance and engage in learning in context that shapes the apprentice's growing perception of what constitutes good practice. Rather than learning skills in isolation as is done with much of school learning, learning in a real-world setting provides more signals and reminders, or what some call affordances, about how to apply the skills that have been learned.

The Apprentice Model of Learning in Context

Apprentices start out working on small pieces of the final product with assistance from the experts and advance to more difficult tasks and products that successively approximate the final product. Because they learn in context, apprentices have access to experts who provide both modelling and coaching and offer examples of both finished products and work-in-progress. Through observation of the experts' successful techniques (and also the errors of other apprentices) apprentices can create internal models of the final product, which they can use to guide their developing skills.

A basic tenet of Lave and Wenger's theory of situated cognition is that the interaction of observation, coaching and scaffolding provided by the expert and the increasingly skilled performance of the apprentice allows the apprentice to shape a productive mental model that can guide their progress. Contrast this with typical decontextualized schooling methods that try to build up knowledge and skills in a sequence of small pieces where the learner does not get to observe the final product for a considerable amount of time. Not only is the learner deprived of any guiding model with which to direct their developing skills in this scenario, the lack of context for their learning hampers them in the development of the self-monitoring and-correction skills that come with having continual access to expert techniques and problem-solving skills.

Finally, by developing their skills in context, apprentices develop not just a set of skills and knowledge about tasks, they also develop a practice informed by social learning principles (modelling, group-learning) into what some have called a habitus, or habits of mind that guide practitioners in that profession. Apprenticeship learning then, is learning for practice. Situated learning, the idea that learning in context produces knowledge through activity connects this perspective to apprenticeship learning and leads the way to a new pedagogy for producing reflective practitioners whose knowledge and skills are blended in a complex, network of skilled practice.

Cognitive Apprenticeship

Cognitive researchers such as Alan Collins, John Seely Brown and others extended Lave and Wegner's characterizations of apprenticeship and situated cognition and applied them to attempts to improve teaching by focusing on cognitive skills in school subjects such as math, reading and writing. Collins, et al., (1987) established a set of principles for what they called 'cognitive apprenticeship' or the application of apprentice learning to the teaching of cognitive skills in applied settings.

The term cognitive apprenticeship was used to stress two issues: First, as with traditional apprenticeships, teaching methods attempt to express explicitly expert's mental processes and strategies used in solving problems in a domain such as math or reading and domain knowledge is always taught in service of carrying out actual tasks rather than as isolated, decontextualized knowledge. Second, although cognitive apprenticeship teaching uses the same modelling, coaching and scaffolding techniques as traditional apprenticeships, the focus is cognitive and metacognitive skill development (Collins, Brown and Newman, 1987).

In a follow-up article, Collins, Brown, and Holum (1991) using the principles of apprenticeship derived from Lave and Wenger and their own previous work, outlined a cognitive apprenticeship instructional methodology comprised of modelling, coaching, scaffolding, articulation, reflection and exploration. In their methodology, modelling, coaching and scaffolding are social learning methods that are used to help students develop the cognitive and metacognitive skills that are the target of cognitive apprenticeship.

Modelling is the technique of learning from observing expert performance, coaching is where the expert provides feedback to guide the development of expert performance and scaffolding is the technique of providing support for performance at first but then reducing that support until which time the learner can successfully perform the task without support.

The next two methods are articulation, where the instructor aims to encourage the students to express their knowledge or strategies and reflection, which is a comparison of the student's critical processes and those of the expert. Exploration, the last technique in cognitive apprentice instruction, is an attempt to move the student to independently execute expert problem solving and to seek out and define new problems that can be solved with the newly acquired skills and strategies.

The idea that learning in context produces knowledge through activity has been applied to health science education and points the way to a new instructional paradigm for producing reflective practitioners whose knowledge and skills are blended in a complex, network that results in skilled practice.

Pedagogies to Produce Reflective Practitioners

Many health care educators (Slavin, et al., 2014; Dyrbye, 2010; Benner and Sutphen, 2007) have written about the need for more effective pedagogical elements that foster effective professional health care practice. For instance, it has been suggested that teaching students to practice reflection is critical for making professional and humanistic qualities more clinically salient for students (Shrank, Reed & Jernstedt, 2004). Teaching the importance of reflection develops collaborative learning and fosters lifelong learning through habits of inquiry (Puvanendran, Vasanwala, Kamei, Hock, & Lie, 2012). One method to teach reflection within the medical learning environment is to teach the knowledge, skills and professional comportment in reflective health care practice (Stalmeijer, Dolmans, Wolfhagen, & Scherpbier, 2009) using an apprenticeship model derived from social cognitive learning theory as describe previously. This approach can, in theory, lead to a more humanistic and connected type of medical education learning environment.

The Three Professional Apprenticeships

The idea of applying apprenticeship principles to education was picked up by the Carnegie Foundation (2007) in their studies that identified the important components of professional education. Because of the need to teach both knowledge *and* skills in professions, there is a need for educational techniques that help students integrate not only knowledge and skill but also another aspect of professionalism that some equate to ethical practice, which is identity or thinking like a member of the profession. Out of this work came the notion of teaching to three high-level sets of skills and knowledge called cognitive apprenticeships. The Carnegie studies identified three dimensions, which they labelled high-end apprenticeships for professional education:

- A knowledge apprenticeship that includes teaching the academic knowledge base and habits of mind important to the profession
- A skill-based apprenticeship that relates to practice, and includes professional practice judgment
- An ethical practice apprenticeship that addresses teaching and learning of ethical standards, ethical comportment, social roles, and responsibilities of the profession.

One of the issues of concern for Muzafar, et al., (2015) was the finding that many medical students not only had worries about future competence and professional endurance but also had lost confidence in the medical profession in general. This can be seen as a failure to develop a proper professional identity and is a factor that may be related to burnout. The development of a professional identity can be addressed directly in situative learning environments with specialized pedagogies for professional development implemented in the framework of the three high-end apprenticeships.

Pedagogies of Interpretation

A more humanistic or civic form of professionalism calls for a more contextualized interpretation informed by the ability to filter science and theory through personal experiences and consider the unique nature of the elements that make up the current situation under examination (Benner & Sutphen, 2007). Students being educated for professional practice must develop a certain level of critical interpretation to be able to analyse situations and the methods they use. This type of interpretation is not bad in itself but it can cause the student to become overly critical or analytical of what is being taught and may leave them with restricted forms of action. Instead students need to be prepared to reflect critically on their profession's best practices, theories and techniques but still maintain a solid foundation that allows them to act and practice in a self-reflective way that is grounded in the current situation.

Foster, et al., (2006) have called this type of practice 'passionate engagement' which refers to a type of professional practice that includes the practitioner's ability to situate their learning and practices within their own experience and world view, a contextual awareness of the critical elements of the situation and the knowledge of best practices in their profession. The pedagogy of interpretation requires experiential learning and integrative learning experiences that combine knowledge of theories and techniques so that students will have a repertoire of experiences to bring to bear on the professional situations they face.

Pedagogies of Contextualization

Standard scientific approaches to practice taught in professional education are general and not necessarily linked to any specific situation. But research in the learning sciences points out that knowledge and cognition are situated and therefore practice must be adapted to the given context. Problem solving in practice is practical reasoning and requires that the practitioner select the elements of professional knowledge most relevant to the given context. Again there is an interactive element to reasoning in context and it requires a more self-reflective, personal demeanour then if one were viewing the situation from a decontextualized, scientific perspective that tends to objectify situations and participants.

According to Brookfield and Hess (2008) the pedagogies of contextualization help students to

- Develop a consciousness of the context
- Participate constructively in their encounters with contexts, and
- Engage in social and systemic change

Pedagogies of Formation

Faculty in professional education are used to communicating beliefs, values and attitudes held by the profession as part of helping to socialize students into a profession (Benner & Sutphen, 2007). These are components of professional identity but they are separate from another important aspect of professional identity which has been called habitus or habits of practice and are said to guide practice on a less conscious level then beliefs, values and attitudes (Bourdieu, 1990). The developing habitus comes to define the practitioner's habits of practice and although they do not operate at a conscious level they guide the practitioner's professional activities. The skills and actions guided by the unconscious habitus actually shapes and frames the practitioner's professional perceptions and approaches to practice. Taken together with attitudes, values and beliefs, the skilled practice of habitus can actually enhance the professional's perception of events in practice and provide a constantly improving frame of reference.

Unlike the traditional methods of socialization, which might be communicated didactically, habitus develops through activity and as the skills of the profession are learned they create a keener professional focus and enhance abilities to make finer and finer distinctions. Therefore, habitus or habits of practice are an interactive process whereby a new identify is formed so that students begin to see themselves as members of the profession rather than just acting the part. There is a social aspect to the development of habitus because this development requires activity and activity in most professions requires interaction with other people. The teaching of identify formation can be built into instruction by providing students with opportunities to reflect on practices during problem-based or clinical learning so that we produce practitioners who continually refine his or her abilities of discernment.

Pedagogies of Performance

A strictly scientific or analytic professional perspective may lead students to believe they can practice unconnected to others in the professional situation if they are just dutifully analytical enough. Professional action is situated in the sense that the professional must interact with others in the course of the performance of his or her duties. Performance is where a professional integrates what has been gained from pedagogies of interpretation, formation and contextualization. Performance is embodied theory in practice.

Adapting the curriculum to address issues such as burnout need to address situated learning principles. This requires a design model that integrates the cognitive, skill and comportment components of apprenticeship learning and specifies the identity development elements that will be addressed in the situated learning environment.

FUTURE TRENDS

An important trend in medical education is the increasing use of instructional technology (Colbert & Chokshi, 2014; George, Dumenco, & Dollase, 2013) and medical education needs to examine the merging of instructional technology systems with the situated learning methods described in this chapter to create what Rosenheck (2013) called Cognitive Apprenticeship 2.0. Unfortunately, like so many additions to the medical curriculum, instructional technology is often implemented piecemeal resulting in a fragmented learning experience for students (Hamlin, 2015).

As Colbert and Chokshio (2014) have stated, 'First, any innovation in technology must be integrated with innovation in pedagogy' (p. 1584).

Situated learning methods identified in this chapter address the three high-level apprenticeships that the Carnegie Foundation studies have deemed important for producing reflective practitioners. Implementation studies that merge situated learning techniques with instructional technology need to determine how to extend the range of instruction, from place-based settings to the delivery of instruction wherever students might need to learn. The more information technology driven learning activities can be linked with situative clinical learning experiences the more students can benefit from the power of situated learning principles.

CONCLUSION

Gracey, et al., (2005) stated that many physicians recall a training experience that influenced and changed their practice of medicine. The influence of one experience within the learning environment can have long lasting consequences on the development of the medical student. Learning to practice empathically and reflectively from faculty and clinicians can enable students to develop new ways to relate when presented with similar or unique situations. If the goal of medical education is to produce competent, reflective practitioners who can integrate knowledge, skills and comportment, then apprenticeship-like teaching, coaching and modelling become instrumental in the medical school-learning environment.

Slavin, Schindler, and Chibnall (2014) have demonstrated a significant reduction in burnout occurs after addressing the medical school-learning environment. Without sacrificing critical educational components, the medical programme removed unnecessary stressors in the learning environment itself while teaching students to develop skills in resilience and mindfulness This and other studies have supported the suggestion by Drybye, et al., (2010) that aspects of the learning environment related to burnout are malleable.

This chapter proposes that an apprentice type of mentoring programme among medical students can assist with positive feelings of self-perception. In addition, social learning theory and the apprenticeship model suggests that the level of competence that people attribute to a role model will affect their attitude toward their career decisions (Savickas, 2001). A student with a strong role model relationship will be a satisfied and motivated learner (Lockwood, Jordan & Ziva, 2002). A students' perception of their relationship with their role model is strongly associated with their motivation level and achievement (Maulana, Opdenakker, Den Brok, and Bosker, 2012). Previously, research has shown that there is a strong correlation between the belief of one's abilities and the amount of motivation and performance

(Redmond, 2014). This is important since a positive perception affects motivation and the disposition for self-learning (Wallsten, Pleskac, & Lejuez, 2005). A strong mentoring relationship can be used to reduce burnout among medical students.

Using the cognitive apprenticeship model to create learning experiences that integrate observation, guided-experience, reflection and independent practice (Collins, Brown & Newman, 1987) provides for the development of a professional identity and allows students to think like a physician. The ability of an educational institution to integrate observational learning, apprenticeship-like experiences, cognitive skills training and student reflection is instrumental in influencing the professional competencies that form the reflective practitioner. Viewed within the cognitive apprenticeship framework, the relationship built between learner and faculty shape the future of the practitioner.

REFERENCES

Alshehri, S. A., Alshehri, A. F., & Erwin, T. D. (2012). Measuring the medical school educational environment: Validating an approach from Saudi Arabia. *Health Education Journal, 71*(5), 553–564. doi:10.1177/0017896912450875

Anfosi & Numico. (2014). Empathy in the Doctor-Patient Relationship. *Journal of Clinical Oncology, 22*, 12258–12259. Retrieved from http://jco.ascopubs.org/content/22/11/2258.1.short PMID:15169824

Astrom, S., Nilsson, M., Norberg, A., Sandman, P., & Winblad, B. (1991). Staff burnout in dementia care relations to empathy and attitudes. *International Journal of Nursing Studies, 28*(1), 65–75. doi:10.1016/0020-7489(91)90051-4 PMID:1856035

Back, A., & Arnold, R. (2013). "Isn't there anything more you can do?": When empathic statements work, and when they don't. *Journal of Palliative Medicine, 16*, 1429–1432. doi:10.1089/jpm.2013.0193

Beating burnout: Confidential access to health services for trainees. (n.d.). Retrieved from https://wire.ama-assn.org/life-career/beating-burnout-confidential-access-health-services-trainees?utm_source=Selligent&%3Butm_medium=email&%3Butm_term=%25m%25d%25y&%3Butm_content=Med%2BEd_addr1_12-14-16&%3Butm_campaign=Med%2BEd&%3Butm_uid=8710492&%3Butm_effort

Benbassat, J. (2014). Changes in wellbeing and professional values among medical undergraduate students: A narrative review of the literature. *Advances in Health Sciences Education: Theory and Practice, 19*(4), 597–610. doi:10.1007/s10459-014-9500-1 PMID:24615278

Benner, P. (1984). *From Novice to Expert: Excellence and Power in Clinical Nursing Practice*. Menlo Park, CA: Addison-Wesley Publishing Company.

Benner, P., & Sutphen, M. (2007). Learning across the professions: The clergy, a case in point. *The Journal of Nursing Education, 46*, 103–108. Retrieved from http://search.proquest.com/docview/203971539?accountid=14376 PMID:17396548

Berragan, L. (2013). Conceptualising learning through simulation: An expansive approach for professional and personal learning. *Nurse Education in Practice, 13*(4), 250–255. doi:10.1016/j.nepr.2013.01.004 PMID:23402772

Blasi, Z. D., Harkness, E., Ernst, E., Georgiou, A., & Kleijnen, J. (2001). Influence of context effects on health outcomes: A systematic review. *Lancet, 357*(9258), 757–762. doi:10.1016/S0140-6736(00)04169-6 PMID:11253970

Bourdieu, P. (1990). Structures, habitus, practices. *The Logic of Practice*, 52-65.

Brazeau, C. M., Schroeder, R., Rovi, S., & Boyd, L. (2010). Relationships between medical student burnout, empathy, and professionalism climate. *Academic Medicine, 85*, S33–S36. doi:10.1097/ACM.0b013e3181ed4c47 PMID:20881699

Carnegie Foundation for the Advancement of Teaching. (2007). *Preparation for the Professions Program*. Retrieved January 3, 2015, from http://www.carnegiefoundation.org/publications/new-agenda-higher-education-shaping-life-mind-practice

Carr, S. E., & Johnson, P. H. (2013). Does self-reflection and insight correlate with academic performance in medical students?. *BMC Medical Education, 13*, 113. doi:10.1186/1472-6920-13-113

Chang, E., Eddins-Folensbee, F., & Coverdale, J. (2012). Survey of the prevalence of burnout, stress, depression, and the use of supports by medical students at one school. *Academic Psychiatry, 36*(3), 177–182. doi:10.1176/appi.ap.11040079 PMID:22751817

Cohen, M. J. M., Kay, A., Youakim, J. M., & Balacius, J. M. (2009). Identity transformation in medical students. *American Journal of Psychoanalysis, 69*, 43-52. doi:10.1057/ajp.2008.38

Colbert, J. A., & Chokshi, D. A. (n.d.). Technology in Medical Education-Osler Meets Watson. *Journal of General Internal Medicine, 12*, 29.

Collins, A., Brown, J. S., & Holum, A. (1991). *Cognitive Apprenticeship: Making Thinking Visible*. Retrieved from: http://elc.fhda.edu/transform/resources/collins_brown_holum_1991.pdf

Collins, A., Brown, J. S., & Newman, S. E. (1987). *Cognitive Apprenticeship: Teaching the craft of reading, writing and mathematics*. Center for the Study of Reading, Technical report No. 403. University of Illinois. Retrieved from: http://files.eric.ed.gov/fulltext/ED284181.pdf

Coulehan, J. L., Platt, F. W., Egener, B., Frankel, R., Lin, C., Lown, B., & Salazar, W. H. (2001). Let Me See If I Have This Right …: Words That Help Build Empathy. *Annals of Internal Medicine*, *135*(3), 221–227. doi:10.7326/0003-4819-135-3-200108070-00022 PMID:11487497

Coulter, M. A., & Abney, P. C. (2009). A study of burnout in international and country of origin teachers. *International Review of Education*, *55*(1), 105–121. doi:10.1007/s11159-008-9116-x

Deosthalee, P. G. (2002). Job satisfaction of teachers in comparison with non-teachers. *Pakistan Journal of Psychological Research*, 17.

Derksen, F., Bensing, J., & Largo-Janssen, A. (2013). Effectiveness of empathy in general practice: A systematic review. *The British journal of general practice. The Journal of the Royal College of General Practitioners*, *63*(606), 76–84. doi:10.3399/bjgp13X660814

DiLalla, L. F., Hull, S. K., & Dorsey, J. K. (2004). Effect of Gender, Age, and Relevant Course Work on Attitudes Toward Empathy, Patient Spirituality, and Physician Wellness. *Teaching and Learning in Medicine: An International Journal*, *16*, 165-170. Retrieved from: http://www.tandfonline.com/doi/abs/10.1207/s15328015tlm1602_8

Dyrbye, L. N., Power, D. V., Stanford Massie, F., Eacker, A., Harper, W., Thomas, M. R., & Shanafelt, T. D. (2010). Factors associated with resilience to and recovery from burnout: A prospective, multi-institutional study of US medical students. *Medical Education*, *44*(10), 1016–1026. doi:10.1111/j.1365-2923.2010.03754.x PMID:20880371

Dyrbye, L. N., Thomas, M. R., Harper, W., Massie, F. S. Jr, Power, D. V., Eacker, A., & Shanafelt, T. D. et al. (2009). The learning environment and medical student burnout: A multicentre study. *Medical Education*, *43*(3), 274–282. doi:10.1111/j.1365-2923.2008.03282.x PMID:19250355

Eckleberry-Hunt, J., Van Dyke, A., Lick, D., & Tucciarone, J. (2009). Changing the Conversation From Burnout to Wellness: Physician Well-being in Residency Training Programs. *Journal of Graduate Medical Education*, *1*(2), 225–230. doi:10.4300/JGME-D-09-00026.1 PMID:21975983

Foster, C. R., Dahill, L. E., Goleman, L., & Tolentino, B. W. (2006). *Educating clergy: Teaching practices and pastoral imagination*. San Francisco, CA: Kossey-Bass.

Galán, F., Sanmartín, A., Polo, J., & Giner, L. (2011). Burnout risk in medical students in Spain using the Maslach Burnout Inventory-Student Survey. *International Archives of Occupational and Environmental Health*, *84*(4), 453–459. doi:10.1007/s00420-011-0623-x PMID:21373879

Gelhaus, P. (2012). The desired moral attitude of the physician (I): Empathy. *Medicine, Health Care, and Philosophy*, *15*(2), 103–111. doi:10.1007/s11019-011-9366-4 PMID:22167298

George, P., Dumenco, L., & Dollase, R. (2013). Introducing technology into medical education: Two pilot studies. *Patient Education and Counseling*, *12*, 93. PMID:23684367

Ghetti, C., Chang, J., & Gosman, G. (2009). Burnout, psychological skills, and empathy: Balint training in obstetrics and gynecology residents. *Journal of Graduate Medical Education*, *1*(2), 231–235. doi:10.4300/JGME-D-09-00049.1 PMID:21975984

Gracey, C. F., Haidet, P., Branch, W. T., Weissman, P., Kern, D. E., Mitchell, G., & Inui, T. et al. (2005). Precepting humanism: Strategies for fostering the human dimensions of care in ambulatory settings. *Academic Medicine*, *80*(1), 21–28. doi:10.1097/00001888-200501000-00007 PMID:15618087

Greeno, J. G. (1997). On claims that answer the wrong questions. *Educational Researcher*, *26*, 5–17.

Greeno, J. G., & Van De Sande, C. (2007). Perspectival understanding of conceptions and conceptual growth in interaction. *Educational Psychologist*, *42*(1), 9–23. doi:10.1080/00461520709336915

Gresalfi, M. S., & Cobb, P. (2011). Negotiating identities for mathematics teaching in the context of professional development. *Journal for Research in Mathematics Education*, *42*, 270–304.

Hamlin, M. D. (2015). Technology in transformative learning environments. In C. Halupa (Ed.), *Transformative Curriculum Design in Health Sciences Education* (pp. 126–140). Hershey, PA: IGI Global. doi:10.4018/978-1-4666-8571-0.ch004

Hellstén, M., & Prescott, A. (2004). Learning at University: The international student experience. *International Education Journal*, *5*, 344–351.

Henderson, A., Twentyman, M., Eaton, E., Creedy, D., Stapleton, P., & Lloyd, B. (2010). Creating supportive clinical learning environments: An intervention study. *Journal of Clinical Nursing, 19*(1-2), 177–182. doi:10.1111/j.1365-2702.2009.02841.x PMID:19686319

Hewson, M. G., & Little, M. L. (1998). Giving Feedback in medical education: Verification of recommended techniques. *Journal of General Internal Medicine, 13*(2), 111–116. doi:10.1046/j.1525-1497.1998.00027.x PMID:9502371

Hirsch, E. M. (2007). The role of empathy in medicine: A medical student's perspective. *The Virtual Mentor, 9*, 423. Retrieved from: http://journalofethics.ama-assn.org/2007/06/pdf/medu1-0706.pdf

Hojat, M. (2009). Ten Approaches for Enhancing Empathy in Health and Human Services Cultures. *Journal of Health and Human Services Administration, 31*, 412–450. Retrieved from http://search.proquest.com/docview/199974037?accountid=14376 PMID:19385420

Hojat, M., Mangione, S., Nasca, T. J., Rattner, S., Erdmann, J. B., Gonnella, J. S., & Magee, M. (2004). An empirical study of decline in empathy in medical school. *Medical Education, 38*(9), 934–941. doi:10.1111/j.1365-2929.2004.01911.x PMID:15327674

IsHak, W., Nikravesh, R., Lederer, S., Perry, R., Ogunyemi, D., & Bernstein, C.. (2013). Burnout in medical students: A systematic review. *The Clinical Teacher, 10*(4), 242–245. doi:10.1111/tct.12014 PMID:23834570

Koparan, Ş., Şahin, E., & Kuter, F. (2010). A comparison on of self-efficacy perception and social physical anxiety levels of teacher candidates at physical education department. *Procedia: Social and Behavioral Sciences, 2*(2), 3932–3937. doi:10.1016/j.sbspro.2010.03.619

Larson, E. B., & Yao, X. Y. (2005). Clinical empathy as emotional labor in the patient-physician relationship. *Journal of the American Medical Association, 293*(9), 1100–1106. doi:10.1001/jama.293.9.1100 PMID:15741532

Lave, J. (1988). *Cognition in practice: Mind, mathematics, and culture in everyday life.* Cambridge, UK: Cambridge University Press. doi:10.1017/CBO9780511609268

Lave, J., & Wenger, E. (1991). *Situated Learning: Legitimate Peripheral Participation.* Cambridge, UK: Cambridge University Press.

Liaison Committee on Medical Education. (2014). *Accreditation Standards.* Retrieved from: http://www.lcme.org/publications.htm#standards-section

Linzer, M., Levine, R., Meltzer, D., Poplau, S., Warde, C., & West, C. P. (2014). 10 bold steps to prevent burnout in general internal medicine. *Journal of General Internal Medicine*, *29*(1), 18–20. doi:10.1007/s11606-013-2597-8 PMID:24002633

Lockwood, P., Jordan, C. H., & Kunda, Z. (2002). Motivation by positive or negative role models: Regulatory focus determines who will best inspire us. *Journal of Personality and Social Psychology*, *83*(4), 854–864. doi:10.1037/0022-3514.83.4.854 PMID:12374440

Lupo, M. K., & Strous, R. D. (2011). Religiosity, anxiety and depression among Israeli medical students. *The Israel Medical Association Journal, 13*, 613-618. Retrieved from: http://touro.summon.serialssolutions.com/search?s.q=religiosity%2C+anxiety+and+depression+among+Israeli+medical#!/search?q=religiosity,%20anxiety%20and%20depression%20among%20Israeli%20medical

Maslach, C. (2003). Job burnout new directions in research and intervention. *Current Directions in Psychological Science*, *12*(5), 189–192. doi:10.1111/1467-8721.01258

Maslach, Schaufeli, & Leiter. (n.d.). Job Burnout. *Annual Review of Psychology, 52*, 397–422. Retrieved from: http://www.annualreviews.org/doi/pdf/10.1146/annurev.psych.52.1.397

Matthews, D. A., Suchman, A. L., & Branch, W. T. (1993). Making Connexions: Enhancing the Therapeutic Potential of Patient Clinician Relationships. *Annals of Internal Medicine*, *118*(12), 973–977. doi:10.7326/0003-4819-118-12-199306150-00010 PMID:8489112

Maulana, R., & Opdenakker, C. (2012). Teacher–student interpersonal relationships and academic motivation within one school year: developmental changes and linkage. *School Effectiveness and School Improvement: An International Journal of Research, Policy and Practice, 23.* Retrieved from: http://www.tandfonline.com/doi/abs/10.1080/09243453.2011.619198

McKenna, K. M., Hashimoto, D. A., Maguire, M. S., & Bynum, W. E. IV. (2016). The missing link: Connection is the key to resilience in medical education. *Academic Medicine*, *91*(9), 1197–1199. doi:10.1097/ACM.0000000000001311 PMID:27438155

Mezirow, J. (2003). Transformative learning as discourse. *Journal of Transformative Education*, *1*(1), 58–63. doi:10.1177/1541344603252172

Monrouxe, L. V. (2010). Identity, identification and medical education: Why should we care? *Medical Education*, *44*(1), 40–49. doi:10.1111/j.1365-2923.2009.03440.x PMID:20078755

Monrouxe, L. V., Rees, C. E., & Hu, W. (2011). Differences in medical students explicit discourses of professionalism. *Medical Education*, *45*(6), 585–602. doi:10.1111/j.1365-2923.2010.03878.x PMID:21564198

Murinson, B. B., Klick, B., Haythornthwaite, J. A., Shochet, R., Levine, R. B., & Wright, S. M. (2010). Formative experiences of emerging physicians: Gauging the impact of events that occur during medical school. *Academic Medicne, 85*, 1331-1337. Retrieved from: http://journals.lww.com/academicmedicine/Abstract/2010/08000/Formative_Experiences_of_Emerging_Physicians_.18.aspx

Muzafar, Y., Khan, H. H., Ashraf, H., Hussain, W., Sajid, H., Tahir, M., Ahmad, W. (2015). Burnout and its Associated Factors in Medical Students of Lahore, Pakistan. *Cureus,* 7. 10.7759/cureus.390

Nedrow, A., Steckler, N. A., & Hardman, J. (2013). Physician resilience and burnout: Can you make the switch? *Family Practice Management*, *20*, 25. Retrieved from https://www.ncbi.nlm.nih.gov/pubmed/23418835 PMID:23418835

Neumann, M., Edelhauser, F., Tauschel, D., Fischer, M. R., Wirtz, M., Woopen, C., & Scheffer, C. et al. (2011). Empathy decline and its reasons: A systematic review of studies with medical students and residents. *Academic Medicine*, *86*(8), 996–1009. doi:10.1097/ACM.0b013e318221e615 PMID:21670661

Noone, J. (2009). Teaching to the three apprenticeships: Designing learning activities for professional practice in an undergraduate curriculum. *The Journal of Nursing Education*, *48*, 468–471. Retrieved from http://search.proquest.com/docview/203967665?accountid=14376

Puvanendran, R., Park, C., Lee, Y. J., Hong, M., Jung, C.-H., Synn, Y., & Bahn, G. H. et al. (2016). A Multicenter Study Investigating Empathy and Burnout Characteristics in Medical Residents with Various Specialties. *Journal of Korean Medical Science*, *31*, 590–597. doi:10.3346/jkms.2016.31.4.590

Puvanendran, R., Vasanwala, F. F., Kamei, R. K., Hock, L. K., & Lie, D. A. (2012). What do medical students learn when they follow patients from hospital to community? A longitudinal qualitative study. *Medical Education Online*, 17. PMID:22791959

Ramani, S., & Krackov, S. K. (2012). Twelve tips for giving feedback effectively in the clinical environment. *Medical Teacher*, *34*(10), 787–791. doi:10.3109/0142159X.2012.684916 PMID:22730899

Redmond, B. F. (2014). *Self-Efficacy and Social Cognitive Theories*. Retrieved March 24 2014 from https://wikispaces.psu.edu/display/PSYCH484/7.+Self-Efficacy+and+Social+Cognitive+Theories

Roff, S., McAleer, S., Harden, R. M., & Al-Qahtani, M. (1997). Development and validation of the Dundee ready education environment measure (DREEM). *Medical Teacher, 19*, 295-299. Retrieved from http://search.proquest.com/docview/233249246?accountid=14376

Rogers, C. R. (1975). Empathic: An unappreciated way of being. *The Counseling Psychologist*, *5*(2), 2–10. doi:10.1177/001100007500500202

Rose, G. L., & Rukstalis, M. R. (2008). Imparting medical ethics: the role of mentorship in clinical training. *Mentoring & Tutoring: Partnership in Learning, 16*, 77-89. Retrieved from: http://www.tandfonline.com/doi/pdf/10.1080/13611260701801031

Rosen, I. M., Gimotty, P. A., Shea, J. A., & Bellini, L. M. (2006). Evolution of sleep quantity, sleep deprivation, mood disturbances, empathy, and burnout among interns. Academic Medicine. *Journal. Association of American Medical Colleges*, *81*(1), 82–85. doi:10.1097/00001888-200601000-00020

Rosenthal, J. M., & Okie, S. (2005). White coat, mood indigo - depression in medical school. *The New England Journal of Medicine*, *353*(11), 1085–1088. doi:10.1056/NEJMp058183 PMID:16162877

Savickas, M. L. (2001). A developmental perspective on vocational behavior: Career patterns, salience, and themes. *International Journal for Educational and Vocational Guidance*, *1*(1/2), 49–57. doi:10.1023/A:1016916713523

Serwint, J. R., Bostwick, S., Burke, A. E., Church, A., Gogo, A., Hofkosh, D., & Osta, A. (2016). The AAP Resilience in the Face of Grief and Loss Curriculum. *Pediatrics*, *e20160791*. Retrieved from http://pediatrics.aappublications.org/content/early/2016/10/06/peds.2016-0791 PMID:27940771

Shrank, W. H., Reed, V. A., & Jernstedt, C. (2004). Fostering professionalism in medical education: A call for improved assessment and meaningful incentives. *Journal of General Internal Medicine*, *19*(8), 887–892. doi:10.1111/j.1525-1497.2004.30635.x PMID:15242476

Slavin, S. J., Schindler, D. L., & Chibnall, J. T. (2014). Medical student mental health 3.0: Improving student wellness through curricular changes. *Academic Medicine*, *89*(4), 573–577. doi:10.1097/ACM.0000000000000166 PMID:24556765

Social Cognitive Theory. (2014). University of Twente. Retrieved from: http://www.utwente.nl/cw/theorieenoverzicht/Theory%20Clusters/Health%20Communication/Social_cognitive_theory.doc/

Stalmeijer, R. E., Dolmans, D., Wolfhagen, I., & Scherpbier, A. (2009). Cognitive apprenticeship in clinical practice: Can it stimulate learning in the opinion of students?. *Advances in Health Sciences Education: Theory and Practice, 14*, 535. Retrieved from: http://link.springer.com/article/10.1007/s10459-008-9136-0#page-1

Stepien, K. A., & Baernstein, A. (2006). Educating for Empathy. *Journal of General Internal Medicine, 21*(5), 524–530. doi:10.1111/j.1525-1497.2006.00443.x PMID:16704404

Suchman, A. L., Williamson, P. R., Litzelman, D. K., Frankel, R. M., Mossbarger, D. L., & Inui, T. S. (2004). Toward an Informal Curriculum that Teaches Professionalism Transforming the Social Environment of a Medical School. *Journal of General Internal Medicine, 19*(5), 501–504. doi:10.1111/j.1525-1497.2004.30157.x PMID:15109312

Turner, J. C., & Nolen, S. B. (2015). Introduction: The relevance of the situative perspective in educational psychology. *Educational Psychologist, 50*(3), 167–172. doi:10.1080/00461520.2015.1075404

Vasanwala, F. F., Kamei, R. K., Hock, L. K., & Lie, D. A. (2012). What do medical students learn when they follow patients from hospital to community? A longitudinal qualitative study. *Medical Education Online, 17*, 1–8. Retrieved from http://www.ncbi.nlm.nih.gov/pmc/articles/PMC3395028/ PMID:22791959

Wallsten, T. S., Pleskac, T. J., & Lejuez, C. W. (2005). Modeling behavior in a clinically diagnostic sequential risk-taking task. *Psychological Review, 112*(4), 862–880. doi:10.1037/0033-295X.112.4.862 PMID:16262471

Wayne, S. J., Fortner, S. A., Kitzes, J. A., Timm, C., & Kalishman, S. (2013). Cause or effect? the relationship between student perception of the medical school learning environment and academic performance on USMLE step 1. *Medical Teacher, 35*(5), 376–380. doi:10.3109/0142159X.2013.769678 PMID:23444883

Weiner, B. (2000). Attributional thoughts about consumer behavior. *The Journal of Consumer Research, 27*(3), 382–387. doi:10.1086/317592

West, C. P., & Shanafelt, T. D. (2007). The influence of personal and environmental factors on professionalism in medical education. *BMC Medical Education, 7*, 1. Retrieved from http://bmcmededuc.biomedcentral.com/articles/10.1186/1472-6920-7-29

Wilczek-Ruzyczka, E. (2011). Empathy vs. professional burnout in health care professionals. *Journal of US - China Medical Science, 8*. Retrieved from http://search.proquest.com/docview/1465056775?accountid=14376

KEY TERMS AND DEFINITIONS

Apprenticeship Learning: Traditional method of training people into a profession that has powerful features for learning. Researchers such as Jean Lave, Allan Collins and John Seely Brown have identified effective learning and teaching techniques from apprenticeship learning and applied them to classroom learning.

Burnout: A psychological syndrome of emotional exhaustion, depersonalization, and reduced personal accomplishment.

Clinical Empathy: A predominantly cognitive (rather than emotional) attribute that involves an understanding (rather than feeling) of experiences, concerns and perspectives of the patients, combined with a capacity to communicate this understanding.

Cognitive Apprenticeship: Extension of apprenticeship training techniques to the teaching of cognitive and metacognitive skills.

Contextualization: Practical reasoning and requires that the practitioner select the elements of professional knowledge most relevant to the given context.

Formation: A pedagogy that produces habits of mind or what some have labelled habits which is the ability to think in context and perform like a member of the profession.

Situative Learning: The perspective that learning and cognition are distributed over activity systems and communities of practice and looks at learning, cognition, motivation and achievement as social activities and applies the sociocultural view to research in classroom learning.

Social Cognitive Learning Theory: The learning theory that learning is a social activity and that people learn from one another, via observation, imitation, and modelling.

Chapter 5
Deliberate Self-Harm and Suicide Ideology in Medical Students

Vinod Gopalan
Griffith University, Australia

Erick Chan
Griffith University, Australia

Debbie Thao Thanh Ho
Griffith University, Australia

ABSTRACT

The risk of deliberate self-harm (DSH) and suicide ideology in medical students is a pertinent issue that has received a surge in attention over recent years. Medical students are at risk of normalisation of DSH and suicide ideology despite their mental health literacy levels and are still susceptible to the stigma of help-seeking for their mental wellbeing. This chapter will explore assessment, preventative and management strategies to improve education, awareness and ultimately reduce the rates of DSH and suicide risk. A comprehensive review of practices and techniques that medical training community and their family members could utilise to aid medical students to adequately and safety manage DSH and suicide ideology. This will assist in identifying crucial areas for future research to aid students, professionals, family and friends in supporting medical student health to optimise mental health overall wellbeing of medical students.

DOI: 10.4018/978-1-5225-2811-1.ch005

BACKGROUND

The risk of deliberate self-harm (DSH) and suicide ideology in medical students is a pertinent issue that has received a surge in attention over recent years (Wu et al., 2016, Rotenstein et al., 2016). Rates of suicide among general adolescents are increasing at staggering rates. This population of young adults are considered 'at risk' in 33% of countries around the world (Miletic, Lukovic, Ratkovic, Aleksic, & Grgurevic, 2014). Rotenstein et al. extracted suicidal prevalence data from 24 cross-sectional studies from 15 countries resulting in a pooled prevalence of suicidal ideation of 11.1% in medical students. Wu et al. conducted a cross-sectional study of over 4000 students from 22 Chinese medical universities, and found that prevalence of DSH was 9.6% over 12 months. It is, therefore, important for medical students, professionals, parents, and friends to understand the impact of DSH and suicide ideology on an academic and psychosocial level. Furthermore, because DSH and suicide ideology prevalence can be reduced with early intervention, it is all too important to know how to screen for early signs and symptoms as well as provide appropriate intervention (Downs et al., 2014).

Medical students are a unique population as they are learning about the organic and psychosocial impacts of mental health, including factors that may contribute to poor mental health, whilst being exposed to these exact factors. Stressors that are prominent in medical students include increased contact hours, high academic pressure, assessments, exposure to high-intensity workloads, high-performance expectations, strained social balance and workplace bullying (Chan, Batterham, Christensen, & Galletly, 2014; Osama et al., 2014; Wu et al., 2016). There are multiple factors contributing towards negative mental health sequelae among medical students and it can lead to undeniably anxious and stressful times during their academic and clinical career. These sequelae may involve more common psychiatric presentations such as anxiety and depression, to more formidable presentations such as DSH and suicidal ideology (Wege, Muth, Li, & Angerer, 2016).

Medical schools have an inherent requirement to produce safe working graduates and they must also ensure that students are primed to cope with stress, burnout, and failure. Addressing the negative mental health sequelae is therefore in the best interest of every medical school. Promoting and enhancing medical student well-being will be beneficial for each trainee throughout their career, with benefits in overall education, physician resilience, personal fulfilment, professionalism and of course patient care (Dunn, Iglewicz & Moutier, 2008).

DSH is most commonly associated with borderline personality disorder and is often associated with major depression, antisocial personality disorder, dissociative identity disorder, posttraumatic stress disorder, eating disorders, autism, developmental disabilities and Lesch-Nyhan syndrome (Stanley et al., 2010). At a molecular level, serotonergic and dopaminergic dysfunctions do not appear to be related to DSH, however, it has been demonstrated that those who self-harm have lower levels of CSF ß-endorphins and met-enkephalins, both of which are opioids involved in emotion-induced and physical pain analgesia (Stanley et al., 2010). This is an important distinguishing factor as serotonergic and dopaminergic dysfunctions are usually associated with suicidal behaviour and depression, whereas endogenous opioid deficiency plays a more prominent role in DSH without suicidal intent (Stanley et al., 2010). This relationship will be discussed further in the following sections.

For the purposes of addressing medical student stress, this chapter refers to medicine as traditional Western medicine, not inclusive of any alternative medicine fields.

DEFINING DELIBERATE SELF-HARM

Deliberate self-harm may seem to be a straightforward definition in and of itself, however, many more aspects must be considered, including the frequency and time-period that DSH may occur, the purpose or expectations by the individual and the associations that DSH may have with concurrent moods, feelings, and thoughts. This section will discuss various definitions of DSH, the types of self-harm and its relation to other mental health disorders.

The definition of deliberate self-harm has been argued in the scientific community without a resolute definition for many years. This phenomenon has also been known as self-harm, self-injurious behaviour, repeated self-injury, self-wounding, para suicide, self-mutilation, episodic and repetitive self-injury and autodestructive behaviour (Mangnall, 2008). Current literature has conflicting definitions including the intention to kill and intention to not kill, which convolutes the distinction of DSH from suicide ideology, as discussed later in this chapter. Based on the literature, DSH may be defined as a 'direct behaviour that causes minor to moderate physical injury, that is undertaken without conscious suicidal intent and that occurs in the absence of psychoses and/or organic intellectual impairment' (Mangnall, 2008).

This definition addresses both cause and purpose of DSH and this is further expanded upon in the Diagnostic and Statistical Manual of Mental Disorders (DSM-5) criteria for diagnosis (See Figure 1) (Diagnostic and statistical manual of mental disorders, 2013). Key diagnostic features focus around repeated infliction of shallow yet painful injuries with a purpose to reduce negative emotions, such as tension, anxiety, self-reproach and/or to resolve an interpersonal difficulty though with an absence of suicidal intent. The individual may exhibit a behavioural pattern resembling an addiction or describe a compulsive nature due to an immediate sensation of relief during the self-harming process.

Figure 1. Proposed Criteria for Non-Suicidal Self-Injury
Source: Adapted from Diagnostic and Statistical Manual of Mental Disorders, 2013

NONSUICIDAL SELF-INJURY

Proposed Criteria

A. In the last year, the individual has, on 5 or more days, engaged in intentional self-inflicted damage to the surface of his or her body of a sort likely to induce bleeding, bruising, pain (e.g. cutting, burning, stabbing, hitting, excessive rubbing), with the expectation that the injury will lead to only minor or moderate physical harm (i.e. there is no suicidal intent.)
NOTE: The absence of suicidal intent has either been stated by the individual or can be inferred by the individual's repeated engagement in a behaviour that the individual knows, or has learned, is not likely to results in death.

B. The individual engages in the self-injurious behaviour with one or more of the following expectations:
   1. To obtain relief from a negative feeling or cognitive state
   2. To resolve an interpersonal difficulty
   3. To induce a positive feeling state

C. The intentional self-injury is associated with at least one of the following:
   1. Interpersonal difficulties or negative feelings or thoughts, such as depression, anxiety, tension, anger, generalised distress, or self-criticism, occurring in the period immediately prior to self-injurious act.
   2. Prior to engaging in the act, a period of preoccupation with the intended behaviour that is difficult to control.
   3. Thinking about self-injury that occurs frequently, even when it is not acted upon.

D. The behaviour is not socially sanctioned (e.g. body piercing, tattooing, part of a religious or cultural ritual) and is not restricted to picking a scab or nail biting.

E. The behaviour or its consequences cause clinically significant distress or interference in interpersonal, academic, or other important areas of functioning.

F. The behaviour does not occur exclusively during psychotic episodes, delirium, substance intoxication, or substance withdrawal. In individuals with a neurodevelopmental disorder, the behaviour is not part of a pattern of repetitive stereotypes. The behaviour is not better explained by another mental disorder or medical condition (e.g. psychotic disorder, autism spectrum disorder, intellectual disability, Lesch-Nyhan syndrome, stereotypic movement disorder with self-injury, trichotillomania (hair-pulling disorder), excoriation (skin-picking) disorder.

Self-harm may present in a multitude of ways and can be divided into two broad groups: self-injury and self-poisoning (Lilley et al., 2008). Self-injury most commonly presents by cutting oneself, whilst less commonly presenting as swallowing objects, putting objects inside the body, burning, self-bruising or breaking bones. On the other hand, self-poisoning involves overdosing with medicine(s), often over-the-counter medication or swallowing a poisonous substance (Lilley et al., 2008). It should be noted that there are no specifications as to whether the self-harming act is planned or unplanned and infrequent or frequent.

Unfortunately, the large majority of individuals who engage in self-harm do not seek clinical attention, although people who self-poison are most likely to seek professional medical assistance (Diagnostic and statistical manual of mental disorders, 2013; Lilley et al., 2008). It is hypothesised that the positive experiences gained by an individual who is self-harming may deter them from seeking treatment, whilst the absent suicidal intent is apparent in those who self-poison yet present to the emergency department (Diagnostic and statistical manual of mental disorders, 2013; Mangnall, 2008). These positive experiences may include a separation or disconnection from the individual's feelings or pain, and can develop as a method of coping with overwhelming situations or feelings.

DEFINING SUICIDE AND SUICIDE IDEOLOGY

The World Health Organisation defines suicide as the act of deliberately killing oneself. Suicidal ideology encompasses the contemplation of suicide, ranging from a detailed plan to a fleeting consideration. A suicide attempt is defined as a self-inflicted, potentially injurious behaviour with intent to die, however not resulting in death (Wasserman et. al. 2011). The DSM-5 further specifies a proposed criterion for Suicidal Behaviour Disorder, which makes a clear distinction from deliberate self-harm (See Figure 2).

Suicidal behaviour can be categorised into violent and non-violent behaviours. For example, some violent behaviours include jumping from a life-threatening height and firearms, whilst non-violent behaviours may include overdosing with legal or illegal substances (Ajdacic-Gross, 2008). Suicidal behaviour can be associated with a wide variety of mental disorders, including bipolar disorder, major depressive disorder, schizophrenia, anxiety disorders and eating disorders to name a few (Diagnostic and statistical manual of mental disorders, 2013).

Wasserman et al. discuss suicide from the perspective of the Stress-Vulnerability model which explains that genetic make-up and acquired susceptibility both contribute to a person's predisposition or vulnerability to suicidal behaviour. This suicidal process involves an interaction of biological, psychological, environmental

Figure 2. Proposed criteria for Suicidal Behaviour Disorder
Source: Adapted from Diagnostic and statistical manual of mental disorders, 2013

SUICIDAL BEHAVIOUR DISORDER

Proposed Criteria

A. Within the last 24 months, the individual has made a suicide attempt.
NOTE: A suicide attempt is a self-initiated sequence of behaviours by an individual who, at the time of initiation, expected that the set of actions would lead to his or her own death. The 'time of initiation' is the time when a behaviour took place that involved applying a method

B. The act does not meet criteria for nonsuicidal self-injury – that is, it does not involve self-injury directed to the surface of the body undertaken to induce relief from a negative feeling or cognitive state or to achieve a positive mood state

C. The diagnosis is not applied to suicidal ideation or to preparatory acts.

D. The act was not initiated during a state of delirium or confusion.

E. The act was not undertaken solely for a political or religious objective

Specify if

- **Current:** Not more than 12 months since the last attempt.
- **In Early Remission:** 12-24 months since the last attempt.

and situational factors. The vulnerability may be increased due to early traumatic life experiences, chronic illness, alcohol and drug use and environmental and social factors (Wasserman et al., 2011). The reasons for why people may attempt suicide include, though are not limited to, severe depression, impulsivity, psychosis, lack of help or social support and philosophical desire. Most importantly, many suicidal processes decline and subside by means of individual coping or treatment strategies (Wasserman et al., 2011).

THE RELATIONSHIP BETWEEN DELIBERATE SELF-HARM AND SUICIDE IDEOLOGY

Based on the definitions outlined thus far, the key distinction between deliberate self-harm and suicide ideology is that suicidal intent is absent in deliberate self-harm actions. Despite this difference, evidence suggests that those who engage in self-harm are at an increased risk of likelihood of attempting suicide (Wan, Y., Gao, R., Tao, X., Tao, F., & Hu, C., 2012; Whitlock et al., 2013). Whitlock et al. conducted a longitudinal study of 1466 students across five colleges in the United States and concluded that a history of deliberate self-harm among students significantly leads to concurrent or later suicide ideology. The risk of suicide ideology is usually predicted by the occurrence of >20-lifetime non-suicidal self-injurious incidents and by the history of mental health treatments. The act of self-harm has two important risk factors for suicide; the experience of emotional distress and the experience of self-inflicted pain/injury (Klonsky, May, & Glenn, 2013). This is particularly important because addressing the risk factors, protective factors, finding an appropriate method of screening and determining effective treatment should take consideration of the relation between DSH and suicide ideology.

EPIDEMIOLOGY OF DELIBERATE SELF-HARM AND SUICIDE IDEOLOGY AMONG MEDICAL STUDENTS

Deliberate self-harm and suicide ideology are increasingly common in young adolescents, with particular prevalence in medical students. This section will detail the epidemiology of DSH and suicide ideology amongst the general public and medical students.

According to the World Health Organisation, ‘self-inflicted injury [defined as deliberate self-harm and suicide] is the fourth leading cause of death and sixth leading cause of morbidity and disability amongst people aged 15-44 years’ around the world (Wu et al., 2016). This is evidently a serious public health concern, although, can be prevented with timely, evidence-based and often low-cost interventions (Wasserman et. al. 2011).

Deliberate Self-Harm

Prevalence of DSH is difficult to ascertain as individual concealment and unwillingness to seek help can substantially underestimate the true prevalence of DSH. Higher prevalence of DSH amongst general population of students is a universal finding with 12-month prevalence of 7% and lifetime prevalence of 17% in American students, life-time prevalence of 15% in Turkish students, 12-month prevalence of 33% in Indian students and 11-33% in Chinese students (Wu et al., 2016). According to the Royal College of Psychiatrists, 1 in 3 people who self-harm for the first time will have a repeat episode in the following year, whilst 3 in 100 people who self-harm over 15 years will actually kill themselves (Bateman, 2014). The short-term recurrence and long-term consequences further highlight the importance of assessment and treatment.

In a recent study that examined deliberate self-harm among Chinese medical students, the 12-month prevalence was found to be 9.6%. This was lower in comparison to the general student population, however, is possibly due to their 'academic background' which may increase their understanding and implementation of self-care (Wu et al., 2016). Despite this the prevalence being lower than the general population of students, this remains to be an important issue that needs to be addressed. Previous studies from the UK and the USA have found that the amount of self-reporting in medical students is indeed higher than other college students, thereby increasing their likelihood of receiving treatment (Wu et al., 2016). Amongst medical students, male students reported a higher prevalence of DSH than females with one study finding that 11.51% of males self-reported DSH compared to 8.71% of females. The most common types of DSH being hitting in males and scratching among females (Wu et al., 2016).

Several key demographics are found to be linked to DSH including age, academic background and household income (Wu et al., 2016). DSH has become more prevalent among adolescents, young adults and college students, with DSH prevalence highest among freshmen and receding with progression through college. Also, low socioeconomic status has also been associated with higher prevalence of DSH (Wu et al., 2016). DSH appears to be higher amongst students in general, due to both their psychosocial stage of development as an adolescent and added pressures of higher education which predispose them to significant stressors of physical separation from parents, academic demands, independence and new social networks making them more vulnerable to self-harming acts (Amiri et al., 2013; Wu et al., 2016).

Suicide

On a global scale it is estimated that over 1 million people die due to suicide annually (Wasserman et. al. 2011). In fact, suicide itself is the second leading cause of death amongst 15 - 29-year-olds, which is, of course, the key age group of students (Wasserman et. al. 2011). Stressors for students include information and input overload, lack of leisure time, financial indebtedness and work pressures (Amiri et al., 2013).

Worldwide statistics show that medical students and even doctors are at a higher risk of suicide than the general population (Chan, Batterham, Christensen, & Galletly, 2014; Downs et al., 2014). In Australia, 14% of medical students have been found to experience suicidal ideation (Chan, Batterham, Christensen, & Galletly, 2014). In the United States of America, 4% of medical students considered committing suicide during their studies in the medical school (Schwenk, Davis, & Wimsatt, 2010). Additionally, the lifetime prevalence of suicide was between 16.8% and 51.5% and suicide attempts between 1.4 to 5.9% in Norwegian, Austrian, Indian and Turkish medical students (Eskin et al., 2011; Etzersdorfer, Vijayakumar, Schöny, Grausgruber, & Sonneck, 1998; Tyssen et al., 2001). Studies in developing countries such as Pakistan have also found that '35.6% medical students have considered suicide in the past 12 months and 4.8% had attempted suicide in their lifetime' (Osama et al., 2014).

RISK FACTORS

Deliberate self-harm and suicide ideology are associated with a number of risk factors, some of which are common across both domains and a few of which are specific for medical students. A multitude of biological, social, psychological, economic and cultural factors influence both suicide and deliberate self-harm in young people (Miletic, Lukovic, Ratkovic, Aleksic, & Grgurevic, 2014; Osama et al., 2014).

Generally, major risk factors for deliberate self-harm and suicidal ideology include psychiatric disorders, hopelessness, and impulsivity. Other general factors that have been found to be precipitating factors including male gender, young age, short duration of illness, multiple admissions, recent discharge from hospital, previous and recent suicide attempt, comorbid depression, drug abuse, poor medication compliance, poor treatment adherence, adaptation to new environments, high IQ and suicidal ideations, (Miletic, Lukovic, Ratkovic, Aleksic, & Grgurevic, 2014; Osama et al., 2014). Social exclusion in the form of being institutionalised, imprisoned or homeless, as well as parental neglect, has also been noted as contributing factors (Osama et al., 2014). It should be noted that presence of these risk factors increase the risk of DSH and suicide, however, other internal factors, resilience and coping strategies may influence whether that suicide ideology or DSH eventually manifests (Dunn, Iglewicz & Moutier, 2008).

In medical students, there is increased the risk of DSH and suicide ideology due to specific risk factors which can be classified into medical student stressors, self-care and the culture of medicine (Dunn, Iglewicz & Moutier, 2008). Medical students must withstand more overwhelming levels of psychological stress compared to others of similar demographic in the general population (Chan, Batterham, Christensen, & Galletly, 2014). Medical student stressors arise from various sources including transition into medical school, high-self expectations, time and energy demands, internal conflict and negative personal life events. Most unique to medical students is the transition from being a high academic achiever in secondary school to being surrounded by similarly talented students in medical school (Dunn, Iglewicz & Moutier, 2008). This creates a competitive atmosphere in which they may no longer be able to meet their high self-expectations – this is a major shift which may predispose to increased anxiety and depression.

The time and energy required to maintain a strong academic portfolio alongside high expectations can take a toll on students' physical and mental stamina. The constant drive for knowledge and performance through independent study or extracurricular activities minimises the opportunity for health promoting and socialising activities, not to mention physical and mental fatigue and sleep deprivation. This consequently results in a lack of self-care which further increases the risk of DSH and suicidality. Because medical career paths are arduous in nature, students may often feel ambivalent, conflicted and, even at times, dysphoric about their career path. This internal conflict can drain their emotional reservoir and hinder their ability to cope with the sheer stress of medical training and may even drive them towards utilising negative coping mechanisms, such as substance abuse (Dunn, Iglewicz & Moutier, 2008). Substance abuse was found to increase the risk of suicide among medicals students by 28 fold due to impaired verbal intellectual ability, poor psychomotor processing, and problematic behaviour. Parental neglect in these students is also thought to be associated with increased risk possibly due to lack of internal resources to cope with difficult times and situations (Osama et al., 2014).

In addition to the stressors already outlined, students are often at the age where negative life events can arise (Chan, Batterham, Christensen, & Galletly, 2014). These may include family breakdown, sickness or death, relationship issues which may compromise their ability to cope, and impact their academic performance (Dunn, Iglewicz & Moutier, 2008). Overall, such risk factors make them more vulnerable to DSH and suicidal tendencies (Wu et al., 2016).

Due to the 'Culture of Medicine', seeking help is often viewed as a sign of weakness rather than empowering act, resulting in stigma and pressure when vulnerable students need support (Dunn, Iglewicz & Moutier, 2008). Furthermore, medical students tend to withhold from help-seeking behaviour due to fear of career implications', 'physician heal thyself' culture, time pressures and concerns for confidentiality (Chan, Batterham, Christensen, & Galletly, 2014; Downs et al., 2014; Yousuf, Beh, & Wong, 2013). Another factor that influences help-seeking behaviour is attitudes towards suicide. Permissive attitudes are associated with more help-seeking behaviour where stigmatisation and sanctioning of suicide leads to the deterrence of help-seeking behaviour (Yousuf, Beh, & Wong, 2013). Attitudes vary among countries with some cultures being more restrictive and others more permissive (Amiri et al., 2013). For example, students in India were found to be more restrictive than Austrian students and Japanese students were more likely to normalise suicide than American medical students (Amiri et al., 2013). Additionally, clinical experience and exposure to suicidal patients may improve knowledge but lead to more negative attitudes to informal help-seeking (Chan, Batterham, Christensen, & Galletly, 2014). Avoidance of and barriers to help-seeking behaviour can, therefore, increase the risk of DHS and suicidal ideations (Wasserman et. al. 2011).

PROTECTIVE FACTORS

Whilst there are numerous factors that precipitate an increased risk of deliberate self-harm and suicide in general, there are also common protective factors. These protective factors range from lifestyle factors such as maintaining a good diet, good sleeping hygiene and keeping an active lifestyle, to personality factors such as one's coping strategy, sense of personal value, confidence, ability to seek help and communicate (Wasserman et. al. 2011). Other protective factors such as social support and family connectedness are also valuable (Goldsmith, 2002).

Similarly, in medical students, general protective factors for mental well-being include psychosocial support and activities, internal characteristics and coping strategy as well as mentorship and intellectual stimulation. (Dunn, Iglewicz & Moutier, 2008). Presence of psychosocial support from family, friends, peers, medical school administration, therapists and religious affiliations and social activities, either spontaneous or structured, act as protective factors which may prevent or reduce DSH and suicide ideations. (Dunn, Iglewicz & Moutier, 2008).

Internal characteristics such as students' personal traits, temperament, and coping style are built upon the developmental task of young adulthood, gender-specific issues, and cultural/ethnic role expectations. Internal characteristics describe students coping reserve and resilience, which may vary between students, can be adaptive and protective. (Dunn, Iglewicz & Moutier, 2008).

Uniquely to medical students, the presence of mentorship from clinical preceptors, research mentors, assigned faculty mentors and/or peers may serve as role models and as one that students may be comfortable to disclose personal information or issues (Dunn, Iglewicz & Moutier, 2008). Additionally, intellectual stimulation whereby students start to appreciate the clinical significance and correlation of the basic sciences may serve as protective factors. This may be through enhancing enthusiasm for their career path (Dunn, Iglewicz & Moutier, 2008).

The factors mentioned above are general protective factors that relate to overall mental health and well-being. Unfortunately, as there is limited information in the literature, specific protective factors for DSH and suicide in medical students was not available. Further research in this area would be of interest and yield worthwhile information.

SOLUTIONS AND RECOMMENDATIONS

In this section, the authors explore assessment, preventative and management strategies to improve education, awareness and ultimately reduce the rates of DSH and suicide risk. Presented is a comprehensive review of practises and techniques that medical professionals and medical educators could utilise to aid medical students to adequately and safely manage DSH and suicide ideology. This will include highlighting the benefits of using surveys and questionnaires to assess and identify at-risk medical students, counselling and educational group programmes to increase education and literacy as well as referring for further treatment (Yousuf, Beh, & Wong, 2013). The solutions and recommendations will aim to improve mental health literacy, alleviate the stigma and normalisation of suicide that exists amongst medical students as well as increase self-care principles (Chan, Batterham, Christensen, & Galletly, 2014).

As discussed previously, medical students are at risk of normalisation of DSH and suicide ideology despite their mental health literacy levels and are still susceptible to the stigma of help-seeking for their mental well-being (Yousuf, Beh, & Wong, 2013). Medical students receive minimal training in suicide and DSH prevention (Yousuf, Beh, & Wong, 2013).

Both DSH and suicidal behaviour can be prevented with timely, evidence-based and often low-cost interventions (Wasserman et al., 2011; Muehlenkamp, Walsh, & McDade, 2009). Current approaches towards the prevention of DSH and suicidal ideology targets early screening programmes and psychoeducational interventions.

Primary Prevention

Focusing on preventing DSH and suicidal ideology in medical students should begin with targeted psychoeducational interventions early in their career. The purpose of this is to raise mental health literacy, reduce stigmatising attitudes, limiting normalisation/ glorification of suicide (Chan, Batterham, Christensen, & Galletly, 2014).

Suicide prevention and education modules can lead to positive attitudes towards understanding suicide and are well received by medical students (Yousuf, Beh, & Wong, 2013). Specifically, it can reduce negative attitudes towards and stigmatisation of suicide (Yousuf, Beh, & Wong, 2013). For example, a 2-week special studies module (SSM) on suicidology and suicide prevention for undergraduate medical students resulted in reduced negative appraisal, reduced stigmatisation and increased sensitivity towards suicide literacy, all of which are positive attitudes towards suicide (Yousuf, Beh, & Wong, 2013). The course itself covered a variety of topics from risk assessment to prevention and intervention strategies, suicide among health professionals, life, and death as well as skills for overcoming stress through a diverse range of teaching modalities such as presentations, discussions, skills-based training sessions and films.

DSH primary prevention should idealistically work in the same manner as suicide primary prevention, unfortunately, no specific studies currently exist for medical students. There are, however, prevention programmes which have been trialed in adolescents in a school-based prevention program. Muehlenkamp, Walsh & McDale discuss the use of the Signs of Self-Injury (SOSI) programme which is designed for both staff and students. The programme is divided into two modules, with the staff module providing psychoeducational material about DSH as well as warning signs and methods of response. The student module utilises multimedia presentation to overview DSH signs and symptoms and how to approach for help. This is followed by a group discussion to consolidate all the information. The results indicated that students had improved help-seeking attitudes and intentions and preliminary data demonstrated that the programme may be an effective prevention programme for schools (Muehlenkamp, Walsh, & McDade, 2009). This may be a viable option if adapted for medical students as well as medical teaching faculty.

Secondary Prevention

There is insufficient data to support that suicide screening of the general population in primary care will reduce mortality (LeFevre, 2014; O'Connor, Gaynes, Burda, Soh, & Whitlock, 2013). Despite this, identification of cases based upon risk factors, sensitivity to high-risk situations in depressed patients, and assessment of suicidality in patients treated for depression is appropriate and can reveal occasional patients with suicidal intent and can benefit from interjection and intervention (LeFevre, 2014; O'Connor, Gaynes, Burda, Soh, & Whitlock, 2013).

For medical students, secondary and tertiary prevention strategies should be utilised to ensure early intervention. One example of a screening and referral system is The Healer Education Assessment and Referral (HEAR) programme. This encompassed a two-tiered programme involving educational models followed by anonymous screening using 9-item Patient Health Questionnaire (PHQ-9) to identify affective disorders and suicide risk in medical students (Simon et al., 2013). Students who were found to be at risk were then assessed further and referred for care if necessary (See Figure 3) ("The Patient Health Questionnaire (PHQ-9)", 1999). This study found that a significant number of 'at-risk' students were not in treatment (Downs et al., 2014). Programmes like this have the potential to identify, refer and treat 'at-risk' students with depression and increased suicide risk with the ultimate goal of reducing suicide behaviour, death from suicide, deliberate self-harm, education, treatment, screening, engagement, and follow-up. The Royal College of Psychiatrists actually endorses repeated assessments and screening, as they can actually increase engagement in treatment (Self-harm, suicide, and risk: a summary, 2010).

Screening for deliberate self-harm has proven more challenging due to aforementioned reasons of individual concealment and unwillingness to seek help. Despite this, the Columbia-Suicide Severity Rating Scale (C-SSRS) has been

Figure 3. 9-Item Patient Health Questionnaire (PHQ-9)
Source: Adapted from The Patient Health Questionnaire (PHQ-9, 1999)

Over the past 2 weeks, how often have you been bothered by any of the following problems?	Not At All	Several Days	More Than Half the Days	Nearly Every Day
1. Little interest or pleasure in doing things	0	1	2	3
2. Feeling down, depressed or hopeless	0	1	2	3
3. Trouble falling asleep, staying asleep or sleeping too much	0	1	2	3
4. Feeling tired or having little energy	0	1	2	3
5. Poor appetite or overeating	0	1	2	3
6. Feeling bad about yourself – or that you're a failure or have let yourself or your family down	0	1	2	3
7. Trouble concentrating on things, such as reading the newspaper or watching television	0	1	2	3
8. Moving or speaking so slowly that other people could have noticed. Or, the opposite – being so fidgety or restless that you have been moving around a lot more than usual	0	1	2	3
9. Thoughts that you would be better off dead or off hurting yourself in some way	0	1	2	3

developed to assess suicidal ideation, lethality, and severity of suicide attempt as well as DSH without suicidal intent (Wasserman et al., 2011). The C-SSRS differs from the PHQ-9 in that it more thoroughly assesses suicidal intent, a key factor in differing suicide ideation and deliberate self-harm (Viguera et al., 2015). Unfortunately, neither the C-SSRS or the PHQ-9 have been evaluated for their sensitivity or specificity in identifying deliberate self-harm in medical students.

Tertiary Prevention

Any acute, life-threatening incidences of suicide attempts or self-harm should be managed promptly by appropriately trained staff and acute psychiatric services (Carter et al., 2016; Hirschfeld & Russell, 1997). Ongoing treatment and follow up should be conducted by a health professional unrelated to the medical school to prevent any conflicts of interest. Any discussion between the medical school and treating team about a medical student's mental health should only be made with explicit consent of the patient.

According to the Royal College of Psychiatrists, there is insufficient evidence to clearly define the best therapy for those who have self-harmed or plan to self-harm (Bateman, 2014). This is further supported by the Royal Australian and New Zealand College of Psychiatrists, who define clinical practise guidelines for specific population sub-groups, none of which focus on medical student demographics (Carter et al., 2016). There is limited randomised controlled trial evidence to support pharmacological treatment for DSH, in fact, it has demonstrated an unfavourable risk-benefit ratio (Carter et al., 2016; Suarez & Saunders, 2012). Psychological or psychosocial interventions such as problem-solving therapy, cognitive-behavioural therapy and psychodynamic interpersonal therapy have been effective in reducing the number of recurrent DSH events (Carter et al., 2016). A health professional should make a tailored approach based on each individual's problems.

Suicidal behaviour is a serious psychiatric emergency with complex treatment. This treatment strategy serves as tertiary prevention to prevent progression of condition or a successful attempt. In acute cases, patients require evaluation and either inpatient or outpatient care (O'Connor, Gaynes, Burda, Soh, & Whitlock, 2013). The decision whether to admit patients to psychiatric ward is difficult due to the circumstances of each case, use of economic resources as well as negative effects of hospitalisation (Wasserman et al., 2011).

In acute suicidal cases, the early phase is when patients are most at risk (Wasserman et al., 2011). An empathetic and supportive approach should be taken and encompass symptomatic, pharmacological treatment. Medications prescribed should be supervised by family or community services and given in small packages (Wasserman et al., 2011). Adequate monitoring and follow-up are of paramount importance as the risk of suicide increases in days and initial weeks after discharge (Hirschfeld & Russell, 1997).

Long-term management should be commenced immediately and include follow-up consultations e.g. active involvement of family members, telephone contacts, appointments and social network evaluation (Wasserman et al., 2011). Prevention of suicidal behaviours is achieved by treating underlying psychiatric disorders and symptoms. The treatment regime varies and depends largely on the specific cause which will not be discussed here as it is beyond the scope of this chapter.

Psychological treatment includes cognitive behavioural therapy (CBT) which is the evidence-based method of treatment, however this is not specific to medical students (O'Connor, Gaynes, Burda, Soh, & Whitlock, 2013). Other forms of psychological treatment which may be useful includes dialectical behaviour therapy, in-home interpersonal psychotherapy, family psychotherapy developmental group therapy and psycho dynamic therapy however further research is needed to confirm effectiveness of these treatment methods. Irrespective of psychotherapy employed, effective strategies require a good therapeutic relationship between patient and therapist, treatment fidelity, compliance, targeting identifiable skills and emphasis on personal responsibility (Wasserman et al., 2011).

Community resources are recommended as patients struggle with existential crises. These may involve support from family and friends, helplines, crisis centres, mental health centres, religious counsellor (Wasserman et al., 2011). The goal of elevating psychosocial support is to enhance sense of meaning in life. Such strategies can be implemented into medical school policies for both students and educators, as discussed in the following section.

Recommendations for Medical Schools and Educators

Implementation of prevention strategies to reduce suicide and deliberate self-harm amongst medical students requires an integrated and committed effort from both medical schools and educators (Hughes, Kent, & Bowman, 2008). Such entities have important roles in ensuring the success of intervention strategies and therefore reduce stigma and barriers seeking health services (Thornicroft et al., 2016).

Whilst no current literature supports any specific mental health interventions in medical students, a multitude of research has been conducted regarding guidelines for tertiary education institutions in support students with a mental illness. A 2013 Delphi consensus study conducted with 74 Australian professionals and 35 consumers supported 155 strategies that addressed mental illness in all students at tertiary institutions. These strategies encompassed generating policies in a variety of domains to assist students such as promotion, enhancement and accessibility of support services, education, and training of staff as well as funding, research and evaluation (Reavley, Ross, Killackey & Jorm, 2013). The authors will continue to discuss methods through which medical schools and educators can promote awareness and implement strategies in their institution, specifically with regards to university policy, support services and staff and student education.

University policies should address the promotion of mental health awareness, prevention of mental illness and provide the foundation for services for students with a mental illness (Reavley, Ross, Killackey & Jorm, 2013). Mental health awareness should be employed by leading executives and professors of the faculty in conjunction with student associations and representatives from external services. Most importantly, institutions should develop a plan for communicating this mental health policy to all staff and students. A report from the Australian Medical Students' Association in 2013 outlined several student-based initiatives such as mentoring programmes, wellbeing events including guest speakers on self-care, yoga and meditation as well as providing student-friendly external services such as general practitioners and psychologists. A collaborative approach from students and staff is essential in ensuring student participation (Australia Medical Students' Association Student Mental Health and Wellbeing Committee, 2013; Reavley, Ross, Killackey & Jorm, 2013).

Institution support services such as student counsellors, telephone counselling, online services and support groups should be made available to all staff and students. As discussed previously, barriers to seeking help play a large role in a medical student's decision and universities should adopt an easy access, non-judgemental approach to entry for assessment and treatment, a method that Hughes, Kent & Bowman address as the 'no wrong door' policy (Hughes, Kent, & Bowman, 2008).

As discussed in primary prevention, psychoeducational modules would be beneficial in conveying information to staff and students. This should clearly detail signs, symptoms, causes, treatment and the benefits of early intervention and prevention (Reavley, Ross, Killackey & Jorm, 2013). Staff should also be trained to use non-judgemental listening skills, respond appropriately when a student discloses a mental illness to them, techniques for motivating students and raising self-esteem and most importantly how to handle a mental health crisis (Reavley, Ross, Killackey & Jorm, 2013). These skills can be taught to staff over on-going professional development sessions and online training, to be accessible and thorough, yet not create a high burden of work. The university and staff should also provide 'reasonable adjustments' for assessments to encourage and assist students in coping with their mental illness and to ensure that high workload demands or expectations do not negatively impact an already stressed student (Hughes, Kent, & Bowman, 2008). Furthermore, this process should be made open and transparent for the fairness of all students.

Major limitations to these prevention strategies are due to lack of funding and resources. Despite this, medical schools should endeavour to allocate adequate funds and seek funding opportunities to enhance student mental health services to benefit their students. Additionally, these services should be followed up and evaluated in ongoing research to monitor the efficacy of such interventions.

The combination of university policy support services and staff and student education is a useful intervention strategy but an area that still requires further research in the medical school domain. As discussed in the sections above, implementation of intervention strategies is vital as they target all facets of prevention to ultimately reduce the risk of suicide and self-harm in this vulnerable population (Wasserman et al., 2011).

FUTURE RESEARCH DIRECTIONS

Deliberate self-harm and suicide ideology is an important, emerging issue amongst medical students. Current literature on this issue only scratches the surface of a deeper problem and requires further research to explore the depth and breadth of the issues. Future research is needed to quantify the severity and predisposing factors contributing to this issue, to ascertain student perspectives and engage students in finding solutions. Similarly, the perspectives and roles of medical educators and administrators in medical schools should also be examined. The downstream impact of deliberate self-harm and suicide ideology during medical school on well-being and performance in future clinical practise could also be explored. Implementation of the proposed solutions and recommendations can be a stepping stone to addressing deliberate self-harm and suicide in medical students and will also serve as future research opportunities to evaluate the usefulness and effectiveness of such strategies.

CONCLUSION

Deliberate self-harm and suicide ideology are pertinent issues amongst medical students. The relation between deliberate self-harm and suicide ideology is important and helpful for understanding the risk factors and preventative factors behind both diagnoses. Early screening assessment and intervention are evidence-based and often low-cost, meaning their implementation can be quick and effective.

REFERENCES

Ajdacic-Gross, V. (2008). Methods of suicide: International suicide patters derived from the WHO mortality database. *Bulletin of the World Health Organization, 86*(9), 726–732. doi:10.2471/BLT.07.043489 PMID:18797649

Amiri, L., Voracek, M., Yousef, S., Galadari, A., Yammahi, S., Sadeghi, M., & Dervic, K. et al. (2013). Suicidal Behavior and Attitudes Among Medical Students in the United Arab Emirates. *Crisis, 34*(2), 116–123. doi:10.1027/0227-5910/a000170 PMID:23195458

Australia Medical Students' Association Student Mental Health and Wellbeing Committee. (2013). *Student Based Mental Health Interventions: Australian Medical Schools*. Canberra: AMSA. Retrieved from http://mentalhealth.amsa.org.au/wp-content/uploads/2015/09/AMSA-SMHW-Australian-Medical-Student-Report-2013.pdf

Bateman, A. (2014). *Self-Harm. Royal College of Psychiatrists*. Retrieved 1 October 2016, from http://www.rcpsych.ac.uk/healthadvice/problemsdisorders/self-harm.aspx

Carter, G., Page, A., Large, M., Hetrick, S., Milner, A., Bendit, N., & Christensen, H. et al. (2016). Royal Australian and New Zealand College of Psychiatrists clinical practice guideline for the management of deliberate self-harm. *The Australian and New Zealand Journal of Psychiatry, 50*(10), 939–1000. doi:10.1177/0004867416661039 PMID:27650687

Chan, W., Batterham, P., Christensen, H., & Galletly, C. (2014). Suicide literacy, suicide stigma and help-seeking intentions in Australian medical students. *Australasian Psychiatry, 22*(2), 132–139. doi:10.1177/1039856214522528 PMID:24526795

Diagnostic and statistical manual of mental disorders. (2013). Washington, DC: Academic Press.

Dieserud, G., Roysamb, E., Ekeberg, O., & Kraft, P. (2001). Toward an Integrative Model of Suicide Attempt: A Cognitive Psychological Approach. *Suicide & Life-Threatening Behavior, 31*(2), 153–168. doi:10.1521/suli.31.2.153.21511 PMID:11459248

Downs, N., Feng, W., Kirby, B., McGuire, T., Moutier, C., Norcross, W., & Zisook, S. et al. (2014). Listening to Depression and Suicide Risk in Medical Students: The Healer Education Assessment and Referral (HEAR) Program. *Academic Psychiatry, 38*(5), 547–553. doi:10.1007/s40596-014-0115-x PMID:24705825

Dunn, L., Iglewicz, A., & Moutier, C. (2008). A Conceptual Model of Medical Student Well-Being: Promoting Resilience and Preventing Burnout. *Academic Psychiatry*, *32*(1), 44–53. doi:10.1176/appi.ap.32.1.44 PMID:18270280

Eskin, M., Voracek, M., Stieger, S., & Altinyazar, V. (2011). A cross-cultural investigation of suicidal behavior and attitudes in Austrian and Turkish medical students. *Social Psychiatry and Psychiatric Epidemiology*, *46*(9), 813–823. doi:10.1007/s00127-010-0254-7 PMID:20563550

Etzersdorfer, E., Vijayakumar, L., Schöny, W., Grausgruber, A., & Sonneck, G. (1998). Attitudes toward suicide among medical students: Comparison between Madras (India) and Vienna (Austria). *Social Psychiatry and Psychiatric Epidemiology*, *33*(3), 104–110. doi:10.1007/s001270050029 PMID:9540384

Goldsmith, S. (2002). *Reducing suicide*. Washington, DC: National Academies Press.

Hirschfeld, R., & Russell, J. (1997). Assessment and Treatment of Suicidal Patients. *The New England Journal of Medicine*, *337*(13), 910–915. doi:10.1056/NEJM199709253371307 PMID:9302306

Hughes, P., Kent, A., & Bowman, D. (2008). Medical students and mental health: The UK perspective. *The Clinical Teacher*, *5*(2), 83–87. doi:10.1111/j.1743-498X.2007.00196.x

Klonsky, E., May, A., & Glenn, C. (2013). The relationship between nonsuicidal self-injury and attempted suicide: Converging evidence from four samples. *Journal of Abnormal Psychology*, *122*(1), 231–237. doi:10.1037/a0030278 PMID:23067259

LeFevre, M. (2014). Screening for Suicide Risk in Adolescents, Adults, and Older Adults in Primary Care: U.S. Preventive Services Task Force Recommendation Statement. *Annals of Internal Medicine*, *160*(10), 719. doi:10.7326/M14-0589 PMID:24842417

Lilley, R., Owens, D., Horrocks, J., House, A., Noble, R., Bergen, H., & Kapur, N. et al. (2008). Hospital care and repetition following self-harm: Multicentre comparison of self-poisoning and self-injury. *The British Journal of Psychiatry*, *192*(6), 440–445. doi:10.1192/bjp.bp.107.043380 PMID:18515895

Mangnall, J., & Yurkovich, E. (2008). A Literature Review of Deliberate Self-Harm. *Perspectives in Psychiatric Care*, *44*(3), 175–184. doi:10.1111/j.1744-6163.2008.00172.x PMID:18577123

Miletic, V., Lukovic, J., Ratkovic, N., Aleksic, D., & Grgurevic, A. (2014). Demographic risk factors for suicide and depression among Serbian medical school students. *Social Psychiatry and Psychiatric Epidemiology*, *50*(4), 633–638. doi:10.1007/s00127-014-0950-9 PMID:25205334

Muehlenkamp, J., Walsh, B., & McDade, M. (2009). Preventing Non-Suicidal Self-Injury in Adolescents: The Signs of Self-Injury Program. *Journal of Youth and Adolescence*, *39*(3), 306–314. doi:10.1007/s10964-009-9450-8 PMID:19756992

OConnor, E., Gaynes, B., Burda, B., Soh, C., & Whitlock, E. (2013). Screening for and Treatment of Suicide Risk Relevant to Primary Care: A Systematic Review for the U.S. Preventive Services Task Force. *Annals of Internal Medicine*, *158*(10), 741. doi:10.7326/0003-4819-158-10-201305210-00642 PMID:23609101

Osama, M., Islam, M., Hussain, S., Masroor, S., Burney, M., Masood, M., & Rehman, R. et al. (2014). Suicidal ideation among medical students of Pakistan: A cross-sectional study. *Journal of Forensic and Legal Medicine*, *27*, 65–68. doi:10.1016/j.jflm.2014.08.006 PMID:25287803

Reavley, N., Ross, A., Killackey, E., & Jorm, A. (2013). Development of guidelines for tertiary education institutions to assist them in supporting students with a mental illness: A Delphi consensus study with Australian professionals and consumers. *Peerj*, *1*, e43. doi:10.7717/peerj.43 PMID:23638380

Rotenstein, L., Ramos, M., Torre, M., Segal, J., Peluso, M., Guille, C., & Mata, D. A. et al. (2016). Prevalence of Depression, Depressive Symptoms, and Suicidal Ideation Among Medical Students. *Journal of the American Medical Association*, *316*(21), 2214. doi:10.1001/jama.2016.17324 PMID:27923088

Schwenk, T. L., Davis, L., & Wimsatt, L. A. (2010). Depression, stigma, and suicidal ideation in medical students. *Journal of the American Medical Association*, *304*(11), 1181–1190. doi:10.1001/jama.2010.1300 PMID:20841531

Simon, G., Rutter, C., Peterson, D., Oliver, M., Whiteside, U., Operskalski, B., & Ludman, E. (2013). Does Response on the PHQ-9 Depression Questionnaire Predict Subsequent Suicide Attempt or Suicide Death? *Psychiatric Services (Washington, D.C.)*, *64*(12), 1195–1202. doi:10.1176/appi.ps.201200587 PMID:24036589

Stanley, B., Sher, L., Wilson, S., Ekman, R., Huang, Y., & Mann, J. (2010). Non-suicidal self-injurious behaviour, endogenous opioids and monoamine neurotransmitters. *Journal of Affective Disorders*, *124*(1-2), 134–140. doi:10.1016/j.jad.2009.10.028 PMID:19942295

Suarez, N., & Saunders, K. (2012). Assessment and management of self harm. *Student BMJ, 20*. http://dx.doi.org.libraryproxy.griffith.edu.au/10.1136/sbmj.e511

The Patient Health Questionnaire (PHQ-9). (1999). Centre for Quality Assessment and Improvement in Mental Health. Retrieved 1 October 2016, from http://www.cqaimh.org/pdf/tool_phq9.pdf

Thornicroft, G., Mehta, N., Clement, S., Evans-Lacko, S., Doherty, M., Rose, D., & Henderson, C. et al. (2016). Evidence for effective interventions to reduce mental-health-related stigma and discrimination. *Lancet*, *387*(10023), 1123–1132. doi:10.1016/S0140-6736(15)00298-6 PMID:26410341

Tyssen, R., Vaglum, P., Grønvold, N. T., & Ekeberg, O. (2001). Suicidal ideation among medical students and young physi- cians: A nationwide and prospective study of prevalence and predictors. *Journal of Affective Disorders*, *64*(1), 69–79. doi:10.1016/S0165-0327(00)00205-6 PMID:11292521

Viguera, A., Milano, N., Laurel, R., Thompson, N., Griffith, S., Baldessarini, R., & Katzan, I. (2015). Comparison of Electronic Screening for Suicidal Risk with the Patient Health Questionnaire Item 9 and the Columbia Suicide Severity Rating Scale in an Outpatient Psychiatric Clinic. *Psychosomatics*, *56*(5), 460–469. doi:10.1016/j.psym.2015.04.005 PMID:26278339

Wan, Y., Gao, R., Tao, X., Tao, F., & Hu, C. (2012). Relationship between deliberate self-harm and suicidal behaviors in college students. *Zhonghua Liu Xing Bing Xue Za Zhi = Zhonghua Liuxingbingxue Zazhi, 33*(5), 474-477.

Wasserman, D., Rihmer, Z., Rujescu, D., Sarchiapone, M., Sokolowski, M., Titelman, D., & Carli, V. et al. (2011). The European Psychiatric Association (EPA) guidance on suicide treatment and prevention. *European Psychiatry*, *27*(2), 129–141. doi:10.1016/j.eurpsy.2011.06.003 PMID:22137775

Wege, N., Muth, T., Li, J., & Angerer, P. (2016). Mental health among currently enrolled medical students in Germany. *Public Health*, *132*, 92–100. doi:10.1016/j.puhe.2015.12.014 PMID:26880490

Whitlock, J., Muehlenkamp, J., Eckenrode, J., Purington, A., Baral Abrams, G., Barreira, P., & Kress, V. (2013). Nonsuicidal Self-Injury as a Gateway to Suicide in Young Adults. *The Journal of Adolescent Health*, *52*(4), 486–492. doi:10.1016/j.jadohealth.2012.09.010 PMID:23298982

Wu, D., Rockett, I., Yang, T., Feng, X., Jiang, S., & Yu, L. (2016). Deliberate self-harm among Chinese medical students: A population-based study. *Journal of Affective Disorders*, *202*, 137–144. doi:10.1016/j.jad.2016.05.030 PMID:27262635

Yousuf, S., Beh, P., & Wong, P. (2013). Attitudes towards suicide following an undergraduate suicide prevention module: Experience of medical students in Hong Kong. *Hong Kong Medical Journal, 19*(5), 377–385. doi:10.12809/hkmj133950 PMID:24088587

KEY TERMS AND DEFINITIONS

Deliberate Self-Harm: Direct behaviour that causes minor to moderate physical injury, that is undertaken without conscious suicidal intent and that occurs in the absence of psychoses and/or organic intellectual impairment.

Primary Prevention: Intervention or action that aims to prevent disease or injury before it ever occurs.

Psycho-Educational Intervention: A broad range of activities, combining education, counselling and support interventions. These may be delivered individually or in groups, may be tailored or standardised.

Secondary Prevention: Intervention or action that aims to reduce the impact of a disease or injury that has already occurred through screening, early detection or halting.

Suicide: The act of deliberately killing oneself.

Suicide Ideology: Concerns, thoughts about or unusual preoccupation with suicide. Also known as suicide ideation.

Tertiary Prevention: Intervention, action or treatment for disease or injury that prevents complication and/or progression.

Section 3
Graduate Medical Education

Chapter 6
From Medical Student to Medical Resident:
Graduate Medical Education and Mental Health in the United States

Warren G. McDonald
Methoodist University, USA

Matt Martin
Southern Regional Area Health Education Center, USA

Lenard D. Salzberg
Southern Regional Area Health Education Center, USA

ABSTRACT

The transition from medical school to board-certified medical practice includes a period of intense, practical training known as medical residency. Medical residents are at risk for greater mental health distress than the general population. Interns, which are first year residents, are most at risk for, at worst, depression and suicidal ideation, and, at best, negative outlooks on the medical profession. Risk factors include role transition, decreased sleep, relocation, isolation, stigma toward mental health problems and treatment, and health care industry changes. Untreated mental health problems can lead to burnout later during a physician's career. Residents thrive on social and organisational support which can include systematic screening and treatment of mental health problems. Although research regarding best practices for addressing mental health problems during residency is limited, we offer four core strategies for preventing and addressing mental health problems in medical residents: education, screening, treatment, and support.

DOI: 10.4018/978-1-5225-2811-1.ch006

INTRODUCTION

The purpose of graduate medical education (i.e., medical residency) is to cultivate competency, enthusiasm, and confidence within new medical school graduates and prepare these newly minted physicians for a rewarding and successful career in medicine. Residency training in the United States is primarily distinct from medical school education. Residents, unlike medical students, are fully responsible for the treatment of large panels of patients which means they order laboratory and diagnostic tests, perform surgical procedures, make referrals, and design treatment plans. In addition, residents spend long hours during inpatient and outpatient shifts including night rotations and on-call hours. This particular training is necessary for physicians to develop the skills and temperament required for medical practice. However, such training also exposes residents to isolation, role transition, fatigue, and stress.

While it is clear that residents are at greater risk for depression and suicidal ideation than the general population, researchers have not yet identified the best practises for addressing resident mental health (de Oliveira et al., 2013; Goldman, Shah, & Bernstein, 2015; Govardhan, Pinelli, & Schnatz, 2012). Some qualitative data shows that social support is crucial (Mata, Ramos, Kim, Guille, & Sen, 2016). The medical school literature shows promising results for physical activity, organisational changes and support (e.g., pass/fail grading, faculty advisors, and student retreats), and mindfulness training (Drolet & Rodgers, 2010; Kötter, Tautphäus, Obst, Voltmer, & Scherer, 2016; Slavin & Chibnall, 2016). In this chapter, the authors will describe the transition from medical school to residency training, the relationship between residency training and resident mental health, the effect of chronic stress on resident wellbeing, and a four-part programme for supporting resident mental health.

BACKGROUND

Residency selection is a long and cost-intensive process. During the fourth year of medical school in the United States, students apply to multiple residency programmes devoting significant money and time. Concurrently, residency directors and coordinators spend substantial resources recruiting and interviewing students for a limited number of slots. After interviews conclude, faculty members meet and rank all applicants according to programme fit and quality. Osteopathic students match to their respective residency programmes at the beginning of February while allopathic student match in the middle of March. Residency selection is a long and arduous process for both sides. New residents report to their programmes in June or July, complete orientation, and begin their first rotations.

First-year residents (interns) hit the ground running. Even during orientation, interns are signing medical orders and patients charts. They assume responsibility of continuity patients from recently graduated residents and make treatment decisions at the hospital. With a limited patient panel and under the watchful supervision of attending physicians, interns act like fully-functioning physicians. During the first three months of residency, incidences of depression can increase from 4% to 27% while suicidal ideation can increased nearly 400% (Sen et al., 2010).

In an effort to curb resident fatigue and distress, the Accreditation Council for Graduate Medical Education (ACGME) mandated resident duty hour reforms which, among several requirements, capped residents' weekly duty hours at 80 per week (Bolster & Rourke, 2015). There is no doubt that residents work long and hard hours; yet, it is unclear if limiting resident hours is beneficial to patient care and resident well-being (Bolster & Rourke, 2015; Lin, Lin, Auditore, & Fanning, 2016). Under long periods of duress, residents can experience allostatic load (i.e., chronic stress) which puts them at risk for mental health problems like depression (McEwen, 2003). Chronic stress can lead to feelings of isolation and helplessness, social withdrawal, and impaired immunity function. In addition to stress, residents also grapple with mental health stigma and poor work-life balance (Billings, Lazarus, Wenrich, Curtis, & Engelberg, 2011; Mata et al., 2016). These experiences can create negative frameworks of patients and medical practice and lead to future burnout.

Transition From Medical School to Medical Residency

The mental health of residents is partially understood when examining the experience of medical school and the transition to graduate medical education. Life transitions, such as those experienced by new medical students, are times of high stress. The impact of stressors is reduced when people have high levels of mastery, high self-esteem, and/or have social support (Thoits, 2010).

Medical school curricula vary. In most U.S. medical schools, the initial two years of school are taught in the classroom, a familiar setting for students who have recently completed four years of undergraduate education following twelve years of primary education. The structure of medical school is such that there is a high level of social support built into the first two years. All first year students take the same courses together. Synchronised schedules give students time off concurrently, creating an opportunity to socialize, celebrate, and commiserate together. The large medical school class is frequently divided into smaller work groups (e.g. a group of four that share a cadaver; groups of eight to twelve that meet for problem-based learning) that naturally form social networks. These social networks and social support help medical students cope with the increased stresses inherent in medical school.

Medical school is a time of high stress (MacLean, Booza, & Balon, 2016). The pace of medical school is much faster than anything students experienced during college. Prior to medical school most students are the best or brightest in their class. In medical school, these students are surrounded by others who have achieved as much as they have, and are in competition with other high achievers for grades if they desire the most coveted residency positions.

By the end of the second year of medical school, students are required to pass the first of three parts of the United States Medical Licensing Examination (USMLE). The USMLE is designed to assess a physician's ability to apply knowledge, concepts and principles to demonstrate fundamental patient-centered skills. The first step tests classroom knowledge. This test generates anxiety: If students do not pass, they are not promoted to the next year of medical school and may not graduate. If students pass but do not excel, they may not be considered for residency spots in highly competitive medical specialties (e.g. dermatology, ophthalmology, radiology).

During the initial two years of medical school, there is a gradual introduction to patient care. In some U.S. schools, students are first exposed to patients during a physical diagnosis course taught in the latter half of the second year of school. In other schools there is longitudinal exposure to patients beginning in the first year. This controlled exposure to patient care is used to prepare students for the final two years of medical school, the clinical clerkship years. During the third and fourth year of medical school (the clerkship years) students interact with patients in hospitals and in physicians' offices.

The clerkship years bring new stressors. Beginning in the third year of medical school, students are no longer in a single large cohort. Due to the limited ability to provide teaching/learning activities for all the students at once, students rotate through the different clinical disciplines at different times. Each students' peer support group grows much smaller as schedules are no longer synchronised.

The clerkship years are frequently the first-time students are exposed to death and dying (MacLean et al., 2016). There is usually not time to process these new experiences and there is typically no guide or structure to do so. Medical students may not know what to do with their feelings, and may be encouraged to ignore them or bury them, leading to increased stress.

During the preclinical years, students typically have learned that there is a 'right answer' or a 'wrong answer' to questions that are posed regarding medication choice, test ordering, and diagnosis. Once in the clerkship years, students see that there are multiple possible answers to every clinical question. This can be frightening to the learner and can lead to a feeling of lack of control (MacLean et al., 2016). It can be stressful to the learner who does not know if the reason there is no clear answer is because they are inadequate or if there truly is no answer.

Medical Residency Training

Changing roles from medical student to physician is a major life stressor. After spending 20 years as students receiving financial and other support from parents and others, the new resident physician may now be facing life issues for the first time (Coates, Spector, & Uijtdehaage, 2012). College students and medical students typically accrue debt. Once they are graduates, residents are now members of the adult work-force, many for the first time in their lives. While in school the burden of debt felt theoretical; now that loans have started to come due, the debt is real. Financial concerns are atop the list of stress producing situations for new residents (Coates et al., 2012).

For those residents who never held full-time employment prior to residency the reality of work is shocking. Resident hours are long and inflexible. Residents work on weekends, holidays, and special occasions (e.g. birthdays). Calling in sick is not an easy option. Lateness is not excused or overlooked.

The biggest stress for new residents is assuming responsibility for patients' lives. Medical schools give students the opportunity to observe and participate in patient care, but at no point are medical students solely responsible for patient care decisions. They may suggest a diagnostic test or medication, or list potential diagnoses, but ultimately the resident and attending physicians are responsible for making decisions. No medical student orders are taken off the chart unless cosigned in hospitals, and no prescriptions solely signed by a medical student can be filled at a pharmacy. From the first day of residency, residents are given the responsibility of responding to pages, writing patients' prescriptions, writing orders, and making clinical decisions. The realisation that every decision needs to be made and that each of these decisions have implications for patients' wellbeing can be harrowing to the new resident (Abuhusain, Chotirmall, Hamid, & O'Neill, 2009).

When medical students graduate medical school, they are no longer students; they are now 'doctors'. This title change alters perceptions. Faculty, peers, and even family members look at these newly minted physicians as professionals who have sworn an oath to put patients' needs above their own. From day one in residency, these doctors are responsible for their patients' care, and will be held to the same standards as physicians in practice for twenty years. Patients in the hospital and in the office do not distinguish between a resident starting her first day and a resident who has completed her training. Patients look at these new physicians as competent professionals, even if the resident does not feel competent. A new resident can feel like an imposter.

Residents in training are given progressive responsibility. From day one, residents are responsible for their own panel of patients. As they progress through residency training, the size of the resident's panel grows. Early in training residents are directly supervised. As they develop competence and confidence, the residents are directly observed less frequently, and instead report to a preceptor during each patient encounter. During this report, the preceptor gives the resident feedback on presentation skills, thinking and organization, and patient care. Residents are asked to make assessments and plans which are reviewed by the preceptor. The resident-preceptor relationship is integral for developing confidence and competency.

Second year and third year residents have fewer required rotations and more elective rotations. As they progress through training they have increased responsibility in the inpatient and outpatient settings. In outpatient care, their patient panel grows dramatically at the conclusion of their first year. By the end of third year, residents see patients at a pace similar to community physicians. Residents are required to precept all patient encounters during their first year of residency. After successful completion of their first year in residency, residents are no longer required to universally precept, and subsequently have less time allotted into their schedule to see each patient.

In addition to office and hospital-based experiential learning, residents are taught in longitudinal seminar series. Humanism and professionalism are taught by example but also through readings and discussion. Practice management, likewise, is taught by example and through didactics. As residents grow in medical knowledge and develop a professional identity, they develop a sense of mastery which helps to mitigate residency distress. Residents are required to teach themselves, alongside faculty instruction, in order to obtain this competency.

Residency training challenges new physicians on a variety of personal and professional skills. Program directors identify a lack of medical knowledge as only one of the common struggles interns face. Lack of self-reflection and improvement, poor organisational skills, and underdeveloped professionalism were identified as deficits in a study of thirty residency program directors across ten specialties (Lyss-Lerman et al., 2009). These deficits are developmentally appropriate and expected for young residents and can lead to frustration and undue distress when not addressed by the resident and supporting faculty.

Residents are evaluated on each rotation (with both formative, mid-rotation evaluations and summative, end-of-rotation evaluations) and longitudinally. Evaluations allow faculty to measure the progress of residents and identify any deficits in patient care or professionalism. Knowledge is evaluated during rotations and by standardised exams administered annually. Physicians in practise are required to maintain certification once they have been specialty board certified. Residents are introduced to this process during residency and complete certification modules during each of their three years of training.

As residents progress through the training their patient care ability matures. They are treated more as colleagues when they are PGY-3 residents than they were when they were PGY-1 residents. By the time they are allowed to graduate, residents are ready to be independent practitioners.

Medical Residency and Mental Health

Mental health is the combined emotional, psychological, and social well-being of an individual and determines how that individual handles stress, relates to others, and makes choices. Burnout is a state of chronic stress that leads to physical and emotional exhaustion, cynicism and detachment, and feelings of ineffectiveness and lack of accomplishment. Burnout is more common among physicians than other US workers (Shanafelt et al., 2012). Over the past several years, physician burnout has increased with one estimate that more than half of US physicians are experiencing professional burnout (Shanafelt et al., 2015). Mental health support and treatment can help medical residents develop resiliency and alleviate the effects of stress from graduate medical education.

The purpose of graduate medical education (i.e., medical residency) is to cultivate competency, enthusiasm, and confidence within new medical school graduates and prepare these newly minted physicians for a rewarding and successful career in medicine. The process by which residents grow and develop is purposefully intense and, consequently, places residents at risk for experiencing poorer mental health. Compared to the general US population, medical residents are at greater risk for poorer mental health (Dyrbye et al., 2014). The importance of addressing resident mental health cannot be overstated. Untreated mental health can undermine residents' professional development, negatively affect patient care, and lead to mental illness and suicidal ideation (Dyrbye & Shanafelt, 2016).

It not entirely clear why residents are at risk for poorer mental health due to a lack of large, prospective studies. However, it seems that factors within the learning and work environment, rather than individual attributes, are the main drivers of mental health problems (Dyrbye & Shanafelt, 2016). Moreover, resident distress does not seem to be the result of poor medical knowledge and suboptimal clinical performance (Beckman, Reed, Shanafelt, & West, 2012). Rather, it seems that unmitigated burnout and distress lead to increased medical errors (Fahrenkopf et al., 2008; West, Tan, Habermann, Sloan, & Shanafelt, 2009), decreased empathy (West et al., 2006), and unprofessional conduct. One common result of burnout is depersonalisation which causes physicians to act callous or detached towards patients (Dyrbye et al., 2008; Shanafelt, Bradley, Wipf, & Back, 2002).

Risk and Protective Factors

There are several risk factors that can lead to poorer mental health outcomes for medical residents: prior history of mental illness, poor work-life balance, organisational stressors, and health care industry change. The first three apply to all US workers while the latter is unique to physicians. Whether due to family genetics, adverse childhood events, or ineffective coping strategies, residents with a history of depression, anxiety, trauma-related disorders, or serious mental illness (e.g., bipolar disorder, schizophrenia) are at greater risk for poorer mental health during residency training. Mental health stigma in the medical profession can discourage residents from recognising their own mental illness and seeking support and treatment. Some may minimize or veil their personal struggle with mental illness in order to be accepted into and complete residency training (Cooley-Wilder, 2016).

Work-life balance is the sense that one's work schedule allows time for personal and family activities. Dissatisfaction with this balance is a symptom of either an overburdening employer or a resident who does not schedule time for activities outside of work. Most residents are young adults with limited life experience and few if any robust coping strategies for stress. In addition, graduate medical education places residents in a variety of new health care systems with long hours and heavy responsibilities. When not directly taking care of patients, residents spend time completing medical charts, preparing for examinations, and other residency requirements. Residents with a poor work-life balance may not engage in physical activity, nutritious eating, good sleep hygiene, and social and community activities.

Organisational stressors include chronic high workload, lack of training and support, and unclear roles and responsibilities (Kapinos, Fitzgerald, Greer, & Rutks, 2012). The workload of a resident depends on the rotation and medical setting. For example, a resident on a hospital medicine rotation will work long shifts for several days in a row treating very sick patients. Meanwhile, a resident on an outpatient clinic rotation will work a shorter shift and have more time to rest. A high workload is normal in residency training and is offset by the change in responsibilities and stress. For example, the resident who completes a demanding rotation with long hours may then start a new rotation with a lighter load. This oscillation of schedules allows residents to recover and build stamina over time. Chronically high workloads do not allow residents to recover and lead to distress and burnout.

Residents need orientation training (e.g., didactics, shadowing, training modules) to learn electronic medical record systems, clinical policies and protocol, organisational hierarchies, academic requirements, building layouts, and more. Residents also need peer and faculty support to recover from stress, answer questions, and receive feedback. Residents who relocate from far away for residency training may especially need social support. A lack of training and support is a sign that a residency programme has few resources, is disorganised, or is not invested in resident mental health.

The third organisational stressor, unclear roles and responsibilities, is a direct consequence of the second stressor (WHO, 2003). Residents work in multiple health care systems with multiple providers during their training. When residents consider their role and responsibilities as unclear, they feel a lack of control with their environment and experience distress. For example, a resident who does not know which patients are under her responsibility and which attending physician to report to will experience distress. A resident who covers hospital admissions at night but does not know the protocol will experience distress as well. Most residents will quickly learn how to work in various systems but residents who are constantly confused about their place in a system will flounder.

Most of the risk factors listed thus far are not unique to residency training; most individuals are at risk for poorer mental health with mental illness, poor work-life balance, and little social and organisational support (World Health Organisation, 2012). A risk factor that is unique to residents is the constant change in the US health care industry. Residents are beginning a medical profession at a time of massive change and regulation in US health care including pressure from government, payers, and patients. Since the passing of the Affordable Care Act in 2010, physician burnout has increased by 10% compared to the US working population, even after controlling for other factors like number of hours worked, age, sex, and relationship status (Shanafelt et al., 2015). Some medical specialties report burnout rates of well over 50%. This is a concerning trend which may influence medical students to choose medical specialties that are less stressful but sorely needed.

In a large review of nearly 400 meta-analyses, researchers identified three major risk factors as genetic (e.g., multiple gene polymorphisms, gene networks), psychological (e.g., self-esteem, emotional intelligence, learning disabilities, mental health history), and physiological and health (e.g., physiological vulnerabilities and strengths, illness and disability, obstetrical and perinatal factors) (Furber, Leach, Guy, & Segal, 2016). These findings fit with a World Health Organisation report that states, in addition to individual characteristics, mental health is influenced by social circumstances and environment across the life span (World Health Organization, 2012). The worst outcome of resident mental illness is suicide. Residents are at greater risk for suicidal ideation than the general population (Sen et al., 2010). It is not clear how many residency programs screen for depression and suicide much less talk about it as well. Mental health treatment is effective and can help those residents struggling with feelings of hopelessness and helplessness. Residency programmes can even go further by investing in preventive services to help residents manage stress and avoid a journey toward burnout and possible mental illness.

Protective factors for residents include wellness activities that benefit virtually all human beings. Residents need social and organisational support to mitigate the effects of stress and orient themselves to new health care systems. Residents also benefit from a work-life balance that includes activities of self-care like physical activity, restful sleep, and healthy eating habits. Mindfulness training can specifically help residents alleviate the effects of burnout (Krasner et al., 2009).

One of the most significant changes in 21st century graduate medical education is resident duty hour restrictions (DHR). Historically, residents would complete 30 hour shifts and then rest. In 2002 the Accreditation Council for Graduate Medical Education (ACGME) mandated that intern resident shifts be restricted to 16 hour shifts, and a maximum of 80 hours per week (Philibert, Friedmann, & Williams, 2002). In 2011, the ACGME revised the 2002 rules and added more extensive guidelines for resident supervision and patient handoffs. Since the inaugural restructuring, DHRs have remained a source of controversy and empirical inquiry. Despite the numerous publications on the subject, studies on the impact of DHRs suffer from limitations.

It is not clear if DHRs are good or bad for residents (Bolster & Rourke, 2015; Lin et al., 2016). Obviously, the field needs large, prospective studies of interventions over a long period of time to further distil trends. The current research suggests that DHRs have not delivered on their promise for significantly improving resident wellness. Some reforms like night float have the opposite intended result. This suggests that DHRs are not the main strategy for preventing poor mental health outcomes among residents. Indeed, some may intuit that residents need lighter workloads and shorter shifts when perhaps the most effective strategy is an organised programme of resident wellness and support in tandem with a demanding education experience.

The Spectre and Spectrum of Stress

Sound mental health does not equal the absence of stress. Stress is a natural phenomenon and provides the functional benefit of recognizing physical and psychological reactions to external stimuli. This operational view of stress is counterintuitive to many clinicians and to society as a whole who typically perceive stress as a 'killer' that requires elimination. It is impossible to eliminate stress and research shows that a negative perception of stress is harmful. In a large study of nearly 30,000 U.S. adults, 34% of survey respondents perceived that stress affected their health a lot or to some extent (Keller et al., 2012). This negative perception of stress increased the likelihood of worse medical and mental health outcomes. Those who reported high stress and believed stress affected their health a lot had a 43% increased risk of premature death.

There are two implications of this study on resident mental health. First, residents can benefit from a holistic perception of stress as signals that the body is energised and ready to meet a challenge. Residents who perceive stress as a sign of incompetence or failure do not understand the correct role of stress in their lives as well as the nature of residency training. Such residents may attempt to remove or diminish stress using avoidance behaviours (e.g., not collaborating with peers and attending physicians, not seeking feedback and instruction) or creating unrealistic expectations for themselves (e.g., 'I should not feel stress'). Stress is undoubtedly uncomfortable and when experienced at high levels and for long periods of time is detrimental (Schneiderman, Ironson, & Siegel, 2005). Research indicates that a stress-as-enhancing mindset moderates cortisol reactivity and induces a desire for performance feedback (Crum, Salovey, & Achor, 2013).

The second implication is that faculty can teach residents to recognise stress and respond in a healthy manner. Faculty can also set the example by effectively managing their own stress and creating a residency culture that allows safe discussions on stress and wellness. Residents are acutely observant of faculty behaviour and what is known as the 'hidden curriculum' which are unintended messages conveyed by faculty, staff, and senior residents (Billings et al., 2011). A hidden curriculum condones certain behaviours and results in creating a residency culture that may not be intended by the faculty. For example, faculty who disrespect others in front of residents passively excuse such behaviour. Faculty who have a poor work-life balance and complain about work convey unintended messages of poor stress identification and management.

Stress is not a spectre that residents and faculty should fear. Through education, residents can see stress as a vital alert system that connects them to the inherent wisdom of their bodies. This alert system developed over eons of times. From an evolutionary standpoint, the primitive ancestors of the human race who survived the jungles and savannahs of the past were the ones with an effective stress response that alerted them to dangers. Humans today carry that same alert system in relatively safe towns and cities of the modern era. In addition, the cardiovascular response to stress includes an increase in heart rate and blood vessel constriction which is similar to the physiological state of positive emotions like joy and courage. People who view their stress as helpful still experience increased heart rates but without the constriction of blood vessels which is a risk factor for cardiovascular problems. This stress-as-enhancing mindset does not always fit neatly with American ideals like rugged individualism. Through teaching and leading by example, residents can learn to see stress as an ancient ally and not a spectre.

One helpful tool for teaching residents is the spectrum of stress which includes distress, chronic stress, burnout, and mental illness (McEwen, 2003, 2004; see Figure 1). Each stage represents not only the accumulated level of stress but the response of the individual as well. The first stage, distress, is a common experience caused by a sense of real or implied threat that activates involuntary mechanisms (e.g.,

Figure 1. Spectrum of Stress

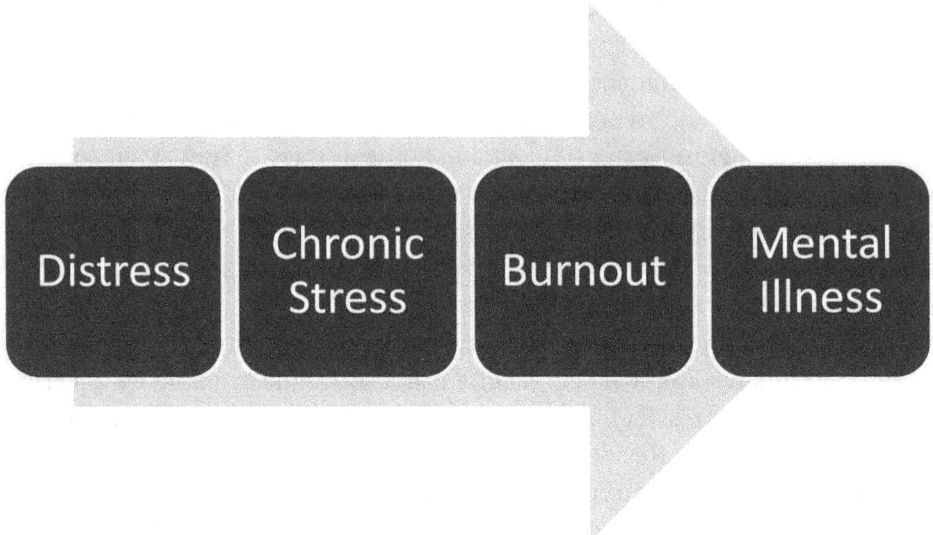

elevated heart and respiratory rates, increased alertness). The sympathetic nervous system becomes active and primes the body for attention and action by increasing the flow of oxygen to vital areas of the body like the brain.

Consider the following example: a resident is paged for a possible hospital admission and upon meeting the patient recognises several distressing personal medical symptoms. Her physiological response to the situation provides energy and focus for the task at hand. As she completes the admission, her parasympathetic system returns her body to a state of rest until the next activation. If the resident feels inadequate to address the patient's health status and does not have peer or supervisory support, then the resident's distress level will increase in both time and intensity. Even this uncomfortable situation has a functional role in that the resident's body is alerting her to the lack of knowledge and support. The resident can actively address the medical knowledge deficit or develop a strategy for collaborating more effectively with peers and supervisors. If the resident does not address the knowledge deficit or avoids collaboration, then the distress can become a prolonged experience and increase the chance of repeating in the future (Gross & Levenson, 1997).

Residents can cope with distress when it comes in short episodes followed by periods of rest. This allows for physical and psychological resources to replenish. Chronic or prolonged states of arousal and alertness can lead to fatigue, burnout, and even mental illness, especially when the individual perceives the stress as bad. The accumulation of stress over time is usually gradual and can include small stresses that combine into a generalized or continuous feeling of distress. Accumulated stress, however, is not the sole cause for chronic stress. The resident's reaction to the daily stress is just as important, if not more so, as the amount of stress (Crum, Salovey, & Achor, 2013). For example, a resident who works in a low income, urban area with a very sick patient population and with few resources may experience daily distress with little alleviation. If the resident has strong social and organisational support and begins a new rotation in a less stressful setting, then he will likely return to a state of respite. If instead he worries about his ability to care for very sick patients, begins avoiding similar patients in the future, and does not disclose his feelings to peers and supervisors, he may begin to experience chronic distress over the issue. His avoidance reaction exacerbates and extends a normal stress experience (Gross & Levenson, 1997).

Chronic stress affects all systems in the body. When the body is stressed, muscles tense to protect the body from injury and pain. Long-term musculoskeletal tension can lead to other problems like headaches and physical pain. Prolonged periods of stress can contribute to cardiovascular problems possibly due to the inflammation of coronary arteries. Cholesterol levels can rise as people develop a sedentary lifestyle and unhealthy eating habits in response to stress. When stress hormones (e.g., cortisol, epinephrine) are released, the liver produces more glucose for energy. People with diabetes are at risk for complications when extra glucose is released due to stress. Chronic stress also affects the gastrointestinal system leading to stomach pain, diarrhoea, and constipation. All of these bodily changes contribute to an overall state of exhaustion as the nervous system is constantly aroused. Residents and faculty can attend to these physical symptoms and prevent chronic stress from developing into burnout and even mental illness (Drolet & Rodgers, 2010).

Burnout is a syndrome of emotional exhaustion, loss of meaning in work, feelings of ineffectiveness, and a tendency to view people as objects rather than as human beings (Maslach, Jackson, & Leiter, 1996). Burnout affects physicians and their families, impacts patient care, and contributes to physician turnover. One study estimates that over half of all US physicians are currently experiencing burnout (Shanafelt et al., 2015).

In regard to residents, one study of 47 Dutch residents found 31% met the criteria for burnout which was significantly associated with work-family conflict, work-related autonomy (amount of control over work activities), and work-engagement (level of vigour, dedication, and absorption at work) (Ringrose, Houterman, Koops, & Oei, 2009). A study of anaesthesiology residents found 41% met burnout criteria (de Oliveira et al., 2013). Risk factors for burnout included working over 70 hours a week, consuming more than five drinks with alcohol a week, and female gender. One large study of over 1,700 residents found a 60% burnout rate, higher than medical students and early career physicians (Dyrbye et al., 2014). Residents were more likely to report high levels of depersonalisation (50%) than medical students (37%) and early career physicians (37%).

Burnout is the result of working with difficult patients or being exposed to patient suffering for extended periods of time without adequate opportunities for recuperation. Physicians can feel a sense of psychological numbness, a disconnection from others, and apathy to the suffering of others. This is similar to symptoms found in trauma-related disorders like post-traumatic stress disorder in which people survive highly stressful events and then experience a debilitation of adaptive abilities.

The most common measure for physician burnout is the Maslach Burnout Inventory (MBI; (Maslach et al., 1996). There are three domains within the MBI: emotional exhaustion, depersonalisation, and personal achievement. Emotional exhaustion includes items like 'I feel emotionally drained from my work' and 'I feel used up at the end of the workday'; depersonalisation includes items like 'I feel I have become more callous toward people'. One major limitation of the MBI is that it was normed for physicians and other US workers, not for residents who are under supervision and moving to and from various medical settings. This raises serious questions about the validity of the MBI in measuring resident burnout. Yet the vast majority of studies on resident burnout use the MBI (Dyrbye & Shanafelt, 2016). Futures studies should develop an inventory normed to the unique experience of graduate medical education.

Another limitation for any burnout inventory is that it does not focus on resilience which is the ability to adapt in the face of significant adversity, past or present. Burnout denotes pathology and deficits in positive adaptability and subtly minimises ways in which residents successfully cope with difficult tasks. Resilience is a resident's ability to struggle well during his or her training. It includes multiple individual and environmental factors that provide a protective benefit to the resident. Resilience incudes periods of accumulation and maintenance and does not necessarily mean that the resident accomplishes every single goal. Rather, resilience helps the resident to persevere even when temporarily failing. Resilience can be taught but must be practised. Resilience can help a resident to recover from burnout and avoid developing a mental health disorder.

Resident mental illness has received national attention in the past few years. In the first two months of the 2014-2015 academic year two medical interns in New York City died from two separate suicides. Soon thereafter, an intern from Yale School of Medicine wrote an op-ed in the *New York Times* about the effects of medical training on mental health (Sinha, 2014). Rates of depression can increase seven-fold for medical interns during the first three months of training while rates of suicidal ideation can increase by 370% (Sen et al., 2010). In one study of paediatric residents, 20% met criteria for depression and were six times more likely to commit medical errors (Fahrenkopf et al., 2008). It is not clear how many residents seek mental health treatment. In one study of 385 medical students, 34% who reported depression or anxiety sought mental health counselling (MacLean et al., 2016).

Whereas burnout is emotional exhaustion from working in a highly stressful environment, mental illness refers to specific diagnosable health conditions in which an individual's capacity to think, behave, and interact with others is affected. Mental illness is correlated with increased rates of morbidity and mortality (Walker, McGee, & Druss, 2015). There is no current literature on pathways between physician burnout and mental illness. Moreover, the genesis of mental health problems for any individual is multiple and varied.

Mental Health Programme for Medical Residents

The goal of a mental health programme for medical residents is to train residents in self-awareness and self-care and develop a culture of wellness and support. Programme directors and faculty play a vital role in ensuring residents are equipped for thriving during residency training. The authors offer a four-part template that residency programmes can use for tailoring their own distinctive programme (see Figure 2).

Support

The most significant mental health benefit a residency programme can offer is a culture of wellness and support which requires a concerted and intentional effort by all faculty, staff, and residents. Organisational support does not happen spontaneously. Residency leaders must diligently structure wellness activities and nurture key

Figure 2. Mental Health Wellness Program

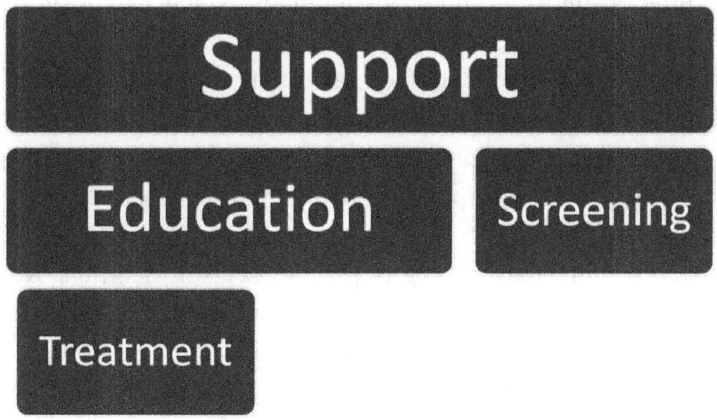

relationships between faculty and residents to generate any mental health benefits. The authors offer four ways to give organisational support.

First, nurture relationships between faculty members and residents. In a highly supportive residency culture, faculty advisors and supervisors take a genuine interest in the lives of their residents, including their experience in residency training and what happens outside of medicine. The same advisors are assigned to residents throughout their entire training and advocate for their wellbeing, including asking direct questions about mental health. Advisors and preceptors give direct, effective feedback and help residents clearly understand what they are doing well and what needs improvement. This feedback is both formative and summative and does not require a request from the resident. Continuous feedback instils confidence and trust between the faculty and the residents.

Second, identify and buffer stress points. Stress is a natural part of graduate medical education. In a highly supportive programme, faculty and staff identify time periods in which residents will experience high levels of stress (e.g., intern year, examinations, demanding rotations, life transitions) and design activities that alleviate the stress as much as possible. For example, a long period of orientation helps interns to fully understand the residency culture, their roles and responsibilities, and resources for support. Orientation helps interns to quickly develop relationships with faculty and upper-level residents. In another example, faculty use weekly didactics during examination periods to prepare residents for upcoming exams (e.g., question banks, exam topics) which supplements the residents' personal study. Finally, faculty assist residents who are experiencing a life event or transition (e.g., marriage, loss of loved one, new-born) to create a rotation schedule that fits the resident's current needs. Programmes that anticipate and acknowledge stressful time periods will more effectively manage the unanticipated events (e.g., faculty departure).

Third, include resident leadership in designing and implementing a mental health programme. Supportive programs include residents in designing activities that promote wellness (e.g., residency retreat, lunch meetings, walking groups, and movie and dinner clubs). Residents feel part of the organisation and believe that their ideas matter. Supportive programmes ask chief residents to regularly report any concerns about residents and even consider assigning upper-level residents as peer-support to incoming interns to help with housing options, orientation, schedules, and more. Faculty request ongoing feedback from residents about the residency culture using online surveys, informal focus groups, and advisor meetings. Residents have the advantage of being newcomers to a residency culture and can provide a fresh perspective on strengths, weaknesses, opportunities, and threats.

Fourth, design formal and informal wellness activities. Supportive programme design formal activities like residency retreats, lunch meetings, and didactics that are fun, engaging, and informative. The benefit of formal activities is that they can be scheduled during normal residency hours which protects the time residents have for themselves. Informal activities can include dinner groups at the home of a faculty member or resident, movie clubs, coffee meetings, and volunteer service projects. Some residents will form social groups and events on their own while other, more reserved residents will benefit from faculty-supported activities.

Volunteer service helps residents to become involved in the community, meet new people, develop empathy for vulnerable populations, and reflect on their own personal and professional values. Service has a stress-buffering effect on health, especially for residents who value the service (Poulin, 2014). Supportive programmes create opportunities outside of residency requirements for residents to serve in the community (e.g., homeless shelter, soup kitchen, school tutoring, sports events, natural disaster relief, free medical clinics, and health fairs). Faculty members lead by example in serving the community and invite residents but do not require they join them.

Education

The second most important mental health benefit a residency program can offer is to educate residents about the spectrum of stress and the importance of self-care. It is ideal that a mental health professional (e.g., psychiatrist, psychologist, or counsellor) use curricular time (e.g., grand rounds, didactic conferences, or small meetings) to discuss signs and symptoms of stress as well as the pathway from distress to burnout to mental illness. Residents learn how unmitigated stress affects themselves and their patients and different types of effective coping strategies. The instructor normalises the experience of stress and explains the functional role it plays in alerting and energizing the body and mind. The instructor also explains that stress by itself is usually not the problem; instead, the reaction to stress is what determines a successful outcome. For example, a resident who seeks collaboration and support during a difficult rotation will cope better than a resident who avoids peer and faculty interaction and who believes that they are incompetent. Residents learn to accept stress as part of their training and identify personal ways to become 'psychologically flexible' in the face of ongoing challenges.

One effective tool for teaching residents how to monitor stress levels and increase self-care is mindfulness which is the ability to focus on the present moment with purpose. One study of 70 physicians who participated in an eight-week intensive program of mindfulness training found improvements in well-being and attitudes associated with patient-centred care (Krasner, Epstein, Beckman, et al., 2009). Mindfulness allows residents to slow down, focus on their breathing and emotional state, and see themselves from a different perspective. For most of residency, a resident is either thinking about the patient she just treated or preparing herself mentally for the next one. The resident lives in the cognitive past and future of her mind on a daily basis. Mindfulness gives the resident permission to step out of the past-future dichotomy, create cognitive space for a moment, and connect with her present physical and emotional state.

Mindfulness also allows residents to develop important skills for monitoring stress. As a resident practices mindfulness on a daily basis, he becomes more in tune with physical and emotional signals of stress which empowers him to respond in healthy ways. Programmes can include mindfulness training as part of resident retreats or didactic conferences. Faculty can lead residents in mindfulness exercises at the beginning or end of a meeting or lecture. More simply, residents can incorporate deliberate moments of quiet reflection into their daily schedule (e.g., turning off the radio or phone while driving to work, spending five minutes in contemplation before leaving work at the end of the day).

Supportive programmes also teach residents how to recognise burnout and mental illness and what resources are available for support and treatment. Residents learn that burnout is a syndrome of emotional exhaustion and can lead to psychological numbness, loss of empathy, and a lack of connection with others. They learn that mental health treatment is effective and private and should not have any repercussions on job security, medical licensure, malpractice insurance, and disability coverage. Residents also learn how to access local-based treatment options and hotline-based mental health resources.

Screening

Mental health and physician wellness screening helps identify those residents at risk for mental health problems. Supportive programmes include a psychiatric and substance use history during required annual occupational health history and physical examinations. Programmes also use validated scales (e.g., Patient Health Questionnaire-9, Alcohol Use Disorders Identification Test, and Drug Abuse Screening Test) within the first three months of residency training, a vulnerable time period for new residents (Sen, Kranzler, Krystal, et al, 2010). Programmes assure residents that screening is confidential, not part of a formal evaluation process, and reviewed by a mental health professional who only discusses results with the resident and the programme director. Programmes encourage wide-spread participation by allowing residents time to complete the screening, using web-based programmes which deliver efficient data collection and analysis. Residents receive feedback about the screening from the web-based programme or a mental health professional who follows up in person. The resident understands the results of the screening and, if appropriate, receives a referral for treatment.

Treatment

The final part of the mental health programme is to make mental health treatment access on par with other medical conditions which includes providing a list of trusted professionals in the community who understand graduate medical education and are connected with residency faculty and staff. Residents also have access to confidential settings where they can discuss the challenges and successes of their training in a group or individual format. Some residents prefer a group format which fosters social connection and support. Groups are led by an experienced mental health professional and offered on a regular basis. Supportive programmes develop protocol for team debriefing when a seminal event occurs (e.g., resident leaves programme, patient's death, medical code situation, or a serious medical error). Team debriefing protects time for a resident to express his concerns and feelings, process his experience aloud while peers listen, and receive support and advice. They occur soon after the event and include an experienced faculty member who provides perspective and wisdom.

SOLUTIONS AND RECOMMENDATIONS

Residency programme directors need strategies for identifying and addressing mental health problems. Most residents will not experience depression or suicidal ideation during residency training. However, many will experience chronic stress which affects interprofessional relationships, patient care, and overall quality of life. The authors recommend that programmes adapt a comprehensive strategy that addresses at least these four domains: education, screening, treatment, and support. First, residents can learn the continuum of distress, from burnout to depression to suicide, ways to self-identity, and strategies for increasing resiliency and wellness. Second, programmes can require annual occupational health history and physical examination to screen for potential distress and depression. Staff should provide timely feedback on screening results including treatment options. Third, residents should have access to mental health treatment including counselling and psychiatric care. Faculty can also address any concerns about the potential repercussions of receiving mental health care on job security, state licensure, malpractice insurance, and disability coverage. Finally, residents can attend group support meeting especially during the first year to discuss the challenges of their experience in a confidential setting. Residents can also meet for team debriefings following the conclusion of a seminal event like a patient's death, a code situation, or a serious medical error.

CONCLUSION

Residency training is a time to prepare young physicians for a rewarding and fruitful career. Although residents will undoubtedly experience stress and be at-risk for mental health problems, programme directors and faculty can create an environment that mitigates the expected strain and pressure of training. The authors recommend that residency mental health programs include support, education, screening, and treatment as four pillars of prevention. If faculty do not have a programme in place, it is suggested that they partner with mental health professionals in the area who can consult with them in building a robust and systematic approach to strengthening residency resiliency and preventing physician burnout.

Residents will experience stress during residency training. Although it is unclear which interventions are best for supporting resident mental health, residency programmes can go a long way in preventing normal stress from turning into psychopathology.

REFERENCES

Abuhusain, H., Chotirmall, S. H., Hamid, N., & O'Neill, S. J. (2009). Prepared for internship?. *Irish Medical Journal*, *102*(3), 82–84. PMID:19489196

Accreditation Council for Graduate Medical Education (ACGME). (n.d.). *Resident Survey – Duty Hours FAQ*. Chicago: USA. Retrieved on January 19, 2017 from https://www.acgme.org/Portals/0/dhfaqsresidents.pdf

Beckman, T. J., Reed, D. A., Shanafelt, T. D., & West, C. P. (2012). Resident physician well-being and assessments of their knowledge and clinical performance. *Journal of General Internal Medicine*, *27*(3), 325–330. doi:10.1007/s11606-011-1891-6 PMID:21948207

Billings, M. E., Lazarus, M. E., Wenrich, M., Curtis, J. R., & Engelberg, R. A. (2011). The effect of the hidden curriculum on resident burnout and cynicism. *Journal of Graduate Medical Education*, *3*(4), 503–510. doi:10.4300/JGME-D-11-00044.1 PMID:23205199

Bolster, L., & Rourke, L. (2015). The effect of restricting residents duty hours on patient safety, resident well-being, and resident education: An updated systematic review. *Journal of Graduate Medical Education*, *7*(3), 349–363. doi:10.4300/JGME-D-14-00612.1 PMID:26457139

Coates, W. C., Spector, T. S., & Uijtdehaage, S. (2012). Transition to life-A sendoff to the real world for graduating medical students. *Teaching and Learning in Medicine*, *24*(1), 36–41. doi:10.1080/10401334.2012.641485 PMID:22250934

Crum, A. J., Salovey, P., & Achor, S. (2013). Rethinking stress: The role of mindsets in determining the stress response. *Journal of Personality and Social Psychology*, *104*(4), 716–733. doi:10.1037/a0031201 PMID:23437923

Davies-Black, Mata, D. A., Ramos, M. A., Kim, M. M., Guille, C., & Sen, S. (2016). In their own words: An analysis of the experiences of medical interns participating in a prospective cohort study of depression. *Academic Medicine*, *91*(9), 1244–1250. doi:10.1097/ACM.0000000000001227

de Oliveira, G. S. Jr, Chang, R., Fitzgerald, P. C., Almeida, M. D., Castro-Alves, L. S., Ahmad, S., & McCarthy, R. J. (2013). The prevalence of burnout and depression and their association with adherence to safety and practice standards: A survey of united states anesthesiology trainees. *Anesthesia and Analgesia*, *117*(1), 182–193. doi:10.1213/ANE.0b013e3182917da9 PMID:23687232

Drolet, B. C., & Rodgers, S. (2010). A comprehensive medical student wellness programdesign and implementation at Vanderbilt school of medicine. Academic Medicine. *Journal. Association of American Medical Colleges*, *85*(1), 103–110. doi:10.1097/ACM.0b013e3181c46963

Dyrbye, L., & Shanafelt, T. (2016). A narrative review on burnout experienced by medical students and residents. *Medical Education*, *50*(1), 132–149. doi:10.1111/medu.12927 PMID:26695473

Dyrbye, L. N., Thomas, M. R., Massie, F. S., Power, D. V., Eacker, A., Harper, W., & Shanafelt, T. D. et al. (2008). Burnout and suicidal ideation among U.S. medical students. *Annals of Internal Medicine*, *149*(5), 334–341. doi:10.7326/0003-4819-149-5-200809020-00008 PMID:18765703

Dyrbye, L. N., West, C. P., Satele, D., Boone, S., Tan, L., Sloan, J., & Shanafelt, T. D. (2014). Burnout among U.S. medical students, residents, and early career physicians relative to the general U.S. population. Academic Medicine. *Journal. Association of American Medical Colleges*, *89*(3), 443–451. doi:10.1097/ACM.0000000000000134

Fahrenkopf, A. M., Sectish, T. C., Barger, L. K., Sharek, P. J., Lewin, D., Chiang, V. W., & Landrigan, C. P. et al. (2008). Rates of medication errors among depressed and burnt out residents: Prospective cohort study. *BMJ (Clinical Research Ed.)*, *336*(7642), 488–491. doi:10.1136/bmj.39469.763218.BE PMID:18258931

Furber, G., Leach, M., Guy, S., & Segal, L. (2016). Developing a broad categorisation scheme to describe risk factors for mental illness, for use in prevention policy and planning. *The Australian and New Zealand Journal of Psychiatry*. doi:0004867416642844

Goldman, M. L., Shah, R. N., & Bernstein, C. A. (2015). Depression and suicide among physician trainees: Recommendations for a national response. *JAMA Psychiatry*, *72*(5), 411–412. doi:10.1001/jamapsychiatry.2014.3050 PMID:25738529

Govardhan, L. M., Pinelli, V., & Schnatz, P. F. (2012). Burnout, depression and job satisfaction in obstetrics and gynecology residents. *Connecticut Medicine*, *76*(7), 389. PMID:23248861

Gross, J., & Levenson, R. (1997). Hiding feelings: The acute effects of inhibiting negative and positive emotion. *Journal of Abnormal Psychology*, *106*(1), 95–103. doi:10.1037/0021-843X.106.1.95 PMID:9103721

Kapinos, K. A., Fitzgerald, P., Greer, N., & Rutks, I. (2012). *The effect of working conditions on patient care: A systematic review*. Academic Press.

Keller, A., Litzelman, K., Wisk, L. E., Maddox, T., Cheng, E. R., Creswell, P. D., & Witt, W. P. (2012). Does the perception that stress affects health matter? the association with health and mortality. *Health Psychology*, *31*(5), 677–684. doi:10.1037/a0026743 PMID:22201278

Kötter, T., Tautphäus, Y., Obst, K. U., Voltmer, E., & Scherer, M. (2016). Health-promoting factors in the freshman year of medical school: A longitudinal study. *Medical Education*, *50*(6), 646–656. doi:10.1111/medu.12987 PMID:27170083

Krasner, M. S., Epstein, R. M., Beckman, H., Suchman, A. L., Chapman, B., Mooney, C. J., & Quill, T. E. (2009). Association of an educational program in mindful communication with burnout, empathy, and attitudes among primary care physicians. *Journal of the American Medical Association*, *302*(12), 1284–1293. doi:10.1001/jama.2009.1384 PMID:19773563

Lin, H., Lin, E., Auditore, S., & Fanning, J. (2016). A narrative review of high-quality literature on the effects of resident duty hours reforms. Academic Medicine. *Journal. Association of American Medical Colleges*, *91*(1), 140–150. doi:10.1097/ACM.0000000000000937

Lygo-Baker, S., Kokotailo, P., & Young, K. (2015). Developing confidence in uncertainty: Conflicting roles of trainees as they become educators in veterinary and human medicine. *Journal of Veterinary Medical Education*, *42*(4), 364–372. doi:10.3138/jvme.1114-107R PMID:26315215

Lyss-Lerman, P., Teherani, A., Aagaard, E., Loeser, H., Cooke, M., & Harper, G. M. (2009). What training is needed in the fourth year of medical school? views of residency programme directors. Academic Medicine. *Journal. Association of American Medical Colleges*, *84*(7), 823–829. doi:10.1097/ACM.0b013e3181a82426

MacLean, L., Booza, J., & Balon, R. (2016). The impact of medical school on student mental health. *Academic Psychiatry*, *40*(1), 89–91. doi:10.1007/s40596-015-0301-5 PMID:25749920

Maslach, C., Jackson, S. E., & Leiter, M. P. (1996). Maslach burnout inventory manual. Mountain View, CA: CPP. Inc.

McEwen, B. S. (2003). Mood disorders and allostatic load. *Biological Psychiatry*, *54*(3), 200–207. doi:10.1016/S0006-3223(03)00177-X PMID:12893096

McEwen, B. S. (2004). Protection and damage from acute and chronic stress: Allostasis and allostatic overload and relevance to the pathophysiology of psychiatric disorders. *Annals of the New York Academy of Sciences*, *1032*(1), 1–7. doi:10.1196/annals.1314.001 PMID:15677391

Philibert, I., Friedmann, P., & Williams, W. T. (2002). New requirements for resident duty hours. *Journal of the American Medical Association*, *288*(9), 1112–1114. doi:10.1001/jama.288.9.1112 PMID:12204081

Poulin, M. (2014). Volunteering predicts health among those who value others: Two national studies. *Health Psychology*, *33*(2), 120–129. doi:10.1037/a0031620 PMID:23566179

Ringrose, R., Houterman, S., Koops, W., & Oei, G. (2009). Burnout in medical residents: A questionnaire and interview study. *Psychology Health and Medicine*, *14*(4), 476–486. doi:10.1080/13548500903012822 PMID:19697257

Schneiderman, N., Ironson, G., & Siegel, S. D. (2005). Stress and health: Psychological, behavioral, and biological determinants. *Annual Review of Clinical Psychology*, *1*(1), 607–628. doi:10.1146/annurev.clinpsy.1.102803.144141 PMID:17716101

Sen, S., Kranzler, H. R., Krystal, J. H., Speller, H., Chan, G., Gelernter, J., & Guille, C. (2010). A prospective cohort study investigating factors associated with depression during medical internship. *Archives of General Psychiatry*, *67*(6), 557–565. doi:10.1001/archgenpsychiatry.2010.41 PMID:20368500

Shanafelt, T., Hasan, O., Dyrbye, L., Sinsky, C., Satele, D., Sloan, J., & West, C. (2015). Changes in burnout and satisfaction with work-life balance in physicians and the general US working population between 2011 and 2014. *Mayo Clinic Proceedings*, *90*(12), 1600–1613. doi:10.1016/j.mayocp.2015.08.023 PMID:26653297

Shanafelt, T. D., Boone, S., Tan, L., Dyrbye, L. N., Sotile, W., Satele, D., & Oreskovich, M. R. et al. (2012). Burnout and satisfaction with work-life balance among US physicians relative to the general US population. *Archives of Internal Medicine*, *172*(18), 1377–1385. doi:10.1001/archinternmed.2012.3199 PMID:22911330

Shanafelt, T. D., Bradley, K. A., Wipf, J. E., & Back, A. L. (2002). Burnout and self-reported patient care in an internal medicine residency program. *Annals of Internal Medicine*, *136*(5), 358–367. doi:10.7326/0003-4819-136-5-200203050-00008 PMID:11874308

Sinha, P. (2014, September 4). Why do doctors commit suicide?. *New York Times*. Retrieved on January 18, 2017 from https://nyti.ms/Wi4ns9

Slavin, S. J., & Chibnall, J. T. (2016). Finding the why, changing the how: Improving the mental health of medical students, residents, and physicians. Academic Medicine. *Journal. Association of American Medical Colleges*, *91*(9), 1194–1196. doi:10.1097/ACM.0000000000001226

Thoits, P. A. (2010). Stress and health: Major findings and policy implications. *Journal of Health and Social Behavior*, *51*(1), S41–S53. doi:10.1177/0022146510383499 PMID:20943582

Walker, E. R., McGee, R. E., & Druss, B. G. (2015). Mortality in mental disorders and global disease burden implications: A systematic review and meta-analysis. *JAMA Psychiatry*, *72*(4), 334–341. doi:10.1001/jamapsychiatry.2014.2502 PMID:25671328

West, C. P., Huschka, M. M., Novotny, P. J., Sloan, J. A., Kolars, J. C., Habermann, T. M., & Shanafelt, T. D. (2006). Association of perceived medical errors with resident distress and empathy: A prospective longitudinal study. *Journal of the American Medical Association*, *296*(9), 1071–1078. doi:10.1001/jama.296.9.1071 PMID:16954486

West, C. P., Tan, A. D., Habermann, T. M., Sloan, J. A., & Shanafelt, T. D. (2009). Association of resident fatigue and distress with perceived medical errors. *Journal of the American Medical Association*, *302*(12), 1294–1300. doi:10.1001/jama.2009.1389 PMID:19773564

World Health Organisation. (2003). *Work organization and stress*. Retrieved on January 19, 2017 from http://www.who.int/occupational_health/publications/en/oehstress.pdf

World Health Organisation. (2012). *Risks to mental health: An overview of vulnerabilities and risk factors*. Retrieved on January 19, 2017 from http://www.who.int/mental_health/mhgap/risks_to_mental_health_EN_27_08_12.pdf

KEY TERMS AND DEFINITIONS

Burnout: A syndrome of emotional exhaustion, loss of meaning in work, feelings of ineffectiveness, and a tendency to view people as objects rather than as human beings.

Chronic Stress: Prolonged states of arousal and alertness in response to stress.

Distress: A sense of real or implied threat that activates involuntary mechanisms.

Graduate Medical Education: Any type of formal medical education pursued after completion of medical school.

Intern: First-year medical resident.

Medical Resident: A physician in graduate medical education who practices medicine under the supervision of an attending physician.

Mental Health: A person's condition with regard to their psychological and emotional well-being.

Mental Illness: A wide range of mental health conditions that adversely affect moods, cognitions, and behaviours.

Section 4
Solutions

Chapter 7
Resident Physician and Medical Academic Faculty Burnout:
A Review of Current Literature

Emma A. Omoruyi
University of Texas Health Science Center at Houston, USA

Fehintola Omidele
Johns Hopkins Bloomberg School of Public Health, USA

ABSTRACT

Physician burnout finds its roots in both undergraduate and graduate medical education and has emerged as an important cause of academic faculty turnover. Recognition of the need for resiliency training has led to the development and implementation of wellness programmes throughout the country and world. This chapter examines the causes and potential solutions of combating resident physician and academic faculty burnout in medical education. The authors reviewed current literature on wellness programmes in medical education, including both traditional and curricular approaches and provide a template for creating a well-rounded wellness programme to promote resident physician and academic faculty wellness.

INTRODUCTION

With the pressure of caring for patients, one can understand the importance of physicians maintaining good health, physically and emotionally. However, physician burnout is alarmingly prevalent in the current day with anywhere from 25%-70% experiencing the 'emotional exhaustion, depersonalisation and decreased feelings of

DOI: 10.4018/978-1-5225-2811-1.ch007

personal accomplishment' (Eckleberry-Hunt, Van Dyke, Lick, & Tucciarone, 2009). At one time, burnout has been present in 'one-third to one-half of US medical students and academic faculty' and also been observed with the same prevalence throughout the world in countries such as Japan, New Zealand and Canada (Benbassat, Baumal, Chan, & Nirel, 2011). When dissected, it is clear that physician burnout finds its roots in both undergraduate and graduate medical education.

BACKGROUND

When examining undergraduate medical education, two unique classifications of burnout predispositions have been studied: exogenous stressors and endogenous stressors. Exogenous or environmental stressors include 'adjustment to medical school, student abuse, witnessing and unwillingly participating in unethical behaviour towards patients and exposure to death and suffering' (Benbassat et al., 2011). Of note, the endogenous stressors were often related to qualities identified in one's personality such as neuroticism and contentiousness.

People who chose the field of medicine are often concrete thinkers and interested scientists, looking for evidence to evaluate the strength of a concept. Incoming students are often not prepared for the uncertainty that lies within medicine, so students struggle with an 'intolerance of uncertainty' also known as a 'perception of ambiguous situations as a threat' often comes as an endogenous stressor. Three different types of uncertainty have been described in literature (Benbassat et al., 2011). The first and most common is an uncertainty of one's personal adequacy; students were concerned that they would not learn all they needed to know to be a successful physician. This uncertainty can also be manifested in the competitiveness associated with undergraduate medical education, though newly addressed with curricular changes (Benbassat et al., 2011; Slavin, Schindler, & Chibnall, 2014). The other two uncertainties concerned the limitation of available medical knowledge and lastly, the uncertainty resulting from being unable to distinguish between the other two uncertainties (i.e. uncertainty of personal adequacy and limitation of one's medical knowledge) (Benbassat et al., 2011).

Naturally, when examining graduate medical education (residency), life satisfaction was the lowest and prevalence of mental health problems was the highest within the first year. In fact, 76% of new doctors reported high levels of burnout. Yet again, with a global impact, it was observed that 30% had anxiety symptoms and 15% had depressive symptoms in Switzerland. In Canada, 14% reported they would change specialty and 22% would not pursue medicine if given the opportunity to relive their career (Benbassat et al., 2011). Interestingly, physicians who attended medical school outside of the United States reported lower emotional exhaustion and depersonalisation (essentially, burnout) than United States medical graduates (Eckleberry-Hunt et al., 2009). The reason for this difference is that the general work culture in the United States is thought to be more stressful than other parts of the world due to a variety factors and when it comes to medical training, work hours are more restricted in other countries compared to the United States (Gander, Briar, Gardner, Purnell, & Woodward, 2014). Regardless, given that thousands of new doctors graduate each year, the magnitude of those statistics is astounding. Due to significant variation in schedules as well as the health of patients, certain specialties such as intensive care, emergency medicine and oncology result in lower life satisfaction (Benbassat et al., 2011). Unmet expectations provide a new stressor to new doctors once formal medical education is completed and they are finally practicing. Sometimes, being inexperienced, some new physicians are discovering that the practise of medicine may not reflect what was expected upon applying and entering medical school. To dig deeper in unmet expectations, these doctors also face discrepancies between what is learned in school and what is experienced in practise. These discrepancies revisit and even confirm the stressors of personal inadequacy as mentioned in undergraduate medical education stressors. Overall, personality issues, such as pessimism, perfectionism and lack of coping skills for stress, persist as one common theme in the development of burnout (Eckleberry-Hunt et al., 2009).

Medical students and doctors have higher rates of substance abuse, anxiety, depression and suicide, which are all effects of burnout (Eckleberry-Hunt et al., 2009). With such high rates of burnout and its sequelae, medical education administration is currently paying more attention to wellness programmes, especially considering that physician burnout leads to lower quality patient care (Eckleberry-Hunt et al., 2009). In that sense, physician burnout could very well be considered a public health problem with huge implications for our society's health. Because of those implications, it is now imperative that administration and medical students are educated in the variety of ways to which wellness can be incorporated into medical education and the culture of the institution.

The aim of this chapter is to educate the administration of undergraduate and graduate medical education about the necessity of creating and promoting a wellness culture amongst the health professionals-from medical student to faculty responsible for training future doctors. The chapter includes a review of current data on wellness programmes and pull from these programmes tenets of strong components needed to develop wellness programmes. The review of the literature contains both traditional and curricular approaches, in order to provide a guideline and template for a well-rounded wellness programme. The availability of a template would give widespread access to administration, allowing them to implement programmes in their institutions with ease. With implementation of wellness programmes throughout the country and world, medical education, the health profession and doctors can further ensure the health of communities by ensuring the health of the physicians in those communities.

MAIN FOCUS OF THE CHAPTER

Wellness Programming Across All Levels of Medical Education

Undergraduate Medical Education Wellness Programs

In 1991, the Kirksville College of Osteopathic Medicine launched its pioneering wellness programme, responding to a need that only 20% of current allopathic and osteopathic medical schools had addressed (Gaber & Martin, 2002). The medical school adopted 'I am my own first patient' as the theme of their programme, a very timely and accurate call to action that still applies to all physicians today. The programme is a voluntary initiative that promotes wellness in multiple areas such as physical, environmental, emotional, intellectual, social, spiritual and professional. As of 2002, there were several benefits associated with participation in the programme, including extra points towards the final grade in a course, free aerobic classes, pre-participation physical examination and 6-month fitness assessment. The latter two still exist today. The programme also boasted benefits for mature and older students; second year students could gain clinical experience by performing pre-participation assessments and also learn how to write a 'fitness prescription' and wellness programmes for incoming first year students. The Still Well programme, an earlier model of best practises, still exists today with large participation of the students each year, as previewed from the growth of 41 of the 290 students in 1991 to the 268 of the 290 students that participated in 1998. A strong connection between changing the grading system and lower student anxiety was noted specifically, on the topic of the extra points towards the final grade in the osteopathic theory and methods courses. Comprehensive seminars were provided to the students ensuring participation would yield higher overall scores (Gaber & Martin, 2002). Considering a large amount of stress in medical education comes from academics itself, an investment in wellness as a means to improve grades in any one course is a sound idea. For example, seminar series topics included: diversity in medicine, interpersonal relationship building, test-taking anxiety, high performance nutrition and resume writing. One unique aspect of the Still Well programme was the emphasis on physical health and the access to resources to aid and assess the students' physical health. The pre-participation physical examination was administered within one month of arrival to the school; physical fitness was then re-evaluated at 6 and 12 months. The physical examination was rather comprehensive and included the traditional components of the actual physical examination with vitals, height/weight screening, vision examination and measurement of blood lipid levels. However, the examination had unique components including screening for cardiovascular risk (through waist-to-hip ratio) and cancer as well as resting electrocardiograms and pulmonary function tests. The Still Well programme offers a comprehensive approach to wellness, based on the very simple principle of a 'first patient', yet, targeting burnout in students from physical health to emotional health and everything in between.

Traditional wellness programmes often rely on the individual to seek out improved access to counselling resources and encourage a wellness-focused lifestyle (Slavin et al., 2014). One unique and recent approach, launched at Saint Louis University School of Medicine in 2009, focused on addressing the curriculum in order to 'balance out the negative aspects of medical education' and ensure healthier individuals (Slavin et al., 2014). The first change instituted was the change of the grading system from a 4 -level grading system to pass/fail, a change to which many medical schools are now adhering. The proposed change aimed to decrease competition for grades and reduce overall stress. In addition, it gave students the liberty to focus on topics that they personally found important as opposed to focusing on learning high volume of material at once. Secondly, there was a reduction in course work to allow for participation in other aspects of the wellness programme including learning communities and longitudinal electives. The electives were expanded so that students had access to them during majority of the first and second years of medical school. The electives gave students more time to explore interests, including service and research, as well as. foster relationships with faculty.

Mentorship and generally relationships with faculty who also advocate for wellness has been shown to be an effective method in maintaining wellness in students (Eckleberry-Hunt et al., 2009). Another aspect of the Saint Louis University wellness programme included five specialised learning communities as mentioned-service and advocacy, research, global health, wellness and medical education-which would give interested students and faculty an avenue to share common interests with one another (Slavin et al., 2014). The communities were aimed at tailoring new electives, developing innovative lectures, identifying faculty mentors and expanding service and research. To enhance the breadth of the curriculum, the administration added a resilience and mediation programme to one of the courses which provided sessions on habits from mindfulness cultivation to character strengths to aid students individually. The Human Anatomy course, the most stressful of the first year, was moved to later part in the year, as opposed to the beginning of the year when students already face high levels of stress adjusting to the rigor. The examinations schedules were altered essentially to set students up for higher scores. Lastly, year-long social events were implemented for medical students; this programmatic change is common across medical education and proves to be highly beneficial for the students and residents. The programme yielded significant decreases in depression and anxiety of students progressively through the years starting from the year of implementation. Another added benefit was the increase in the mean scores of the major licensing examination taken in the preclinical years. Saint Louis University's programme proved that a successful wellness programme must integrate all aspects of medical education, from curriculum to social atmosphere, in order to change the culture of the institution. Overall, this curricular approach, though novel, proves to be promising for medical education in years to come.

Graduate Medical Education Wellness Programmes

As described above, prevention interventions like stress management workshops, mindfulness meditation, and wellness curriculums have had documented positive impact on medical education. However, treatment options are important for those who develop significant levels of depression or suicide risk. In one institution, residents and faculty who participated in an anonymous screening of their mental health were more likely to accept a referral to community based counselling after receiving personalised communication (Moutier et al., 2012). The high rates of burnout among resident physicians suggest a significant number would benefit from therapeutic counselling. The United States Accreditation Council for Graduate Medical Education requires that all residency programmes provide psychological services for residents. Barriers to accessing these services include concerns about confidentiality, accessibility, and potential reporting to licensure boards (Givens & Tjia, 2002; Guille, Speller, Laff, Epperson, & Sen, 2010). While higher education is associated with more positive attitudes to counselling (Vessey & Howard, 1993), depressed individuals are often concerned about the risks of treatment (Kushner & Sher, 1989).

Improving the understanding of motivators and barriers to seeking therapeutic help by residents is important in the development of wellness programmes and outreach efforts. Research documents the fact that female physicians are less likely to seek counselling (Dunn, Moutier, Hammond, Lehrmann, & Roberts, 2008), (Moutier et al., 2009) which is concerning given female medical students and residents are at greatest risk to report significant stress compared to their male counterparts. There is limited evidence supporting whether ethnic or racial differences exist within the pool of physicians that seek counselling. Evidence suggests that residents are more comfortable seeking an academic medical centres counselling services rather than an employee assistance programme (Pitt, Rosenthal, Gay, & Lewton, 2004) and typically rate these services as satisfactory (Dabrow, Russell, Ackley, Anderson, &

Fabri, 2006). Lowering the barriers to accessing these services would be an important step by any medical training programme.

In a single institutional study, residents and fellows were surveyed to determine differences in perceived barriers and receptiveness to accessing on-site wellness programmes (Ey, Moffit, Kinzie, Choi, & Girard, 2013). The researchers hoped to determine if residents were willing to seek counselling on-site and identify potential barriers. A plan to stratify by demographic information to help identify targeted interventions was a part of the study. The Resident Wellness Programme at Oregon Health Science Centre implemented the access of what was the equivalent of a full-time psychologist or psychiatrist experienced in working with medical professionals available 5 days a week to its residents (Ey, Moffit, Kinzie, Choi, & Girard, 2013). The services were free, unlimited, not documented on the hospitals' electronic medical record, and health insurance information was not obtained. Moreover, resident physicians were told that the 'wellness counselling' was not reportable to medical licensing boards. The Oregon Health Science Centre found that most residents knew how to access the resident wellness programme (88%) and only 13% were 'not at all likely' to access the programme.

Time was the biggest barrier for most resident physicians and female physicians were the most concerned about taking time off to access the programme. These findings demonstrate that even when the barriers of cost and knowledge of available counselling services was removed, a culture may exist among residents that limits the ability to take a break off to address personal health needs. Addressing critically troubled resident physicians that may be concerned about the consequences of seeking treatment is of the utmost importance. The same institution, Oregon Health Science Centre, expanded on the results of an earlier study which found that 90% of the residents cited the inability to get off work during business hours as the major barrier to seeking care (Cedfeldt et al., 2015). In July 2010, the institutions' Division of Graduate Medical Education implemented a time off policy that required residency training programmes to provide four half-days off per academic year for health care and wellness. The programme directors were made aware of the policy and the programmes were strongly discouraged from tracking the residents' reasons for use of the policy. The intent of the programme was that directors would assign time off for all residents, this planning was included in a pre-scheduling of each resident's time off allotment.

Upon review of the outcomes of the strategy, it was reported that two years after the policy was instituted almost 90 percent of residents knew about the policy but only 49 percent of resident physicians had actually used it. The majority (73%) of those who took a half-day reportedly used it for preventive health services (Cedfeldt et al., 2015). The most common concern by residents was that their absence during wellness day would impact their peers' schedule (Cedfeldt et al., 2015). Pre-scheduling these days off may have decreased the impact of these barriers and also ensuring that the scheduled days off were provided on rotations where patient care transfers are not necessary.

The impact of residents not seeking wellness days even when assigned means that residents may seek other forms of self-help, some of which are not beneficial. Older literature has looked at patterns of substance use over multiple specialties and found that daily alcohol use was reported in 5% of respondents (Hughes, Conard, Baldwin, Storr, & Sheehan, 1991). Conventionally, anaesthesiology residents are thought to be at highest risk due to proximity and access to potential drugs of abuse (Lutsky, Abram, Jacobson, Hopwood, & Kampine, 1991). Emergency resident physicians are also thought to be at high risk due to shift work patterns of high stress followed by long periods of rest (Hughes et al., 1991). A 2008 large scale study of emergency medicine resident physician substance use and impairment, the researchers found an increasing number of residents reporting substance use as 'self-treatment' or to 'relieve stress' as compared to a similar study done in the early 1990s (McBeth et al., 2008). Paralleling this finding was the significant increases in marijuana use and 73.6% of the marijuana users report using it in order to 'relieve stress'. A large number of residents indicated that the consumption of alcohol increased during residency. One of the more concerning findings of this study was the quantity of residents who initiated substance use during residency, especially those using prescription drugs in a nontherapeutic way; this is another interesting finding that came out of this study and is one that it should make educators rethink the way stress and substance abuse is managed during residency. It also serves as important reminder that simply providing more 'time off' does not equate to 'less stress'. However, time off, especially scheduled time off is an important factor in the successful identification and treatment of an impaired resident.

Time off alone does not create a more resilient resident. Stress management or resilience training may be an important step to mitigate some of the factors that lead to resident burnout. During the period from 2012-2013, Duke University Family Medicine, Psychiatry and Anaesthesiology residents participated in two or three 1 hour sessions of mindfulness-based resilience activities (Goldhagen, Kingsolver, Stinnett, & Rosdahl, 2015). The group sessions were developed by a clinical psychologist and held during protected resident time. The learners were taught about the concept of mindfulness-awareness, meditation, value exploration, and cultivation of positivity. Resident physicians were asked to complete an anonymous survey prior, afterwards, and during a 1-month follow-up of the meditation based training. The survey contained questions that came from the Depression Anxiety Stress Scale, Oldenburg Burnout Inventory, and the Mindful Attention Scale. Results of the survey showed that residents, at baseline, had normal levels of stress, with females having significantly higher levels than males (Goldhagen et al., 2015). Residents had a very good awareness of when they were stressed and a majority of residents had findings suggestive of a high level of burnout based on the Oldenburg Burnout Inventory. In the short term, the mindfulness intervention, did not affect these stress level but, a trend was observed on later, when residents scored positively time points of lower burnout and stress scores. These results suggest that the residents may have used the new knowledge to ease future stress and become more resilient. Resilience training is not a new concept.

Other research groups have studied stress reduction training during residency. One group looked at the outcomes of medicine and paediatric residents who received resilience training as compared to a group of residents that did not receive such training. The researchers found that the group that was trained had noted improvements in emotional exhaustion and depersonalisation scores (McCue & Sachs, 1991). Another research group found a positive effect on emotional exhaustion when residents were taught a meditation practise which combined breathing and repetition for reducing stress (Ospina-Kammerer & Figley, 2003).

Along the lines of graduate medical education, Troy Family Residency programme started a structured and more 'traditional' wellness programme in 2003 (Eckleberry-Hunt et al., 2009). This programme provided tangible evidence-based results that medical education and administrators can use to develop solid wellness programmes. These points provide a framework useful towards the development of a comprehensive wellness programme template that can be implemented throughout the world. Most importantly, choosing a definition of wellness from which a medical or residency programme would function is critical in the design process. While many examples or definitions of wellness exists, the Troy example considered 'wellness' to be more than a lack of impairment. Instead it was 'a dynamic and ongoing process involving self-awareness and healthy choices resulting in a successful, balanced lifestyle' (Eckleberry-Hunt et al., 2009). Along the pathway of creating a wellness programme, a critical first step was to select a faculty wellness champion per incoming class of residents. To share the responsibility of leading the programme, it would be ideal to have multiple champions especially for larger programmes or larger classes of medical schools. The responsibility of the wellness champion is to 'ensure that wellness is incorporated into the daily operations of the residency programme' (Eckleberry-Hunt et al., 2009). The use of technology may be useful in sending out articles and reminding students/residents and faculty about wellness meetings. Another important component of the programme, which should be key in an ideal wellness programme, is the administration of a 'burnout tool' twice a year. This approach was also used in the Saint Louis School of Medicine programme as students were surveyed twice a year (once in the beginning, once at the end of the year) to determine their anxiety and depression levels in relation to the interventions put in place' (Slavin et al., 2014). The burnout tool used at the Troy programme and across many wellness programmes is the Maslach Burnout Inventory (Eckleberry-Hunt et al., 2009). The inventory measures the definition of burnout, as mentioned above, on a qualitative scale of low to high. Further study and expansion of this inventory could become a reliable measure of burnout and effectiveness of interventions.

Other interventions of note include providing lectures on wellness and burnout as well as writing a mission statement for the wellness programme. Across the undergraduate and graduate levels of medical education, it would be beneficial to provide 'difficult patient' panels twice a year to discuss how to manage difficult situations and interactions as a group. To ensure accountability, 'wellness partners' can be assigned between faculty and students or residents, in order to establish wellness goals: emotional, physical, spiritual and social goals. Lastly, like many programmes, bringing the classes together socially, especially to celebrate accomplishments, always proves to foster healthier and happier students and residents.

The Stanford University Department of Surgery's Balance in Life programme was a response to the loss of one recent graduate to suicide in 2010. The goals of the programme were clearly defined as 'help residents cope with daily stress, provide tools to manage challenges after completing residency and reduce the risk of burnout, depression and suicide' (Salles, Liebert, & Greco, 2015). For professional well-being, the programme created a resident mentorship programme where junior residents are allowed to choose their senior resident mentors; the pairs are then funded via the administration's budget to have quarterly lunch meetings. The idea of this mentorship, a continuous and effective theme amongst thriving wellness programmes is that it provides an informal setting where both parties can talk about personal stressors as well as it gives junior residents someone 'older' who can provide guidance. Another aspect of fostering professional well-being was actually building in physical activities in the schedule to encourage leadership and team building, the ropes course or a maze are examples of activities in this area.

Upholding physical well-being during residency, one example, to bolster healthier eating options for residents, especially on nights and weekends is to offer healthy options. To address this issue, an example of what one programme did was to provide a refrigerator that would be properly and consistently stocked with healthy food options. To address psychological well-being, the programme had an expert clinical psychologist meet with residents weekly on a confidential basis. Consistency was built into the schedule to allow the psychologist to meet with the different classes of residents every 6 weeks. Lastly, to address social well-being, there are programmes or activities available outside of the hospital that encourage life beyond the hospital and give the residents an opportunity to support each other and interact socially. The Balance in Life programme is an exemplar of direct and concrete policies to address wellness on different levels of training during medical education.

Academic Medical Faculty Wellness Programmes

Academic medical faculty face increasing pressure and challenges in their work environments (Goitein, 2014). Faced with higher clinical load and pressures to increase clinical productivity, coupled with the desire to be fully committed to teaching and research. The loss of autonomy at work can create a sense of disenfranchisement and diminished sense of meaning. One study found that faculty who spent less than 20% of their time on an activity that is most meaningful to them had higher rates of burnout and the ability to focus on the aspects of their work that brought meaning diminished the risk of burnout (Shanafelt et al., 2009). A 2006 study that surveyed 3,519 academic faculty members at four United States medical schools found 20% of faculty had significant levels of depressive symptoms, with higher levels in younger faculty. Noted in this research is a major relationship between work-related strain and faculty mental health and job satisfaction (Schindler et al., 2006).

Professional vitality battles burnout and builds resilience. Job satisfaction and engagement are important keys to vitality (Dankoski, Palmer, Laird, Ribera, & Bogdewic, 2012). Faculty vitality has been defined as 'the high levels of satisfaction, productivity, and engagement that enables [a] faculty member to maximise her/his professional success and achieve goals in concert with institutional goals' (Dankoski et al., 2012). Another group of researchers determined that faculty who find meaning in their work create that sense of professional vitality and it is important for Academic Health Centres to pay more attention to strengthening relationships, improving the misalignment between faculty and institutional values, and improving work–life integration (Pololi et al., 2015). Presently, few training programmes exist that document positive outcomes related to enhanced academic faculty well-being.

A group at Rochester, New York studied whether an intensive educational programme in communication, mindfulness, and self-awareness is associated with improvement in physicians' well-being, psychological distress, burnout, and capacity for relating to patients. The intervention included an 8-week intensive phase (2.5 hour/week and a 7-hour retreat) was followed by a 10-month maintenance phase (2.5 hour/month). The physician's participation in a mindful communication programme correlated with short-term and sustained improvements in well-being and attitudes associated with patient centred care (Krasner et al., 2009).

In 2011, Mayo Clinic Rochester academic physicians were enrolled in a pilot randomised study. In the study, the intervention group received 90-minute training on Stress Management and Resiliency training (Sood, Prasad, Schroeder, & Varkey, 2011). During the intervention groups' time, participation in facilitated small group conversations with peers which concentrated on learning how to use mindfulness and reflection strategies. Moreover, a statistically significant improvement was found for resiliency, perceived stress, anxiety, and overall quality of life compared to the non-intervention group. A group of researchers later expanded this intervention to involve 19 biweekly facilitated physician discussion groups that included features of mindfulness, reflection, shared experience, and small-group learning for 9 months (West et al., 2014). The doctors received protected time, 1 hour of paid time every other week, for their efforts and thus removed the barrier of having to find time in already busy schedules. A compelling finding from the study revealed that the rates of depersonalisation, emotional exhaustion, and overall burnout decreased substantially in the trial intervention stage of the research (West et al., 2014). These optimistic results were sustained up to 12 months after the study.

Such findings from evidenced-based research hold important implications for administrative and department leadership at academic medical centres. The academic physician is a critical resource for these centre of training, scientific discovery, and medical innovation. It can be inferred, that diminishing burnout and increasing resilience are important for long term success of academic health centres and reduction in employee turnover. Academic health centres that encourage faculty mindfulness may help inspire a culture of support for the humanistic needs of health professionals (Pololi et al., 2015).

Increased awareness of these issues affecting the mental health and well-being of medical academic faculty once proactively addressed should ultimately also positively affect students and resident physicians. Thereby, advancing policies to help facilitate an atmosphere that is essential for research productivity, effective teaching and quality patient care.

SOLUTIONS AND RECOMMENDATIONS

The key recommendations on all levels of medical education include an internal review of existing institutional culture surrounding wellness and identifying areas for improvement. Wellness champions and mentors need to take transformative steps with an early introduction of wellness to the medical audience and consider administering self-assessment burn-out tools to aid in monitoring impact of the interventions rendered. Structured wellness events can be incorporated in the form of lectures, retreats, social events and counselling. Most importantly, structures need to be put in place to reduce the barriers (money, time, etc.) that prevent medical learners and medical faculty from accessing these solutions and recommendations. Academic health centre also need to incorporate into the institution's mission statements, policies that promote a culture of wellness assistance for all members of the medical and medicine communities. Inclusive of faculty, staff, administrators, medical students, residents and physicians.

By reviewing current data on wellness programmes, including both traditional and curricular approaches, this chapter concludes with a table created to provide a guideline and template for building a well-rounded wellness programmes. Table 1 presents a summary of current programmes that have been tested and proven successful in fostering wellness among its medical students and residents. Additionally, Table 1 may serve as a template for administration attempting to address burnout within their respective institutions. With this template, one can use key factors to customized wellness programmes to essentially change the culture at each institution for years to come.

FUTURE RESEARCH DIRECTIONS

Medical educators should continue to study the impact that learning environments have on the well-being of their students and resident physicians. Conscious efforts to educate themselves on the consequences and costs associated with these settings is imperative. Using existing knowledge and offering more evidence- based research can be helpful in garnering public support and awareness. Examination of outcomes on various levels (patient, health care delivery, health care cost) and engagement with the multitude of stakeholders in the area to develop informed guidelines is needed. Best practises need to be studied and implemented in a consistent mode for wellness programmes on all levels of medical education from the beginning medical student to more senior academic faculty. To have successful academic reform in medical schools, it therefore would be beneficial to assess and manage occupational burnout among clinical faculty members. Little research has been conducted to investigate role stress experienced by faculty members in medical schools in developing countries. This becomes even more important when the process of reform in medical education has already taken place in many first world countries. Research to understand the impact of academic faculty on physician and resident research is most needed as changes to policies throughout medical education are on the rise.

CONCLUSION

Stress, burnout and lack of vitality in medical training is prevalent. It is certainly not a new problem, but more attention is being paid to its effects on the quality of patient care, learner mental health and faculty turnover. Most importantly, the culture of medicine needs to change. Lack of resiliency on the faculty level spills down to resident and medical student learners and does not model good behaviour.

Table 1. Wellness programme template

Key Factor of Programme	Support
Internal review of curriculum • Change from level grading system to Pass/Fail • Evaluate 'hardest' courses/rotations and discuss ways to alleviate the stress. Can the order of courses be rearranged? • Incorporation of wellness curriculum (meditation, mindfulness, self -reflection)	Slavin et al., 2014
Prepare for arrival of new class • Delve into new student's interests & career goals to match with student mentor and faculty advisor • Send personalised letter prior to arrival	Drolet and Rodgers, 2010
Introduction of wellness at orientation • Educate on common stressors, realistic expectations for programme, student/resident abuse • Invite established faculty who have faced various forms of distress • Define 'wellness'; expand on 'I am my own first patient' • Administer burnout tool; follow up at 6 months	Gaber et al., 2002 Eckleberry-Hunt et al., 2009 Benbasset et al., 2011
Emphasize mentorship & advising • Faculty mentors • Student/resident mentors • Consistent check ins throughout the year • Confidential space for students/residents to vocalise concerns • Wellness champion	Eckleberry-Hunt et al., 2009 Drolet and Rodgers, 2010 Slavin et al., 2014 Salles et al., 2015
Student leadership & investment • Wellness committees focused to tackle different aspects of wellness	Drolet and Rogers, 2010
Lecture series addressing wellness • Meditation/Yoga • Time management • Financial management • Nutrition • Sleeping habits • Diversity in medicine	Eckleberry-Hunt et al, 2009 Goldhagen, Kingsolver, Stinnett, & Rosdahl, 2015
Designated pre-scheduled wellness days/retreats	Cedfledt et al., 2015 Drolet et al., 2010
Measure physical health • Physical examination and extensive studies done upon arrival with fitness at assessment 6 months	Gaber and Martin., 2002
Scheduled social events • Welcome reception • Colleges & 'College Cup' • Sporting events/ art events • Celebrate milestones (transitions in years, birthdays etc.)	Gaber and Martin., 2002 Eckleberry-Hunt et al., 2009 Drolet and Rodgers, 2010 Slavin et al., 2014 Salles et al., 2015
Breaking wellness down into domains • Mind • Body • Social • Community • Professional	Drolet and Rodgers, 2010 Salles et al., 2015
Reduce barriers to accessing behavioural health care • Offer referrals to community based counselling services • Provide free & easy access to full-time psychologist or psychiatrist experienced in working with medical professionals	Moutier et al., 2012 Ey, Moffit, Kinzie, Choi, & Girard, 2013 Salles, Liebert, & Greco, 2015
Provide time off during weekdays/business hours to ensure time for residents/faculty to seek proper health care & promote overall wellness	Cedfeldt et al., 2015

However, it is the authors' hope that as more medical student and resident learners are given the tools they need to combat burnout, they, in turn, will then develop into more vital medical faculty.

REFERENCES

Benbassat, J., Baumal, R., Chan, S., & Nirel, N. (2011). Sources of distress during medical training and clinical practice: Suggestions for reducing their impact. *Medical Teacher*, *33*(6), 486–490. doi:10.3109/0142159X.2010.531156 PMID:21609178

Cedfeldt, A. S., Bower, E., Flores, C., Brunett, P., Choi, D., & Girard, D. E. (2015). Promoting resident wellness: Evaluation of a time-off policy to increase residents utilization of health care services. *Academic Medicine: Journal of the Association of American Medical Colleges*, *90*(5), 678–683. doi:10.1097/ACM.0000000000000541 PMID:25354073

Dabrow, S., Russell, S., Ackley, K., Anderson, E., & Fabri, P. J. (2006). Combating the stress of residency: One schools approach. *Academic Medicine: Journal of the Association of American Medical Colleges*, *81*(5), 436–439. doi:10.1097/01.ACM.0000222261.47643.d2 PMID:16639197

Dankoski, M. E., Palmer, M. M., Laird, T. F. N., Ribera, A. K., & Bogdewic, S. P. (2012). An expanded model of faculty vitality in academic medicine. *Advances in Health Sciences Education : Theory and Practice*, *17*(5), 633–649. doi:10.1007/s10459-011-9339-7 PMID:22134490

Drolet, B. C., & Rodgers, S. (2010). A comprehensive medical student wellness programdesign and implementation at vanderbilt school of medicine. *Academic Medicine: Journal of the Association of American Medical Colleges*, *85*(1), 103–110. doi:10.1097/ACM.0b013e3181c46963 PMID:20042835

Dunn, L. B., Moutier, C., Hammond, K. A. G., Lehrmann, J., & Roberts, L. W. (2008). Personal health care of residents: Preferences for care outside of the training institution. *Academic Psychiatry*, *32*(1), 20–30. doi:10.1176/appi.ap.32.1.20 PMID:18270277

Eckleberry-Hunt, J., Lick, D., Boura, J., Hunt, R., Balasubramaniam, M., Mulhem, E., & Fisher, C. (2009). An exploratory study of resident burnout and wellness. *Academic Medicine: Journal of the Association of American Medical Colleges*, *84*(2), 269–277. doi:10.1097/ACM.0b013e3181938a45 PMID:19174684

Eckleberry-Hunt, J., Van Dyke, A., Lick, D., & Tucciarone, J. (2009). Changing the conversation from burnout to wellness: Physician well-being in residency training programs. *Journal of Graduate Medical Education*, *1*(2), 225–230. doi:10.4300/JGME-D-09-00026.1 PMID:21975983

Ey, S., Moffit, M., Kinzie, J. M., Choi, D., & Girard, D. E. (2013). If you build it, they will come: Attitudes of medical residents and fellows about seeking services in a resident wellness program. *Journal of Graduate Medical Education*, *5*(3), 486–492. doi:10.4300/JGME-D-12-00048.1 PMID:24404315

Gaber, R. R., & Martin, D. M. (2002). Still-well osteopathic medical student wellness program. *The Journal of the American Osteopathic Association*, *102*(5), 289–292. PMID:12033759

Gander, P., Briar, C., Garden, A., Purnell, H., & Woodward, A. (2010). A gender-based analysis of work patterns, fatigue, and work/life balance among physicians in postgraduate training. *Academic Medicine*, *85*(9), 1526–1536. doi:10.1097/ACM.0b013e3181eabd06 PMID:20736682

Givens, J. L., & Tjia, J. (2002). Depressed medical students use of mental health services and barriers to use. *Academic Medicine*, *77*(9), 918–921. doi:10.1097/00001888-200209000-00024 PMID:12228091

Goitein, L. (2014). Physician well-being: Addressing downstream effects, but looking upstream. *JAMA Internal Medicine*, *174*(4), 533–534. doi:10.1001/jamainternmed.2013.13253 PMID:24515255

Goldhagen, B. E., Kingsolver, K., Stinnett, S. S., & Rosdahl, J. A. (2015). Stress and burnout in residents: Impact of mindfulness-based resilience training. *Advances in Medical Education and Practice*, *6*, 525. PMID:26347361

Guille, C., Speller, H., Laff, R., Epperson, C. N., & Sen, S. (2010). Utilization and barriers to mental health services among depressed medical interns: A prospective multisite study. *Journal of Graduate Medical Education*, *2*(2), 210–214. doi:10.4300/JGME-D-09-00086.1 PMID:21975622

Hughes, P. H., Conard, S. E., Baldwin, D. C., Storr, C. L., & Sheehan, D. V. (1991). Resident physician substance use in the united states. *Journal of the American Medical Association*, *265*(16), 2069–2073. doi:10.1001/jama.1991.03460160047027 PMID:2013925

Krasner, M. S., Epstein, R. M., Beckman, H., Suchman, A. L., Chapman, B., Mooney, C. J., & Quill, T. E. (2009). Association of an educational program in mindful communication with burnout, empathy, and attitudes among primary care physicians. *Journal of the American Medical Association*, *302*(12), 1284–1293. doi:10.1001/jama.2009.1384 PMID:19773563

Kushner, M. G., & Sher, K. J. (1989). Fear of psychological treatment and its relation to mental health service avoidance. *Professional Psychology, Research and Practice*, *20*(4), 251–257. doi:10.1037/0735-7028.20.4.251

Lutsky, I., Abram, S. E., Jacobson, G. R., Hopwood, M., & Kampine, J. (1991). Substance abuse by anesthesiology residents. *Academic Medicine*, *66*(3), 164–166. doi:10.1097/00001888-199103000-00009 PMID:1997028

McBeth, B. D., Ankel, F. K., Ling, L. J., Asplin, B. R., Mason, E. J., Flottemesch, T. J., & McNamara, R. M. (2008). Substance use in emergency medicine training programs. *Academic Emergency Medicine*, *15*(1), 45–53. doi:10.1111/j.1553-2712.2007.00008.x PMID:18211313

McCue, J. D., & Sachs, C. L. (1991). A stress management workshop improves residents coping skills. *Archives of Internal Medicine*, *151*(11), 2273–2277. doi:10.1001/archinte.1991.00400110117023 PMID:1953233

Moutier, C., Cornette, M., Lehrmann, J., Geppert, C., Tsao, C., DeBoard, M. R., & Roberts, L. W. etal. (2009). When residents need health care: Stigma of the patient role. *Academic Psychiatry*, *33*(6), 431–441. doi:10.1176/appi.ap.33.6.431 PMID:19933883

Moutier, C., Norcross, W., Jong, P., Norman, M., Kirby, B., McGuire, T., & Zisook, S. (2012). The suicide prevention and depression awareness program at the university of california, san diego school of medicine. *Academic Medicine: Journal of the Association of American Medical Colleges*, *87*(3), 320–326. doi:10.1097/ACM.0b013e31824451ad PMID:22373625

Ospina-Kammerer, V., & Figley, C. R. (2003). An evaluation of the respiratory one method (ROM) in reducing emotional exhaustion among family physician residents. *International Journal of Emergency Mental Health*, *5*(1), 29–32. PMID:12722487

Pitt, E., Rosenthal, M. M., Gay, T. L., & Lewton, E. (2004). Mental health services for residents: More important than ever. *Academic Medicine*, *79*(9), 840–844. doi:10.1097/00001888-200409000-00005 PMID:15326006

Pololi, L. H., Evans, A. T., Civian, J. T., Gibbs, B. K., Coplit, L. D., Gillum, L. H., & Brennan, R. T. (2015). Faculty vitality-surviving the challenges facing academic health centers: A national survey of medical faculty. *Academic Medicine: Journal of the Association of American Medical Colleges*, *90*(7), 930–936. doi:10.1097/ACM.0000000000000674 PMID:25692560

Salles, A., Liebert, C. A., & Greco, R. S. (2015). Promoting balance in the lives of resident physicians: A call to action. *JAMA Surgery*, *150*(7), 607–608. doi:10.1001/jamasurg.2015.0257 PMID:25992632

Schindler, B. A., Novack, D. H., Cohen, D. G., Yager, J., Wang, D., Shaheen, N. J., & Drossman, D. A. etal. (2006). The impact of the changing health care environment on the health and well-being of faculty at four medical schools. *Academic Medicine*, *81*(1), 27–34. doi:10.1097/00001888-200601000-00008 PMID:16377815

Shanafelt, T. D., West, C. P., Sloan, J. A., Novotny, P. J., Poland, G. A., Menaker, R., & Dyrbye, L. N. etal. (2009). Career fit and burnout among academic faculty. *Archives of Internal Medicine*, *169*(10), 990–995. doi:10.1001/archinternmed.2009.70 PMID:19468093

Slavin, S. J., Schindler, D. L., & Chibnall, J. T. (2014). Medical student mental health 3.0: Improving student wellness through curricular changes. *Academic Medicine: Journal of the Association of American Medical Colleges*, *89*(4), 573–577. doi:10.1097/ACM.0000000000000166 PMID:24556765

Sood, A., Prasad, K., Schroeder, D., & Varkey, P. (2011). Stress management and resilience training among department of medicine faculty: A pilot randomized clinical trial. *Journal of General Internal Medicine*, *26*(8), 858–861. doi:10.1007/s11606-011-1640-x PMID:21279454

Vessey, J. T., & Howard, K. I. (1993). Who seeks psychotherapy? *Psychotherapy (Chicago, Ill.)*, *30*(4), 546–553. doi:10.1037/0033-3204.30.4.546

West, C. P., Dyrbye, L. N., Rabatin, J. T., Call, T. G., Davidson, J. H., Multari, A., & Shanafelt, T. D. etal. (2014). Intervention to promote physician well-being, job satisfaction, and professionalism: A randomized clinical trial. *JAMA Internal Medicine*, *174*(4), 527–533. doi:10.1001/jamainternmed.2013.14387 PMID:24515493

KEY TERMS AND DEFINITIONS

Academic Medicine Centres: A health care organisation often connected to a medical school and hospital system.

Burnout: Physical or mental collapse caused by overwork or stress.

Difficult Patients: Patients who are troublesome, tedious and/or noncompliant with medical provider instructions.

Intolerance of Uncertainty: A perception of ambiguous situations as a threat (Benbassat et al., 2011).

Mindfulness: A mental state achieved by focusing one's awareness on the present moment, while acknowledging and accepting one's feelings, thoughts, and sensations; it is often used as a therapeutic technique.

Resident Physician: A resident physician or house officer is an individual who has completed medical school. A resident physician practices medicine under the supervision of an attending physician. In many countries, a physician must successfully complete residency training before they can fully practice medicine. Post-residency physicians are referred to as attending physicians or consultants.

Resiliency: The ability to recover quickly from disruptive change without being overwhelmed or acting in harmful ways.

Value Exploration: Process in which individuals examine their values, beliefs, motivations, interests and abilities to help guide education and career decisions.

Chapter 8
Developing a Comprehensive Wellness Program for Medical Students

LaTanya Love
The University of Texas Health Science Center at Houston, USA

Dana McDowelle
The University of Texas Health Science Center at Houston, USA

ABSTRACT

This chapter addresses the various components that go into the development of a comprehensive wellness programme. Medical school can be a difficult time for students and some will experience an increase in burnout, stress, and anxiety that can lead to less empathetic physicians, decline in professionalism, and ultimately impact the quality of healthcare. Increased stress, burnout, and anxiety can lead to less empathetic doctors, decline in professionalism, and ultimately impact the quality of healthcare. One way to address these issues is through the development of a comprehensive wellness programme that addresses both academic and non-academic contributing factors. Prior to the development of a comprehensive wellness programme one must identify key stakeholders and assess the factors that are contributing to medical student well-being. Equal consideration must be given to both academic and non-academic factors that contribute to overall student well-being and incorporated into the design of a comprehensive wellness programme.

DOI: 10.4018/978-1-5225-2811-1.ch008

INTRODUCTION

Medical school can be a very exciting time for students. The medical school admissions process is extremely competitive and as a result, many students have an increase in stress in comparison to their peers when they are navigating the medical school admissions process; nevertheless, according to the literature, upon entry into medical school, these students enjoy a similar or better mental health status than age-similar controls (Brazeau, et al, 2014). Pre-medical students dedicate a significant block of time to researching the medical school admissions process in an effort to become the most competitive applicant possible and to improve their chances of matriculating to medical school. In a similar vein, an even greater number of hours is spent on preparation for the Medical College Admissions Test (MCAT) and maintaining a stellar academic record, including an acceptable grade point average, to place them in a competitive range for entry. Outside of the formally assessed academic arena, pre-medical students dedicate innumerable hours shadowing healthcare workers, conducting research, and accruing community service hours. In short, the overwhelming majority of medical student-hopefuls have worked particularly hard to be successful medical school applicants. It is not uncommon for the students who matriculate to medical school to have graduated at the top of their undergraduate classes and as their medical education journey ensues, for the first time they may be surrounded by students who are equally accomplished and who have achieved at similar or higher levels as they have, another potential stressor in the form of crisis of confidence.

The decline in mental health status and well-being in medical students is well documented at this point. There is a clear and definitive relationship between medical training (encompassing undergraduate medical education and residency) and an increase in trainee distress with trainees demonstrating burnout, emotional exhaustion, erosion of empathy, depersonalisation, depression and suicidal ideation at higher frequencies than their non-trainee counterparts (Dyrbye, et al 2014). Plainly, distress among medical trainees and physicians has risen to an alarming rate while programs to instil resilience-fostering behaviours and self-care have remained woefully inadequate. It is noteworthy that research findings demonstrate that students with severe depressive symptoms upon graduation are at risk for depression later in practise and later in life (Seritan, et al., 2015; Strøen Gotmol, et al., 2013). Due to these variances, it is important to thoughtfully and carefully identify the predominating stressors by stage of training. It is clear that interventions must be aimed at all stages of medical training and close attention must be paid to factors that affect trainees at each level of their education, starting with year one of medical school.

First Year

First year medical students are not always prepared for the large volume of content they are expected to learn nor are they accustomed to mastering that amount of information in such a short period of time. It is not uncommon for new students to find that the study methods that led to success during their undergraduate tenures are not as effective from the outset of their medical school educations. During their transition to medical school, they may have to adjust their study habits to successfully comprehend the vast amount of material; in some instances, students must adopt entirely new approaches to broaden their funds of knowledge. The volume of material for which the students are responsible necessitates longer hours of concentrated study and dependent upon the format through which the curriculum is delivered, students may be subjected to frequent assessments of their knowledge of basic science materials. Throughout the first months, students will find themselves constantly studying with little downtime for other activities that previously have helped them to strike an appropriate work-school-life balance, a significant stressor unto itself; however, the lack of free time for leisure activities may make it difficult to maintain important relationships, a compounding variable of the accumulation of stress. Students in the beginning of their medical school education will often find themselves with very little free time while some of their peers, especially outside of medicine, will have much more time to engage in leisure or recreational activities. At times first year medical students might find themselves questioning their decision to commit to the rigours of a medical school education.

It is also important to acknowledge that first year medical curricula across the nation (USA) typically include an intensive gross anatomy course that utilises cadavers. The dissection of the cadaver itself can pose a challenge for a small subset of students as they start to associate medical education with actual human beings. Finally, as first year medical students become fully immersed in the culture of medical school, they must also start to think about their long-term career goals and making the best decisions to help them achieve their residency of choice. All taken, the aforementioned experiences and demands are factors that contribute to an increase in stress, anxiety, and depression and a number of students find the transition to medical school to be quite daunting.

Second Year

The second year of medical school provides a different set of challenges for medical students. At this juncture, students feel comfortable with their study methods and readily identify with their colleagues and with the profession. This is not to say that they do not encounter important and significant stressor at this stage of the undergraduate medical curriculum. Many second-year students move into a stage of hypervigilance regarding their preparation for the United States Medical Licensing Examination (USMLE) Step 1. A large majority of medical schools require students to pass Step 1 near the end of the preclinical/basic sciences years of medical school and prior to the transition to clinical education in which students begin to interact with patients as they become engaged in clinical rotations. USMLE Step 1 is considered to be a high stakes examination since it is frequently used by graduate medical education (GME) programmes (also known as internship and residency) as a measure of a student's competitiveness for certain medical specialties. For many students, it is not enough to simply pass the United States Medical Licensing Examination Step 1, but instead many feel tremendous pressure to perform well above the national average to position themselves as competitive applicants for the most competitive programmes. Unlike the Medical College Admissions Test (MCAT), there is not the opportunity to sit for the Step 1 examination multiple times if dissatisfied with a passing score. There are also state-specific attempt limits on how many times a medical student can take the examination in order to be eligible for their full medical license. Second year students continue to deal with the challenge of finding balance between their academic and personal lives. Second year students will also continue to think about their future careers and specialty choice, which now is a constant reminder of the need to perform well.

Third Year

Third year marks another seminal transition during medical education in that students move from a traditional classroom or lecture setting to the clinical setting. During the clinical years of education—the third and fourth years-- students are faced with long hours on clinical rotations, schedules that are not directly under their control, shift work and overnight call. There is evidence that suggests that shift work, specifically overnight call, may be associated with some chronic diseases such as cancer, and cardiovascular disease and general health problems (Flo et al 2012; Wang et al, 2011). Third year is particularly stressful as some students describe their first service on the wards as heavily laden with stress and anxiety; it is quite an adjustment, and for some it presents a great amount of difficulty. Third year students must work on interpersonal communication skills as they adjust to interviewing 'real' patients on a regular basis (as opposed to standardized patients from clinical encounters in the first and second year) and must master the art of accurately and concisely conveying important patient information to other members of the medical team. Most demanding is the expectation to present patients to their residents and attending physicians. Many students become anxious and nervous when they have to present in front of their peers or to other team members. Third year students are also expected to apply their knowledge and formulate differential diagnosis and begin to think of treatment plans for their patients. They may find themselves not wanting to ask questions or speak up on rounds secondary to fear of not knowing the right answer.

Third year students may also face challenges as they are taking care of a variety of patients, some with complex medical and social issues. Furthermore, third year medical students may face an array of emotions as they are learning to care for their patients. At this stage in training many will experience joy when they assist with the birth of a healthy newborn baby, sadness when they witness the death of a patient, empathy when they hear patients receiving bad news and sympathy when observing a family member trying to cope with a loved one's terminal illness. Coping with such a full range of emotions over a short period of time requires fortitude of character and a great deal of resilience and proves difficult to navigate for a reasonable number of third year students.

Fourth Year

Fourth year medical students find themselves under stress as they are finalising their choice of medical specialty. Some students have difficulty deciding between a few specialties and will generally have to make a decision by the beginning of fourth year. Fourth year medical students will have increased stress related to residency applications as they are asking for letters of recommendations and thinking about programmes that they wish to apply for residency training. Fourth year students often have an increased financial strain as they will have expenses associated with their residency applications and interview-related travel expenses. They must plan for the real possibility that they may not match to the residency programme of their choice alongside making financial plans to relocate and coordinating logistics of becoming a practising physician including completion of national examinations and application for licensure. Fourth year students often find themselves anxious about transitioning to the next stage of their career as an intern.

Based on the aforementioned stressors at each level of medical training, it is imperative that the unique needs of students at every stage of training are adequately addressed within the context of wellness and resilience across/throughout the medical education continuum. Direct and deliberate programming to teach students self-care skills in the context of the medical education continuum will produce physicians who are armed with the proper tools to relieve stress and burnout while avoiding lapses in professionalism and the erosion of empathy. As healthy students are better prepared to learn and practise medicine, paramount to that mission are the efforts to maintain a student community that is well.

BACKGROUND

A career in medicine is a very competitive and highly desirable pathway. Students who ultimately matriculate into medical school have worked very hard to gain medical school admissions and look forward to a career in service to others. Unfortunately, medical school is also a time when some students first experience depression, anxiety, stress, and burnout, each of which has the potential to affect professionalism, to contribute to medical errors, and to lead to suicidal ideations. There is a strong positive correlation between the stressors that plague medical students and physicians in training and substance abuse as well as relationship difficulties (Dyrbye, et al., 2014). The transition to medical school is a difficult one for a significant number of medical students, as they juggle more demanding schedules than their peers and grapple with the decreased time to interact with family and friends. High emotional exhaustion has been found to be more prevalent among medical students and residents than people in the general population. As compared to United States college graduates, medical students have a higher prevalence of emotional exhaustion, depersonalisation, and burnout, data that suggest that burnout is more prevalent among medical trainees than similarly aged U.S. population (Dyrbye, et al., 2014). These findings serve as a catalyst for medical schools to identify ways to support students who may encounter increased stress during medical school and to proceed in an intentional and thoughtful manner to build, promote and sustain a culture of wellness, professionalism, self-care and help-seeking in medical students (Thomas, et al., 2011). Keeping in mind that physicians are charged with the responsibility of encouraging healthy lifestyle choices for their patients, the undergraduate medical education arena is a training ground and 'teachable moment' to ingrain in its students the best practises in this regard. Employing unidimensional stress management strategies is not enough, but instead, a multi-tiered programme with various coping strategies is necessary (Shiralkar, et al., 2013).

MAIN FOCUS OF CHAPTER

Medical school administrators seeking to establish a comprehensive wellness programme to support student wellbeing must first understand their school- and community- specific climates. Anonymous climate assessment surveys or open focus groups are effective tools to gauge the culture of wellness and the need for intentional and thoughtful programming. Ideally, the instrument selected should allow for feedback from as many students as possible to gather feedback from a representative sample/cross section of the student community. When designing a survey keep in mind that the length of survey should be reasonable so that it does not take a significant amount of time for completion, as busy students tend to shy away from participation in time-consuming surveys. In designing a study, it is helpful to capture the stage of training of each participant since the sources of stress vary based on level of training.

It is crucial to engage students in every step of building a culture of wellness from programme inception through implementation. Involving students in change management and in building consensus will buoy the likelihood that the programme will be well received by the collective student community; medical students are much more relatable to other medical students. There should be a select group of students who serve as ambassadors for the programme; it may be most helpful to enlist a cadre of students who have demonstrated a commitment to wellness in previous efforts to serve in this capacity. These students are a key component to gaining buy in from other students and stakeholders. Students should be involved in organising programming and working with administrators on developing content that is relevant, timely and impactful will be well received by other students. Regular focus group sessions should be held to constantly keep students engaged and to hear valuable feedback. During the implementation phase student assistance in the advertisement of various programmes will assure information is publicised broadly to reach the largest possible number of students.

As part of the development of a culture of wellness and comprehensive programming dedicated to the support of the wellbeing of medical students, it is critical to take into account the stigma that has long been associated with mental health related issues such as anxiety and stress. Seeking treatment for these disorders is commonly viewed in a negative light by society and unfortunately, by many physicians, medical school faculty and staff and medical students alike. Some students may delay seeking treatment or neglect to pursue treatment at all because of this stigma. There have been differences noticed between preclinical and clinical medical students in their views of depression, with preclinical students more likely to endorse that depressed medical students provide inferior care to their patients, are unable to cope with medical school stress, and are less intelligent than their peers (Schwenk, et al. 2010).

With all of the above in mind, the landscape that encompasses academic and non-academic factors that affect the well-being of medical students includes transitioning to medical school, increased workload, poor study habits, licensing exam scores, career development and clinical rotations, to highlight only a few. Some examples of non-academic contributing factors include relationship stressors, financial difficulties, poor nutrition, and poor time management. The ability to spot students in distress and to correctly pinpoint their specific source or sources of distress is quite difficult indeed, necessitating an arsenal of tools to help student self-identify, self-report, seek assistance and proactively engage in self-care. Medical schools can consider performing a survey to gain a better understanding of common issues and sources of stress for students. A wellness and resilience programme that can comprehensively and effectively support the student community must include various subcomponents that target each stressor to allow students to participate in that programme which is most appropriate for and focused on their individual situation. Potential areas of focus include academic support, occupational development, professionalism, personal health and self-care, interpersonal development and financial wellness. It is important to recruit students who can be champions of any programming or activities that will be planned. These students can help with the promotion and indoctrination of all activities and can serve as advisors to administrators who are involved.

In 2013, Epstein and Krasner emphasised the importance of resilience in the physician workforce, as a means to enhance not only quality of care, but also to sustain the overall health and well- being of the healthcare workforce. While the ability to 'bounce back' varies from individual to individual, taking the opportunity to teach physicians-in-training mindfulness, limit setting, self-monitoring, self-care and resilience-fostering behaviours has the potential to generate far-reaching and long-lasting positive effects in the form of reduced errors, attrition and burnout.

Academic Support

The enormous amount of material that medical students must master and upon which they will be tested is a large and constant source of stress and anxiety. Students may feel that they need to be competitive among their other classmates in order to be successful and to have an advantage. In designing a comprehensive wellness programme, it is important to evaluate areas in the curriculum that could be potentially stressful to students. Once these areas are identified, key stakeholders must work together to address areas that can be modified. Some models of wellness programmes address direct sources of medical student distress within the curriculum and at the same time introduce opportunities for students to develop better resilience skills within the core curriculum (Slavin, et al. 2014).

Support systems need to be incorporated that address any deficiencies and help to increase student success. Many schools integrate problem-based and team-based learning into the curriculum. Some students find these smaller groups beneficial and prefer this setting over the traditional lecture format. Other schools utilise learning communities that consist of faculty leaders and smaller groups of students. Learning communities formed in the first year of medical school can remain intact for the duration of the degree programme, allowing mentor: mentee or advisor: advisee relationships to mature. Individual schools need to receive feedback from their students about the various options of delivering content. Schools can also look at ways of engaging students through enhanced technology and streaming of information. Educational leadership and faculty must look at innovative ways to deliver relevant content and keep trainees engaged. If students are in a curriculum that allows them to be more engaged then they are less likely to look at the curriculum as an additional source of stress.

As part of the wellness programme schools must reconsider traditional assessment and grading conventions. Each school must decide if they want to utilise traditional numerical or letter grading versus moving to a pass/fail grading system. Numerous students have demonstrated higher levels of stress and emotional exhaustion in schools utilising grading scales with three or more levels as compared with schools using pass/fail grading systems (Reed, et al., 2011). A study conducted by Dyrbye, et al. (2005) specifically cites a traditional 5-level grading schema as a major contributor to peer academic competitiveness and anxiety undermining the fundamental collaboration that will ultimately be needed as a member of a medical team (Rohe, et al, 2006). Adoption of a pass/fail grading system has been shown to provide some relief in that there are students who will feel less pressure since they are not focused on a specific numerical or letter grade. Additionally, in a pass-fail grading system, students have the liberty to select the level at which they want to achieve within the passing grade range without serious ramifications for their long-term ability to be successful. Simply put, many students feel that pass/fail is a less competitive grading model. Multiple schools utilise pass/fail grading schemes for the pre-clinical years and a more stratified scheme for the clinical rotations. Each school needs to assess their learning environment to determine what grading system works best for medical education programme at their institution.

In development of a comprehensive wellness programme a strong support system for students must be in place to ensure student success. Sessions can be incorporated that address study skills and time management. A concrete infrastructure of academic and non-academic resources should be in place to provide assistance when students are having academic difficulty or if they find themselves in need of supplemental guidance or advising. Some resources that can be provided include additional review sessions to clarify material and to provide students ample opportunities to ask questions. These sessions can be regularly scheduled or reserved for periods that are closer to examinations. Another resource that can be considered is the use of tutors for students. Consideration should be given for school funding of tutors so that an additional financial burden is not placed on the student. Tutors utilised can be peers who have already successfully completed coursework or post-doctoral candidates. All support services that are made available must be regularly advertised to all students, faculty, and staff should be reminded to encourage students to utilise them if needed and before they are at such a large deficit, that there is not enough time to recover. It is important to remind faculty and student support staff that many medical students have never been in the position to need academic supplements or additional assistance, thus help-seeking behaviours have not necessarily been honed. Students who are facing academic challenges should be aware of the appropriate people to seek out if they are having any concerns. Typically, Student Affairs or Curriculum Deans are available for students and if they are not, then a designee should be appointed to serve as an initial point of contact. Many schools will utilise faculty to serve in advisory roles and will assign students to faculty so they have a designated advisor/mentor to contact when facing academic concerns. Any person designated to assist students should have knowledge of all available resources.

For second year medical students, an added source of anxiety and stress is preparing for and taking Step 1 of the USMLE. As a high-stake exam, it is imperative that schools consider ways in which they can help their students feel confident and reduce the anxiety associated with preparation for and completion of this major milestone. Each school can consider what resources are available and whether the budget can sustain the provision of the most effective and widely utilised review materials. Schools may want to consider additional board review sessions that cover high yield content. Such review sessions can be organised by local faculty or contracted to commercial review courses; in many instances, schools will enlist the assistance of third and fourth year students who performed exceptionally well on the examination to hold a 'Step Prep' review course. In the event that a commercial vendor is selected, it is often easy to negotiate discount rates for groups of students to help ease the financial burden of review materials and overall course cost. As a complement to a review course, most schools will offer opportunities for students to take practise examinations and to engage in self-assessments so that each individual student can establish his/her readiness for the examination. Practise examinations can be purchased in bulk by the school or independently by each student. On the occasion that the school provides a practise examination for all students, it is strongly suggested that very specific feedback be provided to each student upon scoring of the examination. It is the perfect opportunity to speak with those students who are not performing at a passing equivalent and to suggest specific study resources or to create a study plan that will help them to increase their fund of knowledge prior to sitting for the examination. The practise examinations can provide a detailed report that advisors and faculty can use to outline for the student which content areas need the most work and where he/she should focus effort to improve performance. The results of the practise examination can also be used for designated medical school staff to counsel students on the likelihood of success given their practise results. Some students may have a history of difficulty with standardised examinations and should be offered guidance so that they can know about all available resources and options. Adequate study time should be incorporated into the medical degree curriculum so students have the time they need to prepare. Some students may find that they need additional study time and schools should have options readily available for these students. At a regular interval, schools should evaluate the pass rate that their students achieve on Step 1 to internally reflect on their educational programme and its effectiveness and to guide curricular adjustments to increase student success. Strong academic support is a critical component of a wellness programme and should be addressed accordingly.

During the clinical years, there may need to be academic support incorporated in some unusual ways. Students will learn through taking care of patients and on their clinical rotations. Some students may struggle with transitioning to a different type of learning and thinking. Students should be prepared for the schedule of work hours which will vary depending on the clinical rotation. An orientation to the clinical years usually helps to ease this transition and allow clinical students to feel more comfortable.

At some point, usually during the last year of medical school, students will take Step 2 of the United States Medical Licensing Exam. They will have to take a clinical knowledge component as well as a clinical skills component. These examinations do not typically produce the same amount of stress as the first step of the licensing examination but should still be considered as important. Schools should determine if they are able to provide any resources to aid in the preparation for the clinical knowledge portion. Some schools also have standardised patient examinations they use in preparation for the clinical skills component.

Occupational Development

Symptoms of depression, suicidal ideation, and lower sense of accomplishment are most prevalent during medical school and have been shown to decline with each career stage (Dyrbye, et al., 2014). One of the main stressors that medical students often face is related to specialty selection and concerns about matching into their specialty of choice. Stress related to career choice starts in the first year of medical school and continues until a student has successfully matched into their specialty.

Medical schools must implement robust career counselling from the outset of medical school to help decrease or alleviate the fears about the residency application process. Some schools use advisory or college systems. Others will rely on student affairs deans and other trained faculty or staff to perform counselling. What is most important is that students have a wide range of opportunities to explore the various specialties and subspecialties and that they are given access to specialty advisors who can help them understand the demands of the specialty, the level of achievement needed to be competitive for that specialty or subspecialty and the general advantages and disadvantages of pursing that residency. For those medical schools that do not have preceptorships embedded in the curricular requirements, students can pursue observerships with physicians in practise of their desired specialty during break periods. As an accompaniment to the preceptorships, a comprehensive advising system should be in place that gives students individualised career counselling to ensure they are selecting a specialty for which they are realistically competitive and that will fulfil their career objectives.

Professionalism

It is essential for key stakeholders to be aware that a decline in student well-being can lead to lapses in professionalism. Papadakis et al. (2004) demonstrated that there is a strong positive correlation between problematic behaviour in medical school and subsequent disciplinary action by a state medical board. There is a proven relationship between medical student stress and decline in wellbeing with erosion of empathy, reduced compassion, and decreased humanitarian attitudes, all of which contribute to a decline in professionalism and the potential for increased medical errors and poor patient outcomes (Brazeau, et al. 2010). As a result, there is a renewed focus on professionalism as a competency of medical degree programmes and on real-time remediation of academic and professional deficits (Papadakis, et al, 2009). The creation of a professionalism and wellness curriculum that can be grown to include aspirational and longitudinal elements will allow for early remediation of students at risk for breaches of professionalism. The aspirational elements of the programme will offer formal professionalism and wellness education that encompasses authentic leadership in medicine, emotional intelligence assessment (there is a positive correlation between empathy and clinical competency), and an emphasis on best practices and conduct as a physician-in-training (the deconstruction of the hidden curriculum). The corrective elements of the programme necessitate the creation and formalised reporting and review processes for breaches of professional conduct. Ongoing dialogue is useful during the integration of professional identity formation into the medical school curriculum. Students ought to be made aware early on in their careers about the potential consequences of breaches in professionalism.

Self-Care

The health and well-being of all students is critical in the implementation of a comprehensive wellness programme. There may be a stigma associated with seeking mental health services, a potential barrier when implementing a wellness programme (Schwenk et al., 2010). In development of a comprehensive wellness programme administrators must be thoughtful about programming that brings awareness to common themes among medical students such as increased stress, anxiety, and depression. Any platform that can assist in destigmatising declines in mental health and encouraging treatment for mental health issues should be utilised. It is critical that easy access is provided to students seeking care, including resources that can be utilised after hours and in emergencies. Ideally, the availability of such services affiliated with the school and those not affiliated with the school should be readily available.

School-wide engagement is needed to encourage an on-going dialogue with students that encourages them to seek evaluation and treatment if they are feeling overwhelmed, increased anxiety, or depression. It is important to invest the requisite resources to train key faculty and staff who interact closely with students to identify concerning signs and symptoms of students in distress. These same faculty and staff should also be made aware of the resources available for students so that they can be properly referred for more assistance. All medical services provided to students should be confidential and information should not be shared with medical school administrators without student permission. There are students who are reluctant to take advantage of mental health services provided by the school due to concerns around confidentiality and access to medical records. As programmes work to provide broad, but thorough, mental health services for their students, it is crucial to aggressively manage the confidentiality of all student encounters with mental health professionals affiliated with school. Careful planning on location of services to provide privacy must also be prudently considered.

Incorporating healthy physical activity is also paramount in promoting a healthier lifestyle and to achieve all the benefits of regular exercise. Medical students should be provided with convenient options for recreational activities and getting involved in regular physical activity. Many medical schools include a recreational fee in their student fees that covers the cost for an in-house gym membership or access to a local fitness facility through subsidized cost programmes. Others may offer discounts to local chain gyms where students can purchase a membership. As medical students are interacting with patients they are learning the benefits of regular exercise. These interactions may also encourage medical students to serve as role models and to adapt a healthier lifestyle. Some medical students may even feel the pressure to serve as a role model for patients and might find discouragement when they perceive that they are not a good patient role model. A large number of medical students were actively involved in intramural sports programs at their undergraduate institutions, and it is not uncommon to have a cohort of medical students who were Division 1 athletes, which lends itself to healthy competition and bonding through sport. Competitions between classes, learning communities, colleges or societies are wonderful outlets for students that promote health and well-being while also setting the stage for interpersonal development and relationship/team-building. Many students enjoy participating in intramural sports and these groups can be arranged through students or school representatives. Many students appreciate the opportunity to participate in sporting activities with peers and a variety of intramural teams can be formed.

A mixture of outreach activities should also be incorporated and accessible to all students. Workshops that should be considered include coping skills, stress reduction, time management, financial planning, and healthy eating habits. Other activities that should be considered are yoga, recreational activities, meditation, and pet therapy. It is beneficial to introduce these initiatives early on so that when students are faced with obstacles and feeling overwhelmed they are already familiar with available resources and services offered by the institution and the surrounding community. These activities should be highly publicised and are examples of activities that can be student initiated and/or led.

Interpersonal Development

Medicine involves working in teams to ensure that patients receive quality care. Good interpersonal skills are among several cornerstone elements of strong team dynamics. Interpersonal development is a key component of a wellness programme in that it helps students achieve balance in their lives. Interpersonal development can enrich the medical student experience by building self-esteem, providing leadership opportunities, and improving communication skills. Individual medical schools must explore ways they can promote the development of their trainee's interpersonal skills.

Medical students need to develop strong verbal and non-verbal skills during their training that will last throughout their career. Medical students will interact with a variety of patients and strong interpersonal skills will be vital to creating a strong physician: patient bond leading to the best possible patient outcomes. Physicians have to be good communicators with their patients. They have to be equally good at listening and will need to have ample opportunities to practice their interpersonal skills. Many schools will incorporate multiple standardised patient encounters in which students can practise their interpersonal skills. It is important for students to be given feedback so they can work on ways they can improve their interpersonal skills and also so they are made aware of their strong points. Group service events that involve small or larger groups of peers are another good method to incorporate activities that help improve interpersonal skills. Students will find satisfaction in being of service to others and working alongside their peers. Service provides an additional avenue to address the holistic wellness of students. Incorporating other types of social activities is also a good way to improve networking and interpersonal interaction among peers.

Opportunities to participate in interprofessional educational activities should be considered if logistically feasible. This allows students to work on their communication with other health professionals and feel more comfortable with being a part of an interdisciplinary team. It is prudent to allow students the opportunity to work with other disciplines early on to fully grasp and understand the important roles of each team member.

Financial Wellness

Financial counselling is a key area that is often given only a cursory treatment in the undergraduate medical education curriculum or that is overlooked completely. Medical school must be considered as a full-time job for the student, hence, medical students are generally not able to work while attending school full time. This can create a tremendous financial strain for a significant number of students, many of whom are financial independent or whom serve as heads of households. Furthermore, a good number of medical students enter medical school with a debt burden accumulated at the undergraduate level. Numerous public medical schools offer in-state tuition at a rate that is reasonably affordable, however, of the AAMC's 143 allopathic medical schools, students graduating from a significant number of those institutions will carry into residency a sizeable amount of debt based on tuition fees alone. Based on geographical location of the school, living expenses substantially increase that debt burden.

Financial challenges can be a significant source of stress and anxiety for students, particularly those who are not accustomed to being in debt. For example, if a student has food insecurity or concerns about affording their daily living expenses they will be placed under a tremendous amount of daily stress. To help students anticipate the costs of medical school beyond tuition and fees, schools should designate an appropriate time during each year of the curriculum to inform students about financial resources and funding options. Topics to address include fiscal responsibility, using credit wisely, subsidised and unsubsidised loans, etc. During the first-year students might have to adjust to living on a budget if this is the first time they are not being supported by their parents. During the second-year students will have to cover expenses related to Step 1 of their United States Medical Licensing Examination. They will have to pay registration fees and consider expenses related to test preparation. During the fourth year of medical school there needs to be funds budgeted for residency applications and for traveling to residency interviews. If a student ends up matching to a programme in a different city then they will need to budget funds for relocation.

As part of a comprehensive wellness programme consideration needs to be given on the financial burden that medical students will face during medical school and beyond. Opportunities for scholarships should be visible and shared with all students. Financial aid counsellors must be available and give information on debt management and loan repayment options. Working with students on topics such as budgeting and financial wellness should be incorporated from the beginning of medical school.

Medical students must have an understanding that funds that they have received in the form of loans will have to be paid back and that they will accumulate interest until they are paid off. They need to be taught about forbearance versus deferment of student loan payments and understand the implications of both. Financial aid counsellors must work with medical students to explain the different types of repayment plans and the pros and cons of these different plans. Students should be encouraged to pay off student loan debt as soon as possible after training. Information should be given to students about programmes that offer loan repayment in exchange for service in certain specialties or in underserved populations. Students should familiarise themselves with these programmes and be provided with contact information in the event that they would like to get more detailed information. Students can also be made aware of options such as military scholarships and what is expected of them if they decide to pursue this route.

Another factor related to financial wellness should be resources that are available when a student finds themselves in need of emergency financial aid. Many students have unexpected expenses that might not be budgeted and find themselves in need of emergency financial aid. Others might not be good managers of money and have a hard time sticking to their budget which puts them in a bad financial situation. Financial aid counsellors should be prepared with information for emergency loans or grants. Medical schools can also consider budgeting a small amount of funds to be distributed to students who find themselves with an unexpected need. School administrators can decide if this will be a scholarship or a loan that is expected to be repaid. For many students, it is comforting to know that there is some type of aid available if needed and should be incorporated in a comprehensive wellness programme. It should be a goal to encourage responsible spending and budgeting as a student so that they will have financial wellness well beyond medical school.

SOLUTIONS AND RECOMMENDATIONS

Medical schools should design programming that is proactive and not just reactive in response to increased medical student stress, anxiety, and burnout. The creation and implementation of a comprehensive wellness programme is an example of a proactive initiative. Programming should be constantly evaluated to determine its efficacy. Each school should assess the needs of their individual medical school community and make sure any areas of concern with their students are being addressed. Some of the characteristics of medical education that emphasise outstanding performance might be explored as reinforcing, rather than potentially sabotaging, factors in creating a culture that promotes mental health (Schwenk et al., 2010).

FUTURE RESEARCH DIRECTIONS

Future research of the impact wellbeing programmes has on students would be useful for stakeholders to understand the long-term impact. Longitudinal studies that would follow trainees from medical school to residency to practicing physicians would also be of interest to assess the tools that improved their wellbeing. This type of study would also help to gain a better understanding of the major contributing factors to overall medical student wellbeing.

CONCLUSION

Medical student well-being is an important consideration during medical school. Many factors contribute to the well-being of medical students. Comprehensive wellness programmes should be designed that address both academic and non-academic sources of stress. Areas that can be addressed include academic support, occupational development, professionalism, self-care and interpersonal development. There must be buy in from students, high level administrators, and other key stakeholders. It is important to consider integrating student well-being as a part of the medical school curriculum. Administrators should understand that improving medical student wellness can contribute to more empathetic doctors and in the long term better quality health care.

REFERENCES

Brazeau, C. M. (2010). The Surest Way to Prevent Burnout in Medical School and Beyond. *Academic Medicine*, *85*(4), 569–570. doi:10.1097/ACM.0b013e3181d2d643 PMID:20354360

Dyrbye, L. N., West, C. P., Satele, D., Boone, S., Tan, L., Sloan, J., & Shanafelt, T. D. (2014). Burnout Among U.S. Medical Students, Residents, and Early Career Physicians Relative to the General U.S. Population. *Academic Medicine*, *89*(3), 443–451. doi:10.1097/ACM.0000000000000134 PMID:24448053

Epstein, R. M., & Krasner, M. S. (2013). Physician Resilience: What It Means, Why It Matters, and How to Promote It. *Academic Medicine*, *88*(3), 301–303. doi:10.1097/ACM.0b013e318280cff0 PMID:23442430

Flo, E., Pallesen, S., Magerøy, N., Moen, B. E., Grønli, J., Nordhus, I. H., & Bjorvatn, B. (2012, April). Shift Work Disorder in Nurses – Assessment, Prevalence and Related Health Problems. *PLoS ONE*, *7*(4), 1–9. doi:10.1371/journal.pone.0033981 PMID:22485153

Gaber, R. R., & Martin, D. M., (2002, May). Still-Well osteopathic medical student wellness program. *The Journal of the American Osteopathic Association*, *102*(5), 289–292. PMID:12033759

Jackson, E. R., Shanafelt, T. D., Hasan, O., Satele, D. V., & Dyrbye, L. N. (2016). Burnout and Alcohol Abuse/Dependence Among U.S. Medical Students. *Academic Medicine*, *91*(9), 1251–1256. doi:10.1097/ACM.0000000000001138 PMID:26934693

Kligler, B., Linde, B., & Katz, N. T. (2013, April). Becoming a Doctor: A Qualitative Evaluation of Challenges and Opportunities in Medical Student Wellness During the Third Year. *Academic Medicine*, *88*(4), 535–540. doi:10.1097/ACM.0b013e3182860e6d PMID:23425993

Ludwig, A. B., Burton, W., Weingarten, J., Milan, F., Myers, D. C., & Kligler, B. (2015, August 27). Depression and stress amongst undergraduate medical students. *BMC Medical Education*, *15*(141). PMID:26311538

Reed, D. A., Shanafelt, T. D., Satele, D. W., Power, D. V., Eacker, A., Harper, W., & Dyrbye, L. N. et al. (2011). Relationship of Pass/Fail Grading and Curriculum Structure with Well-Being Among Preclinical Medical Students: A Multi-Institutional Study. *Academic Medicine*, *86*(11), 1367–1373. doi:10.1097/ACM.0b013e3182305d81 PMID:21952063

Schwenk, T. L., Davis, L., & Wimsatt, L. A. (2010, September 15). Depression, Stigma, and Suicidal Ideation in Medical Students. *Journal of the American Medical Association*, *304*(11), 1181–1190. doi:10.1001/jama.2010.1300 PMID:20841531

Seritan, A. L., Rai, G., Servis, M., & Pomeroy, C. (2014, May 20). The Office of Student Wellness: Innovating to Improve Student Mental Health. *Academic Psychiatry*, *39*(1), 80–84. doi:10.1007/s40596-014-0152-5 PMID:24840666

Slavin, S. J., Schindler, D. L., & Chibnall, J. T. (2014). Medical Student Mental Health 3.0. *Academic Medicine*, *89*(4), 573–577. doi:10.1097/ACM.0000000000000166 PMID:24556765

Thomas, S., Haney, M., Pelic, C., Shaw, D., & Wong, J. (2011, March 31). Developing a Program to Promote Stress Resilience and Self-Care in First-Year Medical Students. *Canadian Medical Education Journal*, *2*(1), E32–E36. PMID:21822458

Wang, X., Armstrong, M. E., Cairns, B. J., Key, T. J., & Travis, R. C. (2011, March 25). Shift work and chronic disease: The epidemiological evidence. *Occupational Medicine*, *61*(2), 78–89. doi:10.1093/occmed/kqr001 PMID:21355031

KEY TERMS AND DEFINITIONS

Interpersonal Skills: The ability to work and get along with others.
Mentor: Someone who gives advice to a mentee.
Occupational Development: The process of developing towards a career.
Professionalism: Expected behaviour of a professional.
Stress Management: Methods to cope with one's stressors.
Wellness: A state of being in good health.

Chapter 9
Medical School Wellness Initiatives

Lynda Tierney Konecny
A. T. Still University, USA

ABSTRACT

In this chapter, wellness, and the importance of balance among wellness dimensions for medical students will be defined based on information found in relevant peer-reviewed and/or professional literature. Practical, evidence-based examples of wellness programme and initiatives within medical schools will be discussed. Benefits and challenges of the wellness program examples will be presented; limitations to programme results will be provided. Health education models and/or theory applicable to the needs assessment, development, implementation, and evaluation of medical school wellness programmes will be explored. Recommendations and best practices will be suggested to facilitate the practical implementation of wellness initiatives. A discussion of emerging trends will also be presented for future consideration.

INTRODUCTION

With the intensive demands faced by medical students, the medical education community must have current and relevant information to assist in making informed choices about how to develop and implement the most effective wellness programmes. Throughout their education, medical students often struggle with balance in dimensions of wellness, which contributes to mental health issues. Guidance both inside and outside the classroom to help medical students cope with being separated from families and friends, and the wide-range of personal challenges faced while attending medical training, should be provided. To enhance academic performance,

DOI: 10.4018/978-1-5225-2811-1.ch009

students and those within the medical education community should be taught how to recognise wellness imbalances, along with strategies that can be used to increase wellness equilibrium.

According to Agarwall and Lakel (2016) 'successful medical student wellness and professional development are critical areas in medical student education for students reaching optimal performance' (p. 105). The fact that medical students face challenges to mental health and overall wellness throughout their education is well-known and documented in relevant literature. Studies show medical students have higher rates of imbalances in wellness dimensions than their non-medical school peers in similar age groups. Reports of higher suicide rates among medical students than those within other academic disciplines are also alarming and create a sense of urgency to providing wellness interventions for these high-risk students. Medical students can experience extreme stress, anxiety, and depression which can ultimately affect not only their medical school performance, but also their effectiveness later as a practicing physician.

Wellness programming should be proactive and not only offered as reactive services within counselling departments. Outreach and education efforts should be incorporated into daily activities rather than relying on students to seek help when it may be too late and they are already in crisis. A culture in which students learn about and practice self-care, and care for peers, should be fostered. In addition, services that are available to students should be well-advertised. Not only should students be made aware of available wellness development options, faculty, staff, and administrators should also know what services and programmes are available.

Chapter objectives include:

- Evaluate current wellness initiatives and innovations.
- Describe future wellness initiative trends within medical schools.
- Define wellness and the importance of balance in wellness dimensions specifically for medical students.
- Identify an appropriate wellness model to meet medical student and institutional needs.
- Explain how health education models and theory can be applied to develop, implement, and assess wellness programmes for medical students.

BACKGROUND

Wellness Defined

Offering wellness programmes is not a new concept. Programmes in a variety of formats, some with incentives for participation, have long been available in businesses, educational institutions, and health care facilities. Often, programmes focus mainly on information about physical wellness, while others are more comprehensive considering multiple dimensions of wellness. However, while programme formats may differ greatly, the main goals are generally the same. Wellness programmes are offered to help people develop abilities to improve and maintain balance in dimensions of wellness. For individuals who are diagnosed with an illness, wellness programmes can increase opportunities for healing, and decrease risks associated with the illness. For those who are not experiencing health issues, programmes can improve participants' knowledge and skill-levels related to comprehensive wellness and well-being.

The World Health Organisation (WHO, 1948) defined health as 'a state of complete physical, mental and social well-being and not merely the absence of disease or infirmity' (n.p.). The WHO health definition has not been modified since its development in 1948, and includes what some would consider dimensions or components of *wellness*. There are many wellness models available, and in general they cover dimensions to include maintaining balance in areas such as physical, social, emotional, career/occupational, educational/intellectual, environmental, and spiritual. Medical students, in general, face challenges in balancing school, work, family, and other daily activities or concerns.

Importance of Developing Medical Student Wellness

Dunn, Iglewicz, and Moutier (2008) found that medical students dealing with the stressors related to their education suffer high incidents of depression and substance abuse. When medical students begin their educational journey, their rates of depression are equivalent to students pursuing other majors. Unfortunately, as they advance in their medical education, their rates of depression increase and exceed their nonmedical counterparts. Dunn et al. (2008) reported that as many as 56% of medical students experience depression and anxiety. Often, students continue to experience imbalances in wellness dimensions beyond medical school. Teaching medical students about the importance of balance in wellness dimensions early in their medical school career can help them maintain balance in wellness dimensions during school, into their postgraduate training, and beyond. Dunn et al. (2008) concluded that being a good physician requires the skills to maintain balance in wellness, professionalism, and to demonstrate empathy. To develop these coping skills, students must be taught self-care and awareness. When physicians can care for themselves, they will be more effective at caring for others.

McGrady, Brennan, Lynch, and Whearty (2012) conducted a study over a four-year period including 449 medical students randomly assigned to either an intervention or a control group. The purpose of the study was to determine the effectiveness of a structured wellness programme on levels of anxiety and depression, and physical illness. The programme included eight, 45-minute sessions for first-year medical students. During the sessions, students were taught stress management techniques. Study participants completed three assessments throughout their first year of medical school. McGrady et al. (2012) explained that the first assessment was completed during orientation before students began taking classes and experiencing the stressors of medical school, so improvement of assessment results may have been artificially inflated. The sample included only those students who volunteered and provided informed consent, and the study participants were students from only a single medical school.

According to McGrady et al. (2012), intervention group results were compared to those of a programme mewait-listed control group. In both the intervention and control group, women showed higher instances of illness than men. In addition, illness was more frequent in students experiencing significant, stressful life events. Comparison of findings between the intervention and control groups showed significantly less depression among those who participated in the wellness programme. Although there was no significant effect on anxiety or instances of illness, those assigned to the intervention group experienced less depression. In particular, participants who were identified as high-risk based on assessment results, maintained their level of wellness through the end of the school year. McGrady et al. (2012) concluded that structured wellness programmes can help reduce instances of psychological distress among medical students. Students expressed satisfaction with the stress management wellness programming and indicated they would recommend participation to other first-year students.

In an article by Stark, Hoekstra, Lindstrom Hazel, and Barton (2012), the authors discussed the anticipated shortage of health care providers, and increased work-related stress because of strains placed on the health care system. As the number of older adults increases, the decreasing number of health care professionals face greater challenges in balancing additional work loads and work/life demands. A lack of balance in dimensions of wellness can cause health care providers to experience more stress than ever before. Stark et al. (2012) indicated, in addition to increased health care professional recruitment efforts, focus must also be made on retaining those within the profession. Stark et al. (2012) proposed integration of stress management and wellness programmes within health care education to provide professionals with coping skills before they enter the workforce.

Stark et al. (2012) conducted a study with the purpose of determining the effectiveness of a health promotion programme on health behaviours of students. The health promotion information was integrated into a required course for students. The study consisted of 201 participants, assigned to either an intervention or comparison group, who were enrolled in a variety of the health care majors offered at the institution. The researchers used a pretest/posttest design and compared assessment results of students who participated in the course with the incorporated health promotion information to results of a comparison group of students who took the course without the additional health promotion information. In the intervention, students were taught the value of self-care and how their ability to maintain balance in dimensions of wellness would allow them to be more effective health care providers. Participants were also guided through the development of a personal health care plan based on results of a wellness assessment. In addition, students participated in journaling, reflection exercises, and discussions.

In the study, Stark et al. (2012) defined healthy behaviours as 'self-initiated actions that promote health and well-being' (p. 396). The valid and reliable assessment tool used measured participant's self-perceptions of personal responsibility for health, levels of physical activity, nutrition, spirituality, stress management skills, and interpersonal relationships. Analysis of data showed the comparison group had significantly lower scores in the areas of physical activity and nutrition than the comparison group who participated in the course with incorporated health promotion information. In addition, those in the intervention group showed significant increases in scores related to the area of health responsibility. Although there were several limitations to the study such as small sample size, including students from only one institution, and some participant attrition, researchers concluded that including wellness education in health care curriculum would benefit students throughout their educations and careers.

Drolet and Rogers (2010) advised that there must be both proactive and reactive measures to providing wellness services and meeting wellness needs of medical students. Proactive approaches and prevention are ideal. Students should be taught how to recognise signs of issues caused by imbalances in wellness. In addition, students should learn pre-emptive coping skills, and what resources are available for continued growth and development. Unfortunately, there are times when proactive measures are not enough and reactive programmes and services must be made available. Sometimes, wellness imbalances are not identified until they cause issues academically, socially, spiritually, or in any of the other dimensions of wellness (Drolet & Rogers, 2010).

Wellness Initiatives and Innovations

An early adopter of student wellness initiatives, A.T. Still University's Kirksville College of Osteopathic Medicine (KCOM), established the *Still-Well* student wellness programme in 1991. The programme was originally designed for first- and second-year medical students. The theme of the program is 'I am my own first patient' and emphasises the importance of balance in mind, body, and spirit (Gaber & Martin, 2002, p. 289). The programme developers considered the concept that wellness is important for students to model for patients. Students learn about Still-Well during new-student orientation where they are invited to participate in wellness assessments and join wellness teams. Still-Well initiatives are team-based consisting of student and faculty/staff volunteers. The wellness programme is comprehensive emphasizing balance in seven dimensions of wellness to include: physical, social, emotional, spiritual, environmental, professional, and intellectual (Gaber & Martin, 2002). Wellness teams offer programmes throughout the year specific to their wellness dimension, or offer collaborative programmes developed with members of other teams. Still-Well is still ongoing and programming is offered to all health sciences students enrolled in the University.

The Vanderbilt Medical Student (VMS) Wellness Programme was established in 2005 and designed to be primarily a proactive means of addressing medical student wellness (Drolet & Rogers 2010). The VMS Wellness Program focuses on reaching students at each stage in their medical education and includes information and interventions to address a variety of wellness dimensions. The focus of the programme is mainly on learning the value of self-care, and providing long-term programming to continue delivering the message and services to students. Reports by students indicate the programming efforts are successful and benefit both individuals and the peer cohorts as well. The VMS Wellness Programme is an organised, longitudinal program designed to address 'specific stress points' throughout the medical student's education (Drolet & Rogers, 2010, p. 103). The programme also includes contingencies to address unforeseen events in students' lives which may add stress, such as, death in the family. The VMS Wellness Programme is organised to include involvement and inclusion at the student level, within curriculum, and faculty involvement. At all levels, programming is provided to include mentoring/advising, student leadership, and programming to foster personal growth.

Vanderbilt Medical School Wellness Program includes dimensions defined as intellectual, environmental, physical, emotional/spiritual, and interpersonal. Each dimension has been aligned with a student-run committee designed to develop programmes and interventions for their specific dimension(s) (Drolet & Rogers, 2010). The *Mentoring* committee is associated with intellectual wellness and offers programming such as a student mentor/mentee system, online course reviews, and student-centred orientations. The *Body* committee aligns with physical wellness and offers information about proper nutrition and sleep benefits, classes on healthy meal preparation, online and face-to-face fitness physical fitness options, and various physical dimensions challenges. For emotional and spiritual wellness, the *Mind* committee was formed. The Mind committee includes therapy options, and teaches or provides various means in which students can express themselves. The *Social* group deals specifically with interpersonal wellness and engages both online and residential students in different events. *Community* is broad and, in essence, includes environmental wellness, but in definition includes much more. Through the student lounge, study areas, and various surveys, it is apparent the Community group can actually be applicable to multiple dimensions of wellness beyond the originally intended environmental dimensions. The VMS programme is considered to be quite comprehensive and is referenced in many articles and scholarly works in which student wellness programmes and initiatives are discussed.

Another wellness programme, *WellMed,* intended to address several dimensions of wellness to include: health, mental, spiritual, fitness, nutrition, intellectual, social, and financial, was developed and implemented by Ludwig et al. (2015). The programme was offered to students within one institution, and was designed to enhance services already available to students. Ludwig et al. (2015) reported there has been increased attention to the need for wellness programming to be incorporated into medical education curriculum. The Association of American Medical Colleges and Institute of Medicine have recognised the need, and endorsed efforts to increase programmes designed to promote medical student wellness. Several institutions are incorporating wellness programmes into their medical training, but little evidence of the effectiveness of the programmes is available.

The WellMed programme developed and implemented by Ludwig et al. (2015) was designed to have an effect on students' levels of depression, stress, and wellness behaviours. The researchers first administered a needs assessment to identify wellness behaviour trends between first- and third-year medical students. The needs assessment results showed significant increases in self-reported stress-levels and depression risks between the end of the first year, and the end of the third year of medical school. Based on the results of the needs assessment, researchers created the comprehensive WellMed programme offered to all students within the institution. The initiative included students, faculty, and administrators who provided programming along with processes to link students with appropriate services through WellMed connections. Since its implementation, WellMed has been expanded to include mindfulness training and peer mentoring. Ludwig et al. (2015) reported that programme expansion and evaluation of effectiveness will continue.

Hassed, de Lisle, Sullivan, and Pier (2009) established a wellness programme for medical students at one institution titled the *Health Enhancement Program.*

Hassed et al. (2009) reported that, prior to entering medical school, medical students demonstrate wellness levels equal to their non-medical school bound peers. However, as they enter medical school and progress through their education, their levels of wellness decrease at a higher rate than students studying other majors. Hassed et al. (2009) explained that the programme is based on the ESSENCE wellness model addressing wellness dimensions of:

- *Education: the importance of knowledge and reflection*
- *Stress management: the importance of mental health. Intervention covered in the mindfulness program*
- *Spirituality: the role of meaning and/or spirituality on coping, health and illness*
- *Exercise: the importance and application of physical activity*
- *Nutrition: the role of healthy nutrition and the influences on eating patterns*
- *Connectedness: the role of social support for wellbeing and healthcare*
- *Environment: creating a healthy physical, emotional and social environment* (p. 391).

In addition to the ESSENCE model components, the programme also addressed the concept of mindfulness.

According to Hassed et al. (2009), the Health Enhancement Programme was incorporated into the medical school curriculum and consisted of eight lectures covering each of the ESSENCE elements. In addition, participants attended six, two-hour structured tutoring sessions which were facilitated by trained mentors. Each group consisted of approximately 15 students. During the sessions, elements of the ESSENCE model were explored. The tutors guided the students, but discussions and concepts were based on student input and needs. Between sessions, participants were asked to practice mindfulness and the concepts covered in the sessions. Participants also wrote journal entries documenting their experiences and perceptions. Hassed et al. (2009) reported that the evaluation of journal entries and student assessments showed most students found the programme helpful, but some found it 'philosophically challenging' (p. 392).

Hassed et al. (2009) evaluated the efficacy of the Health Enhancement Programme on influencing psychological factors and quality of life. The assessment used was administered twice to participants and primarily gauged depression, anxiety, and hostility of medical students. The administration of the first assessment occurred halfway through a semester. The second survey administration took place during the week prior to final exams. Even though the programme was incorporated into the medical school curriculum, participation in the study was voluntary. Of a possible 270 participants, 148 completed both assessments for comparison. Analysis of survey results showed most students used mindfulness practises after participation in the wellness programme. Results also showed increased wellness in each of the dimensions assessed. Statistically significant differences were noted in depression, hostility, and psychological areas. The researchers claimed this study was the first to demonstrate the value of wellness programing merged with a curriculum in improving medical student wellness, or at least reducing decreases in wellness during particularly stressful periods of medical school. Limits to the study included a small sample size, lack of control group, and a relatively short research timeframe; however, results show the potential of programmes in enhancing student wellness.

In response to an observed growth in medical student stress, decrease in wellness, and the American Association of Medical Colleges endorsement of increasing wellness initiatives for medical students, Wiles (2015) implemented evidence-based programmes and changes to wellness efforts within a medical school. Wiles (2015) reported, even though medical students have already passed many educational hurdles, the unique challenges of medical school can be alarming. Wiles (2015) asserted there is a hidden curriculum in medical school to press forward regardless of personal difficulties. Students are not encouraged to deal with their personal wellness while learning about and encountering the illness and suffering of others.

Wiles (205) began efforts to enhance medical student wellness by renaming existing mental health offerings to include the term wellness. The goal was to make the services more attractive and accessible to students by focusing on proactive wellness programming rather than just reactive treatment for students already experiencing difficulties. By emphasizing the importance and value of continually maintaining balance in dimensions of wellness, students who sought services increased three times in number over a three-year period. In addition to destigmatising wellness programmes, Wiles (2015) increased the number of interdisciplinary professionals available to provide services such as cognitive behavioural counselling to students.

In addition to renaming the mental health centre and increasing services offered, Wiles (2015) implemented outreach programmes to raise awareness among students not actively seeking treatment or services. Wellness surveys were administered to all incoming students to determine levels of wellness. Wiles (2015) reported that the administration of surveys was also considered a proactive measure to help educate students about the stressors and imbalances that can occur in medical school. Wiles (2015) used a wellness wheel model as a visual to teach students skills to rebalance dimensions of wellness. A mentoring programme was also incorporated into the curriculum each week. During the mentoring sessions, students explored wellness assessment results and shared ideas on ways to maintain their own wellness and how to be available for their peers. Students had input in creating wellness programmes to be offered throughout the year, including a week where activities specific to different dimensions of wellness were offered each day. According to Wiles (2015), one of the most popular programmes was one focused on 'mindful medication' which was given by professionals experienced in the area (n.p.). Wiles (2015) reported that mindfulness mediation is an evidence-based practise shown effective in decreasing stress and student burnout.

In another wellness initiative, Kushner, Kessler, and McGaghie (2011) used behaviour change plans to teach the importance of developing wellness coping self-care skills to medical students. In their study, Kushner et al. (2011), second-year medical students enrolled in a required course completed the behaviour change plan. The programme focused on elements of wellness such as nutrition, physical fitness, hygiene, study skills, emotional wellness, and sleep. The behaviour change plan required students to select an area of wellness they wanted to improve and establish goals. Students monitored their own progress and determined their level of success. Kushner et al. (2011) administered a posttest incorporating both qualitative and quantitative elements to study participants evaluating perceptions about the behaviour change plan experience.

Kushner et al. (2011) reported varied results based on the one-group posttest of the behaviour change plan programme. The study included a sample of 343 students and the majority of students established fitness change goals. In addition, popular dimensions identified as in need of change included nutrition and sleep. Of the 343 students, 139 reported they achieved their goals, while 170 did not. Thirty-four students were unable to determine whether goals were obtained. Kushner et al. (2011) reported that analysis of quantitative data showed the only significant self-reported improvements were in the area of sleep. Analysis of qualitative data showed students felt more knowledgeable about the importance of establishing behaviour change plans and tracking progress.

Interesting case reports were included in results reported by Kushner et al. (2011). For example, researchers shared detailed information from student 1:

Student 1 set his goal as getting 60 minutes of exercise (20 minutes of cardiovascular training and 40 minutes of weight lifting) five times each week at a local gym. He decided on this BCP because "often the first thing that gets cut out of my schedule is exercise because of perceived lack of energy and/or time. However, I believe that exercising 60 minutes a day will help me focus more while studying and also help me get better sleep." His baseline monitoring showed that he went to the gym three times the first week, but only once in the following two weeks. During the six weeks he implemented his BCP, he was able to steadily increase his exercise to five times per week (Figure 1). Student 1 reported, "The most important factor in achieving the goal was my motivation to remain healthy while being busy with my M2 workload. Also, my roommate motivated me to go to the gym with him." Student 1 learned that "it is easier to set a goal than to actually carry it out. While I had an ambitious goal..., I was not 100% successful although I did make improvements" (pp. 93-94)

Almost 80% of students included in the study indicated they felt healthier after participating in the programme. Overall, students reported feeling more competent at maintaining balance in dimensions of wellness and would use the behaviour change plan in the future.

Agarwall and Lakel (2016) conducted a four-year programme to educate medical students about challenges they may face during their careers. In addition, the programme emphasised the development of positive psychology and resilience. Throughout the programme, students were taught the value of self-assessment and self-care, and the importance of caring for their peers. Agarwall and Lakel (2016) stated there was a high risk of drop-out when students began medical school, and throughout their medical training students struggled with burnout and depression. Studies by Agarwall and Lakel (2016) showed the issues were greatest during the first two years of academic training. Based on those findings, the authors developed a wellness programme encouraging a proactive approach to enhancing student wellness by increasing awareness of possible stressors and the potential effects. The authors indicated a belief that medical students are initially unaware of the hidden curriculum in medical school, so emphasized providing information to students on what to expect and how to self-monitor reactions and actions. Through providing wellness education, the authors hoped to have a positive effect on medical student retention and satisfaction extending throughout their careers.

The course implemented by Agarwall and Lakel (2016) included an emphasis on positive psychology. Students were taught how to use positive psychology to 'foster resilience and achieve optimal personal functioning' (p. 105). The authors also included information to enhance cultural awareness of medical school and the medical profession. Students were educated on the prevalence of common concerns among those in the medical profession. By increasing awareness, the hope was a healthier culture where open communication about the need for balance in wellness dimensions was emphasized would be encouraged and increased. If the culture does not promote self-care and help-seeking, wellness initiatives are less likely to be successful (Agarwall & Lakel, 2016).

In their programme, Agarwall and Lakel (2016) incorporated programme goals during each of the four years of the students' medical education. Class cohorts were assigned a faculty member who served as mentor throughout their academic training. Classes of students were also randomly divided into small groups who met for one hour each month. Throughout the course, students followed a structured programme and responded, in online blog format, to pre-determined questions. The topics were designed to promote self-assessment and discussion among peers both online and during the small group meetings. By using blogs, the programme developers hoped to provide avenues for students of varying personality styles and learning types to communicate. The programme implemented by Agarwall and Lakel (2016) focused primarily on psychological aspects of wellness, and did not include other dimensions such as spiritual and physical. Analysis of the programme showed the majority of students (82%) felt the course enhanced their ability to self-reflect and increased knowledge of the necessity to seek assistance if needed. Students reported often feeling isolated during medical school, and the small groups provided opportunities to connect with peers in a safe environment to share experiences. Although most students provided positive feedback about the experience, some expressed discomfort at sharing personal information with assigned peer groups consisting of people they did not know. Efforts continue to enhance the course and improve effectiveness.

Slavin, Schindler, and Chibnall (2014) approached medical student wellness by incorporating information and initiatives into the core curriculum of one medical school. As with some of the other wellness initiatives implemented within medical schools, the focus of the programme was on the mental well-being of students. Programme administrators hoped to create an incorporated, proactive approach to increasing student wellness rather than a supplementary, reactive programme that may not reach all students. Slavin, et al. (2014) stated that changes were made to course content to include how classes were scheduled and graded. Positive psychology and an emphasis on the individual guided the programme design. Mindfulness training was also incorporated with participation required of the students.

Specific curricular changes outlined by Slavin et al. (2014) included changing the grading system from an assigned letter grade, to one of pass/fail. The hope was that removing the letter grade would help reduce stress-levels associated with competition among students. The researchers found the majority of students experienced stress and/or depression during the first two years of medical school. Because of the risks linked with increased stress and depression, the authors also reduced contact hours during the first two years. The reduction in contact hours provided students additional elective opportunities. In terms of electives, the options and lengths were expanded allowing students more freedom to pursue personal areas of interest. Outside the classroom, learning communities were established in which students could interact with a faculty mentor to help design and guide wellness programming (Slavin et al., 2014).

Although the programme presented by Slavin et al. (2014) was not designed as an experiment with intervention and comparison groups for comparison, the programme was considered successful. The method of integrating changes to the academic programme was relatively inexpensive, yet resulted in lower reported rates of depression and stress. Programming and the use of learning communities also enhanced the culture of the medical school when compared to data collected prior to programme implementation. Slavin et al. (2014) stated that incorporating wellness elements into standard curricular requirements can provide a new, unique way to positively affect medical student wellness.

Wellness programming and initiatives within medical schools have been developed using a variety of modes of implementation. Some wellness programmes are ancillary, while others are integrated into the medical school curriculum. As discussed, comprehensive wellness models have been used for some programmes, while others have focused primarily on a few dimensions. Overall, the goals are to increase students' abilities to handle medical school and professional stress, decrease depression, and increase medical professional retention. Students are taught the value of self-reflection and given the opportunity to learn and practice coping skills. Some programmes have been developed based on health education theory and models. Using health education theory and models as a basis upon which to build medical school wellness initiatives, regardless of the mode of delivery, can help with successful planning, preparation, implementation, and evaluation.

APPLICATION OF HEALTH EDUCATION MODELS AND THEORY TO MEDICAL STUDENT WELLNESS PROGRAMMES

Health Education Models and Theory

Health education theory and models serve as frameworks for the development of programmes intended to improve the health and well-being of individuals. Programming can be geared to the individual, or for groups. The effectiveness and value of using structured health education planning for health promotion has often been overlooked. Some of the barriers to using health education stems from a lack of understanding of the purpose, and lack of knowledge about health programme planning and evaluation. In addition, because of the fluid and applied nature of health programming, effectiveness can be difficult to document. However, there are plenty of published, professional articles describing successful programmes supporting the value of implementing health education. Based on the demonstrated value of health education and health promotion, using health education theories and models for the development of wellness programmes is an important part of the process. There are several health education theories and models, but for the purposes of developing wellness programming for medical students some of the most applicable include: The Theory of Planned Behaviour, Transtheoretical Model of Change, and the Health Belief Model.

Stark et al. (2012) discussed the value of using the Theory of Planned Behaviour as a framework when designing wellness programmes for health care students.

According to Stark et al. (2012) the Theory of Planned Behaviour developed by Icek Ajzen in 1985 provides a solid model to guide the development of wellness initiatives. The first step in any wellness programme should be to assess students' perceptions of wellness among the various dimensions. Not only does this serve as a tool of assessment, students also receive a certain amount of education on what is involved in *wellness*.

With the Theory of Planned Behaviour 'intent is influenced not only by the attitude towards behaviour but also the perception of social norms (the strength of others' opinions on the behaviour and a person's own motivation to comply with those of significant others)' with consideration for self-perceptions of control over one's ability to perform specific behaviours (World Health Organisation [WHO], 2012, p. 8). The Theory of Planned Behaviour incorporates variables students experience that may be beyond their control. Within the Theory of Planned Behaviour, a normative belief is described as what people think others expect of them while a subjective norm is the perception of social pressures on performance and behaviours. Control belief is described as the perception of available resources and opportunities, and perceived behavioural control is a determination of how difficult achieving a goal may be.

The Theory of Planned Behaviour has been applied to wellness initiatives in a variety of settings to include educational institutions and work places. To be successful, the wellness programmes must be designed so students have positive perceptions of their own expectations and subjective norms regarding wellness. Medical students are often very scheduled and motivated. The Theory of Planned Behaviour works well as a framework for programme development because of the emphasis on the individual's ability to control his or her behaviours (Simons-Morton, McLeroy, & Wendel, 2012). When using the Theory of Planned Behaviour, student attitudes and how factors such as age, gender, race, cultural norms, and other environmental influences affect intentions are considered. When individuals believe they are in control, they are more likely to participate in programmes to work toward behaviour change and balance in dimensions of wellness (Simons-Morton et al., 2012).

The Transtheoretical Model, initially developed by Prochaska and DiClemnete in 1983, is described by the WHO (2012) as promoting behaviour change by 'a progression through a series of five stages: pre-contemplation, contemplation, preparation, action and maintenance' (p. 8). Each stage represents different needs of the individual. Being well-versed in the stages of change can guide programming and provide information for individuals based on where they are in the progression through stages. An interesting concept to consider when using the Transtheoretical Model is that students can move back and forth between stages at any point in life. Teaching self-reflection and the importance of self-awareness are vital to the success of wellness programmes and maintenance of wellness behaviours.

A lot of literature and research exists in which the application and effectiveness of the Transtheoretical Model is described. Learning about what happens at each stage of change helps ensure programme information is comprehensive and inclusive. Knowing behaviour change is fluid and individualised helps guide strategies to accommodate students at each stage. The Transtheoretical Model emphasises self-efficacy, and the ability of participants to make well-informed decisions. Attempts of progression from one stage to the next without adequate information can often result in regression. Table 1 includes definitions of each stage, and strategies that can be used to promote change.

The Health Belief Model is 'one of the earliest behaviour change models to explain human health decision-making and subsequent behaviour is based on the following six constructs: perceived susceptibility, severity, benefits and barriers, cues to action and self-efficacy' (WHO, 2012, p. 7). According to McKenzie, Neiger, and Thackeray (2013), the Health Belief Model is very often used when examining health behaviors. The Health Belief Model, which was created in the 1950s, is considered a 'value-expectancy theory' (McKenzie et al., 2013, p. 173). Value-expectancy theories are those for which individuals who are involved assume that behaviour change will result in some sort of consequence. The expectation can be either various negative consequences based on lack of change, or positive consequences resulting from change. Participants determine their own level of significance to the results of change or lack of change and base decisions on self-perceptions (McKenzie et al., 2013).

McKenzie et al. (2013) asserted that taking steps toward change is dependent on at least three areas of concern. The first area includes a component of relevance.

Table 1. Transtheoretical Model

Stage	Definition	Change Strategy
Precontemplation	No intention of taking action within the next six months.	Provide information about the need for change to include benefits and risks.
Contemplation	Intends to take action within the next six months	Offer inspiration and encourage goal setting.
Preparation	Intends to take action within the next 30 days and has taken some behavioural steps in this direction.	Make available resources to develop and implement wellness plan. Teach self-assessment techniques.
Action	Has changed behaviour for less than six months.	Encourage on-going self-evaluation. Provide individualised and peer group support services.
Maintenance	Has changed behaviour for more than six months.	Aid student when coping with challenges. Establish a system of reminders and a variety of wellness options.

Note: Transtheoretical Model of Change. Adapted from: (World Health Organisation, 2012)

In implementing a wellness programme, students must be educated about the concerns or risks associated with lack of balance in dimensions of wellness. There must be sufficient information to help motivate students to change unhealthy, and/ or incorporate positive behaviours. The second area addresses knowledge about vulnerability. Students must be made aware of why they are at risk for depression, stress, or anxiety during medical school. Programmes should include information about the many stressors of medical school and why the environment can cause imbalances in wellness. The third area includes educating individuals about why the programmes and services offered would be beneficial in reducing risks associated with medical school. Medical students should be educated about the importance in fully participating in wellness programmes. During this awareness process, barriers to student participation must be addressed and solutions offered. Barriers can be internal, such as lack of self-efficacy, or external, such as scheduling, so solutions must be broad-based and inclusive (McKenzie et al., 2013).

The use of health education theories and models supports the development, implementation, and evaluation of health promotion programmes. Theories help program planners to understand behaviours and beliefs driving decisions. Models provide guidance in developing systematic strategies in designing health education programmes. The theory and models presented in this chapter are those that either have been used and proven effective in wellness programming, or are applicable based on evidence and information in relevant literature. Even with evidence-based success information available, there can be barriers the development and implementation of wellness initiatives within medical schools.

SOLUTIONS AND RECOMMENDATIONS

Application of Health Education Theory and Models for Medical Student Wellness Initiatives

Hobson (2013) reported that about half of medical students showed signs of emotional destress, which can lead to burnout. Burnout can affect how medical students, and then physicians, perform daily functions going as far as the reporting physical examinations without actually conducting them. In Hobson's (2013) article, she confirmed that most medical students consider themselves to be 'type A' and have to be encouraged to consider personal wellness and balance (n.p.). Because of the concerns of medical student wellness, medical schools are required to offer wellness programmes in order to be accredited.

There is a gap of information in related literature and resources about what should or should not be included in medical school wellness initiatives, and programme requirements or specifications are not defined. Most institutions focus on the physical dimensions (Hobson, 2013). Comprehensive wellness programmes may be a hard sell to school administrators and stakeholders who are considering budgets and resource allocation. Presenting an evidence-based, well-designed proposal based on a health education theory or models, and information about successes demonstrated by other programmes can be instrumental in gaining support for the wellness initiatives. However, even if support from administration and stakeholders is earned, students may resist programming efforts for a variety of reasons.

The comprehensive wellness efforts of institutions such as Vanderbilt University School of Medicine are well documented within relevant literature (Hobson, 2013). Overall, there is recognised success of programmes addressing several dimensions of wellness and promoting balance. The most successful programmes appear to be well-planned, grounded in health education theory and models, and evidence-based. Some wellness programmes consist of extracurricular activities available for student participation, and others incorporate changes to the medical school curriculum and mentoring opportunities to promote wellness (Hobson, 2013).

FUTURE RESEARCH DIRECTIONS

Because there are gaps between the wellness of medical students, wellness efforts provided to students, and requirements by accrediting bodies, action needs to be taken to enhance efforts and affect change. Seritan, Hunt, Shy, Rea, and Worley (2012) reported that even though the challenges faced by medical students is well-documented, the interrelation of wellness dimensions is not as understood. School administrators need to be made aware of the need to promote overall wellness and balance among the dimensions. Best practices should be developed based on needs assessments performed at institutions, and guided by appropriate health education theory and models.

Needs assessments should be conducted, and based on findings, decisions can be made about the most appropriate health education theory or model. Following a systematic approach, changes to medical school curriculum can be made, and wellness programmes developed and implemented. Assessments should be developed to provide quantitative and qualitative data for analysis to determine levels of success of wellness interventions. Formative assessment should be incorporated throughout the design and implementation of programmes, and adjustments made as appropriate. There are positive and negatives to any programming efforts, so every effort should be made to identify the weaknesses and continually refine wellness initiatives.

CONCLUSION

Wellness initiatives offered for medical students are gaining attention and popularity. Medical students face challenges during their education, and throughout their career causing high levels of stress, anxiety, and depression. Most wellness programmes do not address a comprehensive wellness model including a variety of dimensions and instead focus only on psychological or physical aspects of well-being. While those are very important aspects of wellness, a more inclusive approach should be adopted to address all aspects of student wellness. By emphasising balance in dimensions of wellness, students will become more self-aware, and learn how imbalance of even one of the dimensions of wellness can have an effect on the others.

Medical school administrators, faculty, staff, and students must determine what type of wellness programme would meet their needs and fit into their culture. During the planning process, health education theory and models should be incorporated to ensure a comprehensive wellness programme is designed and implemented. Following a health promotion structure will allow for easier and more efficient formative and summative assessment of results. Appropriate health education theory and models were described in this chapter, but because one size does not fit all, there are more available in the literature that can be reviewed for appropriateness and applied. Pros and cons of each must be evaluated and a process established incorporating representatives from all areas of the medical school to determine the best fit, and enhance buy-in for programme design and implementation. Regardless of programme type, the wellness initiative should be continually developed and enhanced.

REFERENCES

Agarwall, G., & Lakel, M. (2016). Personal transition to the profession: A novel longitudinal professional development and wellness medical student curriculum. *Academic Psychiatry*, *40*(1), 105–108. doi:10.1007/s40596-015-0463-1 PMID:26742500

Drolet, B. C., & Rodgers, S. (2010). A Comprehensive Medical Student Wellness Programme—Design and Implementation at Vanderbilt School of Medicine. *Academic Medicine*, *85*(1), 103–110. doi:10.1097/ACM.0b013e3181c46963 PMID:20042835

Dunn, L. B., Iglewicz, A., & Moutier, C. (2008). A conceptual model of medical student well-being: Promoting resilience and preventing burnout. *Academic Psychiatry*, *32*(1), 44–53. doi:10.1176/appi.ap.32.1.44 PMID:18270280

Gaber, R. R., & Martin, D. M. (2002). Still-Well osteopathic medical student wellness programme. *The Journal of the American Osteopathic Association, 102*(5), 289–292. Retrieved from http://jaoa.org/article.aspx?articleid=2092752 PMID:12033759

Hassed, C., de Lisle, S., Sullivan, G., & Pier, C. (2009). Enhancing the health of medical students: Outcomes of an integrated mindfulness and lifestyle programme. *Advances in Health Sciences Education : Theory and Practice, 14*(3), 387–398. doi:10.1007/s10459-008-9125-3 PMID:18516694

Hobson, K. (2013, March 21). New medical school programmes help students battle burnout. *U.S. News & World Report.* Retrieved from http://www.usnews.com/education/best-graduate-schools/top-medical-schools/articles/2013/03/21/new-medical-school-programs-help-students-battle-burnout

Kushner, R. F., Kessler, S., & McGaghie, W. C. (2011). Using behaviour change plans to improve medical student self-care. *Academic Medicine, 86*(7), 901–906. doi:10.1097/ACM.0b013e31821da193 PMID:21617509

Ludwig, A. B., Burton, W., Weingarten, J., Milan, F., Myers, D. C., & Kligler, B. (2015). Depression and stress amongst undergraduate medical students. *BMC Medical Education, 15*(141). doi:10.1186/s12909-015-0425-z PMID:26311538

McGrady, A., Brennan, J., Lynch, D., & Whearty, K. (2012). A wellness programme for first year medical students. *Applied Psychophysiology and Biofeedback, 37*(4), 253–260. doi:10.1007/s10484-012-9198-x PMID:22699926

McKenzie, J. F., Neiger, B. L., & Thackeray, R. (2013). *Planning, implementing, and evaluating health promotion programmes: a primer* (6th ed.). San Francisco: Pearson/Benjamin Cummings.

Seritan, A., Hunt, J., Shy, A., Rea, M., & Worley, L. (2012). The state of medical student wellness: A call for culture change. *Academic Psychiatry, 36*(1), 7–10. doi:10.1176/appi.ap.10030042 PMID:22362429

Simons-Morton, B. G., McLeroy, K. R., & Wendel, M. L. (2012). *Behaviuor theory in health promotion practice and research.* Sudbury, MA: Jones & Bartlett Learning.

Slavin, S. J., Schindler, D. L., & Chibnall, J. T. (2014). Medical student mental health 3.0: Improving student wellness through curricular changes. *Academic Medicine, 89*(4), 573–577. doi:10.1097/ACM.0000000000000166 PMID:24556765

Stark, M. A., Hoekstra, T., Lindstrom Hazel, D., & Barton, B. (2012). Caring for self and others: Increasing health care students' healthy behaviors. *Work (Reading, Mass.), 42*(3), 393–401. doi:10.3233/WOR-2012-1428 PMID:22523027

Wiles, P. (2015, August 18). Wellness and medical school: Aspiration - or pipe dream?. *Psychiatric Times*. Retrieved from http://www.psychiatrictimes.com/major-depressive-disorder/wellness-and-medical-school-aspiration-or-pipe-dream

World Health Organisation. (1948). *WHO definition of health*. Retrieved from http://www.who.int/about/definition/en/print.html

World Health Organisation. (2012). *Health education: Theoretical concepts, effective strategies and core competencies* [pdf file]. Retrieved from http://applications.emro.who.int/dsaf/EMRPUB_2012_ EN_1362.pdf

KEY TERMS AND DEFINITIONS

Balance in Dimensions of Wellness: The ability to self-assess or understand dimensions of wellness and how to ensure equality among dimensions.

Health Education: To develop and provide learning opportunities focused on improving health and wellness for individuals and communities.

Health Education Models: Models that provide guidance for the planning, implementing, and assessing health promotion programmes.

Health Education Theories: Theories that provide guidance in explaining how and why changes may occur.

Health Promotion: Implementing interventions designed to provide individuals with the knowledge and skills needed to make positive, healthy behaviour changes.

Hidden Curriculum: Unwritten expectation of medical students to push through stressors and not complain or seek assistance.

Mindfulness: Being aware of personal levels of wellness.

Positive Psychology: A field focused on emphasizing the meaningful and optimistic aspects of life. A change from the focus on reaction to dysfunction, to the promotion of enhancing personal fulfilment.

Wellness Dimension: A specific aspect of a wellness model such as spiritual, physical fitness, physical health, emotional, environmental, intellectual, occupational, and social.

Wellness Programmes: Structured initiatives designed to educate and promote balance in dimensions of wellness.

Section 5
The Future

Chapter 10
Essentials for Education and Training for Tomorrow's Physicians

Timothy Edward A. Barrett
University of the West Indies, Bahamas

ABSTRACT

Education and training of medical students and postgraduate residents must undergo a critical review in light of the changing times and attitudes. The demands of life in general are enough to provide significant stressors for today's students in addition to coping with pressures of balancing passing exams with meeting the expectations of family and instructors. This chapter will highlight the realities of the effect of the pressures of study on the students' mental health and well-being. It will then describe several changes that can be made to the way medical students are trained which then shifts the focus to personal growth and development and away from the traditional goals of knowledge, skills and competencies for the goal of passing the exams. In the end, this chapter will challenge readers and institutions to pause and reconsider the current approach to training of medical students.

INTRODUCTION

In this chapter, the author will attempt to articulate the concerns about the way medical students are developed into physicians. These concerns have been shared with other colleagues. These concerns have also been discussed with persons in sensitive administration positions over the years. However, even though there is a listening ear, the author does not seem to be able to convince the powers that be to

DOI: 10.4018/978-1-5225-2811-1.ch010

elevate the issues he will discuss to a level of priority that will result in changes to the way we train our medical students or our postgraduate residents. This chapter will focus on the realities of studying medicine today from the perspective of the whole person, as well as include suggestions to ameliorate the current conditions.

BACKGROUND

The demands of today's world are new and complex. The rapid development of technology and specifically computer technology and the internet have revolutionized every aspect of society and most significantly interpersonal dynamics. The glut of information that is readily available and the immediacy of global news are a two-edged sword in that one does not have to wait to be informed while on the other hand we often wish we had not heard some of the bad news. Social media have also had a profound impact on our interpersonal skills, eroding our face-to-face communication skills and the ability to deal with conflict while affecting our academics in that it appears that most people have to use a spell check to spell words.

Medical students and residents are not immune to the effects of this gradual but steady erosion of social skills in the author's opinion and therefore it is imperative to discuss the potential effects on the individual as well as the quality of health care services. The proper practice of medicine requires personal and interpersonal skills in addition to medical knowledge, skills and competencies. In the author's opinion the most beloved and effective doctors are not necessarily going to be the intellectually brilliant who never fail any exam and who are excellent technically, but will be those who embrace the opportunity to relieve suffering and improve the conditions of the *persons that they treat as patients* with warmth and genuineness. These are not the only character traits that are required but are fundamental and will be found consistently in the best physicians.

HISTORICAL CONSIDERATIONS

The author's impression based on over forty years of practice, is that not too many years ago, the physician seemed to occupy a special place in the eyes of the people in the community and in the hospitals. He or she was the undisputed leader of the team and the developer of healthcare services in addition to being trusted to do his or her best for the patient. This unquestioning trust had a healing effect in that once the doctor reassured the patient; the patient would start the process of improvement from that instant on in quite many cases. Over recent years, the profession of medicine has developed the reputation of having physicians who care much more about finances (their own) than the profession of medical practice and even though the sins of a few have stained the reputation of the many, the public perception has changed significantly. This means that the healing component of the doctor-patient interaction, unquestioning trust, may have been compromised based on that perception.

This author has the habit of asking all students of medicine, whether undergraduate or postgraduate, to give him a description of whom they will be when they graduate with a medical degree or to describe whom they are having graduated with a medical degree. The response is always, 'I will be a doctor or physician or I am a doctor or physician' (of some description). The author's response to them is that they described their role and function but not who they are. The author insists that indeed they are *persons who are practicing medicine* and who can decide not to practice medicine at any given point in time but, they do not have the capacity to stop being a person.

This triggers a discussion which reveals an obvious conflict in the acceptance of this new 'awareness' which can only mean that the struggling person had so much invested in the concept of 'being a doctor' or 'being a physician' he or she is now faced with an uncomfortable reevaluation of self. The author proposes that this is fundamentally wrong and needs correction. One's values and self-esteem should not depend on whether one functions in the role of doctor or physician but should be based on more enduring character traits like the ones Stephen R. Covey described in his posthumously published book, *Primary Greatness* (2015). Covey uses the phrase 'rearranging deck chairs on the Titanic', as shorthand for doing pointless or trivial things, instead of the important things in life. He also points out that when we put appearances before reality we are saying that we care more about image than substance and that we have our priorities backward.

CURRENT OBSERVATIONS

Medical students arrive in medical school having been accepted from a normal population for the study of medicine. The qualities that qualified them for acceptance have much more to do with intellectual achievement than with any character traits. The author does not suggest that character traits should be a priority in the acceptance process. Nonetheless, one need only reflect on the emergence of medical schools in disparate places all over the world to realize that many may be businesses first and sites where academic excellence occupies a somewhat lower priority.

The premise that medical students reflect a normal distribution of the population implies that the character traits they bring into medical school, reflect differences in intellectual ability as well as religious, cultural, family, gender and personal experiences. They may be: married or unmarried, younger or older, experienced or naïve. They arrive in different stages of development but all are exposed to the same curriculum and learning environment. However, the most important area that the education and training of today's physician neglects is the wellbeing of the student. As long as the focus remains on passing the exams rather than on who passes the exam (i.e., the character and wellbeing of the student), medical educators will continue to make the same errors- one cannot have the wrong focus and obtain the right results.

Passing exams is an essential area of focus for the student and his or her family or sponsor, but improving the quality of health care service delivery now must include preparing the whole person in a balanced, holistic way. Medical educators cannot continue to have as primary concerns the pass or failure rate, throwing ourselves wholeheartedly into trying to discover, 'what went wrong with our teaching' or 'taking another look at the quality of our students'. Though necessary and important questions, for which we need answers, these are not the most important questions. In the author's estimation, the most important question is, 'Are we providing our students and postgraduate residents with the best opportunities to develop the character traits and understanding of life that would lead to their holistic development and therefore produce better physicians'?

THE IMPORTANCE OF MENTAL HEALTH AND WELLBEING

The mental health and wellbeing of all persons should be paramount among priorities. However, the negative and pejorative associations with mental illnesses have caused a significant sector of even the best educated in society to neglect this aspect and or to relegate it to an afterthought or low priority when pursuing life's goals. The World Health Organization (1948) defines health broadly as 'a state of complete physical, mental, and social well-being and not merely the absence of disease or infirmity'. Furthermore, it defines mental health as 'a state of well-being in which every individual realizes his or her own potential, can cope with the normal stresses of life, can work productively and fruitfully, and is able to make a contribution to his or her community'.

The National Wellness Institute (2017) defines wellness as, 'an active process through which people become aware of, and make choices toward, a more successful existence'. Wellness can also be described as the complete integration of body, soul, and spirit along with the realization that everything we do, think, feel and believe has an effect on our state of well-being. These definitions and descriptions have existed for some time, the result of much discussion and thought following observation. The intention is to provide information for the individual to achieve a better quality of life because of the application of the principles contained in these definitions. The National Wellness Institute has described six dimensions of wellness (Hettler, 1976):

- How a person contributes to his or her environment and community, and how to build better living spaces and social networks;
- The enrichment of life through work, and its interconnectedness to living and playing;
- The development of belief systems, values, and creating a world view;
- The benefits of regular physical activity, healthy eating habits, strength and vitality as well as personal responsibility, self-care and knowing when to seek medical attention;
- Self-esteem, self-control, and determination as a sense of direction;
- Creative and stimulating mental activities, and sharing your gifts with others.

Further, the Institute points out the following:

- Wellness is a conscious, self-directed and evolving process of achieving full potential;
- Wellness is multidimensional and holistic, encompassing lifestyle, mental and spiritual well-being, and the environment;
- Wellness is positive and affirming.

The Hippocratic Oath is a wonderful foundation for excellence and ethical medical practice. Although *primum non nocere* (first do no harm) is not stated in that form in the oath, the principle is a part of the oath. The whole idea of making sure that 'if one cannot help one certainly does not harm' has deep historical roots. However, we must move from that principle into the current understanding of the importance of quality of life. Addressing the need to promote a balanced life, will make possible the best quality of life for both practitioners and the persons in the community they serve, thus reducing the risk of harm.

THE MEDICAL STUDENTS' EXPERIENCE

In 2013, the Australian Medical Students' Association adopted a new Student Mental Health and Well-Being Policy, which is important for the medical community to consider as we focus on improving our current system. The policy says:

Students are less likely to perform well at University when suffering from mental ill health. Psychiatric illness has been shown to be associated with lower educational achievement, decreased employment, low incomes and lower standard of living, and the studies, specifically of university students, have found a correlation between mental health problems and poorer educational outcomes, as well as increased impairment and more days out of the role. (Wang, Lee, & Wahid, 2013, p. 4)

The policy goes on to say:

[T]he Australian Institute of Health and Welfare (AIHW) data shows more than one quarter (26%) of the 16 to 24 age group experienced a mental health disorder in a 12-month period - the highest incidence of any age group. Anxiety disorders are the most common, followed by substance use disorders and then affective disorders. (Wang, et al., 2013, p. 4)

The report indicated that, 'this is a surprisingly neglected area of research which urgently warrants further empirical investigation' (Wang, et al., 2013, p. 4). Billingsley (2015) reported on a small online survey done by the *Student BMJ* noting that:

Of the 1122 UK-based respondents, 30% (343) declared that they had experienced or received treatment for a mental health condition while at medical school. From this group, 80% (276) thought the level of support available to them was either poor or only moderately adequate. Just under 15% (167) of the survey's respondents also revealed that they had considered committing suicide at some point during their studies. (Billingsley, 2015, para. 1)

One of the respondents remarked that, 'The stigma with mental health issues especially comes into focus when exposed to consultants and tutors who referred to it as a weakness' (Billingsley, 2015, para. 12). These are disturbing facts that cannot be ignored.

'This snapshot from the *Student BMJ* survey adds to the small evidence base about the prevalence of medical students' mental ill health' (Billingsley, 2015, para. 5). The report goes on to say that 'medical schools need to work harder at providing open access to support, with signposts to safe and confidential support structures that have clear boundaries around them' (para. 22). Cohen at the University of Cardiff called for medical schools to introduce more teaching 'on "managing your own health and building resilience" into their curriculums' (para. 22).

Conlon (2012), a counsellor at King's College London noted, 'There is now a great deal of research which indicates that mental ill health among doctors is a global phenomenon' (2012, para. 1). Miller (2009) surveyed members of the UK-based Doctors' Support Network finding 68% of the 116 respondents had a diagnosis of depression, along with other diagnoses including bipolar disorder, anxiety, eating disorders and addictions. Conlon notes, 'These findings highlight the essential need to take care of the mental health of medical students' (para. 2). Similar findings were emerging in surveys and studies in the United States of America and Canada.

Given that we cannot prevent students from having problems and becoming depressed, what can be done to reduce unhealthy levels of stress and anxiety, particularly in medical students, and help them prepare for the even more stressful life of the medical practitioner? (Conlon, 2012, para. 18)

Conlon also notes that the rapid expansion of medical schools in the United Kingdom and elsewhere since 1997 has seen a 60% increase in enrolment (para. 18).

Conlon's paper also references an article in the *Journal of Mental Health* which looked at the mental health of doctors (Brooks, Chalder, & Gerada, 2011), concluding that:

Awareness should be raised during medical school and training instituted which focuses not only on how to seek help but on the psychological and emotional obstacles to seeking help such as fear of shame and stigma which still troubles many doctors. (para. 18)

The important fact noted was, 'Asking for psychological help is always a difficult step, but particularly so, it would seem, in medical institutions' (para. 24). The article goes on to say that if the distress is not expressed and is driven underground it 'may then surface through personal, academic and professional difficulties including alcoholism and drug abuse, self-destructive behaviour and even suicide' (para. 24).

STUDENT STRESS

A very interesting experiment was performed which looked at 'A' (high working memory) students versus 'C' (low working memory) students (Beilock & Carr, 2005). This author suggests that we can accept the premise that the former group represents the high-performing students and the latter group represents the average students. They compared the students' performance when placed in a non-pressure situation and given the same academic test. The 'A' students did A work and the 'C' students did C work. The groups were then re-examined linking their performance to a cash reward as well as group evaluation by their professors and thereby introducing the pressure to maintain a certain level of performance. The 'C' students did C work while the 'A' students faltered to the level of the 'C' students. The explanation is that the increased levels of anxiety in the 'A' student group interfered with working memory and this affected performance.

This author often refers medical students to Beilock's research, which shows how smart people choke under pressure. If instructors then assume that the students in medical school represent those who are high performers or smart students and not average performers, then it is important for both students and instructors to understand how stress and anxiety affects performance. But it cannot end there. Once we, the instructors, have exposed the students to the knowledge, then it is incumbent upon us to make sure that we provide them with an understanding of how to manage their stress levels and to do so in a way that makes it a part of their skill set and lifestyle.

This author has had to deal with a wide variety of problems with which medical students and postgraduate residents present, from low self-esteem and lack of confidence to severe psychosis. In almost every case, the problems only came to light after dips in performance, not because some associate lecturer, lecturer or tutor was sensitive and observant enough to notice that there could indeed be some problems and took steps to intervene. This means that we must make sure to provide the medical students with the right learning environment as well as the opportunity to grow and develop as human beings, at a rate that is equal to or ahead of the pace of their acquisition of medical knowledge and skills. In order to achieve that we must address their basic human needs, as well as the needs of the staff there to educate and train them.

THE PATIENTS' VIEWPOINT

When we consider how to prepare our medical students for the role of physician, we cannot ignore what patients want from physicians. A Mayo Clinic survey (Bendapudi, Berry, Frey, Parish, & Rayburn, 2006) highlighted seven traits listed by patients, and included definitions of those traits:

- **Confident:** 'The doctor's confidence gives me confidence'.
- **Empathetic:** 'The doctor tries to understand what I am feeling and experiencing, physically and emotionally, and communicates that understanding to me'.
- **Humane:** 'The doctor is caring, compassionate, and is kind'.

- **Personal:** 'The doctor is interested in me more than just as a patient, interacts with me, and remembers me as an individual'.
- **Forthright:** 'The doctor tells me what I need to know in plain language and in a forthright manner'.
- **Respectful:** 'The doctor takes my input seriously and works with me'.
- **Thorough:** 'The doctor is conscientious and persistent'.

Today's patients have access to an enormous amount of information via the internet and this author has observed a patient take control of her care in such an organised way it impressed and informed the doctors caring for her in ways never before imagined. An internist referred a woman in her late 30s with severe dysphagia (could not even swallow water) to a general surgeon. The surgeon made the appropriate investigations and discovered that the cause of the dysphagia was cancer of the oesophagus. The surgeon informed the patient of the diagnosis, did a pencil drawing to describe the tumour, and indicated that she needed surgery to remove it. The patient then told the surgeon that she would discuss surgical options with him the following day, then asked the surgeon to give the author (a psychiatrist) a call to come and see her. The surgeon was confused and asked if she had a special reason for wanting to see a psychiatrist. Her response was, 'Do you understand that you just told me I have cancer? I have to have somebody to help me deal with that reality'. Amazing woman! That was not the end of the story. She went on the internet and accessed information about surgical procedures for oesophageal cancer. Using the pencil drawing the surgeon had given her, she matched the drawing with one of the conditions described on the website. She then chose a surgery option, downloaded it, and presented it to the surgeon the next day indicating that it was the procedure she wanted to have.

The surgeon was happy to work with her and the author is happy to say that she made excellent recovery with minimal morbidity. Patients do not want doctors who are timid, uncaring, misleading, cold, callous, disrespectful, and hurried (Bendapudi, et al., 2006). On that note, this author was very encouraged to get a request from the staff of the Accident and Emergency department of the Princess Margaret Hospital to present a CME lecture entitled, 'Putting the Care Back into Healthcare'. This author took that opportunity to point out to the healthcare staff, including physicians and nurses, that the word *patient* comes from the Latin word *Patior*, which means 'To suffer, to be afflicted with'. It should be humbling to realize that physicians' livelihood and role in work and life is related to human suffering and its relief. This too is fundamental knowledge for current and would-be physicians.

PROPOSED SOLUTIONS OR THE WAY FORWARD

How do we prepare the physician of tomorrow in a more appropriate way, to manage his or her own well-being in addition to promoting well-being in the patients he or she serves? What must we take into consideration as we accept the reality of today's world, it's pressures, the massive amounts of information coming our way on a daily basis and our ability or inability to balance all this and enjoy a good quality of life?

Let us start with the staff. Too often students hear about how things were done when their lecturers and tutors were in training. They may be put under the pressure of keeping up and performing without any sensitivity to the individual challenges they may encounter as they try to achieve their academic goals. This will vary from place to place and from person-to-person. Some campuses include groups available for student participation and counselling. Nonetheless, this falls short of the knowledge and skills to which students must be exposed and must acquire, to prevent the problems that interfere with their growth and development as well as their intellectual pursuits.

Sensitivity training in how to empathize with today's students is necessary. In this author's estimation, this will make a world of difference in the attitude of the staff towards the students. Additionally, a curriculum must be developed to focus on sessions for the students that would expose them to holistic self-development and building resilience. The staff members should be offered (perhaps even required but at a minimum encouraged), to take the opportunity to sit in on these sessions to assist them in understanding what is being taught and the concepts to which the students are being exposed.

The staff must be prepared to be mentors as well. Homer described a mentor as a 'wise and trusted counsellor'. In academics, 'mentor' often indicates a role synonymous with faculty adviser; however, mentoring is both a personal and a professional relationship. The mentoring relationship develops over an extended period and the student's needs and the nature of the relationship tend to change (National Academy of Science, 1997, p. 1). The mentor is someone who takes a special interest in helping another person develop into a successful professional. This description alone points to the need for those who mentor to be not only willing, but also trained to perform that function.

In The Bahamas, the University of the West Indies School of Clinical Medicine and Research receives students from the other major campuses of the University of the West Indies' medical school (Barbados, Jamaica and Trinidad). The students continue training in the fourth and fifth years and can go on to do residency and postgraduate training in several medical disciplines in The Bahamas. The cadre of students is mainly Bahamian, so now a unique situation now exists for them. They once had to deal with being away from home and parents, family and guardians and with adjusting to autonomy and independent lifestyle choices without the scrutiny of family members. They have now returned home and a new dynamic develops which involves older, well-established interpersonal dynamics that are very challenging for the students. In many cases, it may feel like regression.

This author suggests that medical students must be aware of the broad spectrum of areas of personal growth so that they are not stuck in the arena of academic achievement and the passing of exams. The course design should contain crucial and important elements, in no particular order, and would start in the third year and continue through the fifth year. This course would focus on enhancing and developing the total person. Personal growth and development, fundamental for building the rest of the knowledge base and skills, would be at the top of this author's list.

PROPOSED RECOMMENDATIONS AND CURRICULUM

Personal Growth and Development

In John C Maxwell's book *The 15 Invaluable Laws of Growth* (2012), the first chapter addresses the Law of Intentionality. Maxwell states that growth does not just happen. The epigraph at the beginning of the chapter says, *'Life is now in session. Are you present'?* He asks very important questions at the outset, such as, 'Do you have a plan for your personal growth'? The questions all lead to one conclusion: 'If you focus on growth, you will grow and always hit goals'. Maxwell points out several important 'Growth Gap Traps' which he calls misconceptions and suggests that these could hold one back from being as intentional as one must be:

1. **The Assumption Gap:** 'I assume that I will automatically grow'.
2. **The Knowledge Gap:** 'I don't know how to grow'.
3. **The Timing Gap:** 'It's not the right time to begin'.
4. **The Mistake Gap:** 'I'm afraid of making mistakes'.
5. **The Perfection Gap:** 'I have to find the best way before I start'.
6. **The Inspiration Gap:** 'I don't feel like doing it'.
7. **The Comparison Gap:** 'Others are better than I am'.
8. **The Expectation Gap:** 'I thought it would be easier than this'.

Maxwell points out that intentional growth:

- Insists on Starting Today
- Takes complete responsibility to grow
- Often learns before mistakes

- Relies on hard work
- Perseveres long and hard
- Fights for good habits
- Follows through
- Takes risks
- Thinks like a learner
- Relies on character
- Never stops growing

This author does not encounter medical students until their fourth and fifth years and they are surprised by the approach which focuses intensely on their growth and development as a priority, and secondarily on their acquisition of knowledge and skills in the practice of medicine. The author informs them that while both are important, personal growth and development are more important. The suggestion is, going forward, that they should be exposed not only to foundational courses in personal growth but also courses in development of character, stress management, emotional intelligence and work-life balance or satisfaction in order to attain and maintain well-being.

In his book *Primary Greatness*, Covey posits that one should focus on character over competency. 'Even though people may be technically well educated, if they don't grow in emotional maturity, eventually their skills may be their undoing' (p. 17). He also refers to Goethe's saying: 'Things that matter most must never be at the mercy of things that matter least' (p. xii). Covey says that primary greatness is the kind of success that comes from contribution; by contrast, 'the trappings of success---position, popularity, public image---are secondary greatness….Primary greatness is on the inside. It is about character. Secondary greatness is on the outside' (p. xii) and that, 'A successful life is about primary greatness - a life of duty, honor, integrity, perseverance, self-sacrifice, and service, regardless of material rewards or circumstances' (p. xiii). Covey also points out that many times secondary greatness follows primary greatness.

Covey describes how to 'make that important journey from an obsession with secondary greatness to a focus on primary greatness' (p. xvi). He describes the following as necessary principles to be internalized if we are going to achieve primary greatness:

- Integrity
- Contribution
- Priority
- Personal sacrifice
- Service

- Responsibility
- Loyalty
- Reciprocity
- Diversity
- Continuous learning
- Renewal
- Teaching to learn

What this author found pivotal to his understanding and appreciation of this work was Covey's description of the three lives that we live: the public life that we expose to others when we are in public; the private life that we expose to close family and friends; and the secret life.

The secret life is where your heart is, where your real motives are - the ultimate desires of your life. It is also the source of primary greatness. If you have the courage to explore your secret life, you can honestly question your deepest motivations. (Covey, 2015, p. 3)

Covey then challenges the reader to explore the secret life and to be prepared to re-script the motivations—to realign one's life to the core principles of true success.

Each principle listed above is described as a lever, used to remove the obstacles one discovers on the road to primary greatness. He references humility and courage as the source of virtues and encourages the reader to:

Break with the physical and emotional addictions that hold them down and reduce their quality of life. Until that happens, there can be little progress because the body is controlling the will. Once the break occurs, people then have a path to progress. If they can get some degree of control over their appetites, they can have some degree of control over their passions, and even begin to restructure their motivations and desires. (Covey, 2015, p. 20)

Another important bit of advice from Covey's (2015) book is the caveat that in the absence of a crisis or significant negative event in our lives:

We tend to live in numbed complacency—so busy doing good, easy, or routine things, that we do not even stop to ask ourselves if we are doing what really matters. The good, then, become the enemy of the best. (p. 27)

He describes humility and courage as the mother and father of all virtues, noting that the humble progress because they willingly submit to and try to live in harmony with natural laws and universal principles, while we need courage to lead our lives by correct principles and to have integrity in the moment of choice.

When we set up our own self-generated or socially validated value systems, and then develop our missions and goals based on what we value rather than on principles, we tend to become laws unto ourselves, proud and independent. Pride hopes to impress; humility seeks to serve others. Just because we value a thing doesn't mean that having it will enhance our quality of life. (Covey, 2015, p. 27)

Last, but not least, Covey points out that 'Nothing sinks people faster in their careers than arrogance. Arrogance shouts, *'I know best!'* In the uniform of arrogance, we fumble and falter; pride comes and goes before the fall. But dressed in humility, we make progress' (p. 27).

Emotional Intelligence

The second foundational course I would include in the curriculum would be a course in emotional intelligence, also known as EQ (distinct but related to 'IQ') or EI (Daniel Goleman, 2006, prefers EI). This author considers it a tragedy when emotional reactions rather than careful, dispassionate consideration control any person of any level of intelligence, or any status. Nothing is wrong with intuition. As we go through life we develop 'gut feelings' about things of all description based on our experience. Gut feelings are good to take into consideration and should not be ignored as they form part of the wisdom accumulated over the years. However, emotional reactions are automatic and unconscious and as Dr. Rudy Tanzi neurologist and author expressed so eloquently, 'I am not my brain, I am not my mind. I manage my brain and I manage my mind.'

Everything about human interaction and reaction is emotional. These emotions do not last but they do trigger thoughts and have a connection with behaviours. Cognitive therapy relies on an understanding of the connection between thoughts, feelings (emotions) and behaviour to assist persons experiencing a variety of conditions (most notably depression and anxiety). Lessening the disability that causes the condition to persist, while improving one's understanding of an internal locus of control which then leads to an enhanced quality of life. Brackett, Rivers and Salovey (2011) from Yale University produced an excellent paper called 'Emotional Intelligence: Implications for Personal, Social, Academic, and Workplace Success'. A portion of the abstract says, 'We describe what is known about how emotionally intelligent people function both intra and interpersonally and in both academic and workplace settings' (Bracket, et al., 2011, p. 88). Additionally, Grant (2007) showed that training can improve emotional intelligence.

This author attended a wonderful presentation at a continuing medical education (CME) session of the University of the West Indies School of Clinical Medicine and Research Bahamas in 2015, 'Perspectives on Emotional Intelligence for Health Professionals'. The presenter's learning objectives included explaining the four scales that are involved in emotional intelligence: the ability to practice greater awareness, ownership and management of one's feelings (emotions), and a commitment to work on continued improvement of the practice of emotional intelligence in our personal and professional relationships. He pointed out that as physicians we are at risk of succeeding in some areas but not in others and asked, 'Do the persons who come top of the class make the most successful practitioners'? The presenter also posed the question, 'Could it be that we have placed too much emphasis on IQ?' Emotional intelligence (EQ or EI) is complementary to IQ and it is the ability to know and manage oneself along with an awareness and ability to manage one's relationships with others.

Four attributes define emotional intelligence (EQ or EI):

1. **Self-Awareness:** The ability to recognize one's own emotions and the effect they have on thoughts and behaviour. It leads to an understanding of your strengths and weaknesses and to the development of confidence.
2. **Self-Management:** The ability to control impulsive feelings and behaviours, manage your emotions in healthy ways, take initiative, follow through on commitments, and adapt to changing circumstances.
3. **Social Awareness:** The ability to understand the emotions, needs, and concerns of other people, recognize emotional cues, feel comfortable socially, and recognize the interpersonal/power dynamics in a group or organisation.
4. **Relationship Management:** The ability to develop and maintain good relationships, communicate clearly, inspire and influence others, work well in a team, and manage conflict.

Mindfulness

Mindfulness is a key skill to master in the development of one's emotional intelligence. Mindfulness is the practice of purposely focusing your attention on the present moment in a nonjudgmental way. Another important factor is the ownership of one's emotional reactions, which allows the owner to be in control of modifying the reaction as opposed to externalizing the control, which then leads to blame, and loss of the internal locus of control.

The development of resilience through the knowledge and skills of stress management follows naturally from a discussion of stress management. This should also be a foundational course. Stress is very likely the most common subject discussed by modern man, and probably the most misunderstood concept. Whenever this author gives a presentation on stress management the responses from the audience are all negative when asked to describe their concept of stress. As a result, it is easy to orient the presentation to make the audience friendlier with the concept of stress but also understand the reality of distress and its effects. Stress is any change to which one must adapt; it is an essential part of everyday life and, if used wisely, can enhance our performance and lead to optimal results and productivity. Distress, on the other hand, is the negative result of stress that overwhelms our coping capacity. It can also be due to boredom.

The Yerkes–Dodson Law suggests that there is a relationship between performance and arousal or stress. Increased arousal (stress) can help improve performance but only up to a certain point after which performance declines. When the medical student understands the relationship between stress and performance and is aware of one's ability to enhance coping capacity by learning how to recognize and manage stress, a new level of confidence is the result and life becomes more manageable in general. The goal is to incorporate a lifestyle of exercise and good nutrition with rest, relaxation and activities that refresh. Additionally, identification of unique, individual stressors, and how to manage them is essential for one's efforts to obtain and maintain a good work-life balance.

DEVELOPMENT OF WELL-BEING

Students must also learn about well-being. They must become familiar with the variety of constituents involved, and learn how to manage the shifting priorities on their journey through life. The European Union commissioned a qualitative research study of its 15 member states to investigate the issue of well-being among citizens of the European Union (TNS Qual+, 2011). The study was conducted in February and March of 2010 and the results identified nine factors as contributing to well-being:

1. Subjective well-being
2. Economic and employment situation
3. Education and intellectual development
4. Health and nutrition
5. Infrastructure
6. Interpersonal relationships
7. Civic life
8. Cultural and spiritual activities
9. Environment

The author will discuss what he considers the more important of these in relation to considering the universality of the human experience and the essentials for one's well-being.

Subjective Well-Being

Too often, we allow a reflection on the mood we are in to affect our well-being, positively or negatively, and this in turn can affect our mood. This will vary widely, of course, in relation to one's mindset and attitude towards life in general. Nonetheless, clearly a direct relationship exists between the labels that we place on people, places, things and events, along with the values attached to them, and their ability to affect our mood. The report says that, 'While personal growth and development positively influences well-being, so does stability and predictability in one's life and work' (TNS Qual+, 2011, p. 7). However, we must teach that the harsh reality of life will not follow our script nor our expectations. As long as this is accepted, we can exist in harmony with the relative unpredictability of future events. However, when we try to force life into our little boxes, disappointment and frustration result.

Health and Nutrition

This is such an important area, especially considering our sedentary lifestyles, the exploding pandemic of obesity, and the consequent increase in the incidence of disorders that are related to noncommunicable diseases. A few years ago, the author was serving as president of the Medical Association of The Bahamas, attempts were made, in vain, to organise committees to look at the health and well-being of the local physician population and to discuss our role as chief promoters of health and wellness in the country. One can only assume that denial was so powerful, none of the committees ever functioned nor was any data collected. Consequently, we never took a good look at ourselves. Physicians cannot escape the reality of our position in society as the main body of persons who are consulted daily in relation to the health and well-being of the citizens. We owe it to ourselves, and to our fellow citizens, to be the best examples of the effects of the products we sell or promote.

Research has made it abundantly clear that small amounts of daily exercise make a significant difference to many health outcomes (Blair & Morris, 2009). Harvard University now offers two-day workshops on 'prescribing exercise'. Cardiovascular as well as resistance exercises along with portion control (reducing the size of the portions on our plates) comprise the formula for good physical health that also reduces the risk of cardiovascular diseases and type II diabetes, and is of great assistance in maintaining one's energy level, mood, and relaxation.

Managing Relationships

We also cannot underestimate the health benefits of good interpersonal relationships (House, Landis, & Umberson). People are healthier when they have good relationships with coworkers. The quality of a marital relationship is inversely proportional to the incidence of cardiovascular disease and heart attacks not to mention its profound effect on well-being. Friends, family members and children all factor into the relationships equation and 'were considered to be a great source of love which has a strong positive influence on well-being' (TNS Qual+, 2011, p. 9).

This author would also include some advice from Dr. Wayne Dyer's book *Being in Balance: 9 Principles for Creating Habits to Match Your Desires* (2006). He encourages the habit of thinking in alignment with our dreams. He presents a different view of stress and says, 'Stress is an inside job. You cannot fill a container with it because tension is not a physical item or object. There isn't some *thing* that you can point to and say, *there it is, that's stress!*' (Dyer, 2006, p. 17). He goes on to point out that one never really enjoys the life one works so hard to achieve because they spend their life running on an endless treadmill. These concepts are important to introduce to the students, so that they can consider several approaches to use to attain and maintain balance and satisfaction between study or work and life.

Finally, yet most importantly is one's attention to one's spirituality. Religion is important. Church affiliation and attendance is important for many in the community as well as for building society and providing help when help is necessary. Spirituality, on the other hand, which is relationship with God or with the higher being of one's faith, is even more important—without it, we tend to lose our moral compass. However, many of us get busy and successful and neglect the spiritual aspect of our being, to our detriment. We must develop ahead of our patients. We must teach medical students to develop ahead of the patients that they will meet. It is not anyone's role to impose their religious or spiritual viewpoints on anyone else but it is certainly the responsibility of the physician to pay attention to the whole person and to treat patients holistically. This means including spiritual beliefs in the assessment process, which would only be authentic when the physician has developed holistically.

In the same way that getting married does not instantly make you a husband or a wife—just a married person—becoming a doctor or physician does not and will not make you a person of character who is empathetic, considerate, compassionate, and caring. The medical degree has no bearing on one's level of growth and maturity, or one's ability to manage the stresses and strains of life effectively. We must develop that kind of physician, as well as physician leaders. We cannot expect them to emerge from the pack in the Darwinian way and produce good results because we know that this expectation would only lead to more of the same flaws and failings.

Therefore, we must accept the reality of the educational institution's responsibility for recognizing the challenge and creating solutions to the problems it poses.

The suggestions in this chapter are far from idealistic and even though not exhaustive they propose a shift in focus and priority in the medical education and training of the students in medical school. It must be remembered that, even though these are adult students, they have come to our various institutions with a mixed bag of abilities and disabilities and that they are products of this modern information and technological age. If we do not say and show that we consider their well-being and their personal growth and development to be at least as important as the acquisition of medical knowledge, competency, and skills, then we abdicate our responsibility to produce the best person who is going to practice medicine in his or her chosen field.

The General Medical Council of the United Kingdom requires new medical graduates to have a fitness-to-practice certificate in addition to their medical degree. This body understands that more is needed in the development of the physician in training than knowledge, skills, and competency. The four domains of good medical practice are:

1. **Knowledge, Skills, and Performance:** Doctors must develop and maintain their professional performance, must apply their knowledge and experiences and practice within the limits of their competence and must record their work clearly, accurately and legibly. They must have the necessary knowledge of the English language to provide a good standard of practice and care in the UK.
2. **Safety and Quality:** Doctors must contribute to and comply with systems to protect patients, respond to risks safely and protect patients and colleagues from any risk posed by their own health.
3. **Communication, Partnership, and Teamwork:** Doctors must communicate effectively with patients and establish and maintain partnerships with them. They must work collaboratively with colleagues, be willing to contribute to teaching, training, supporting and assessing and must contribute to the continuity and coordination of care for patients transferring between providers.
4. **Maintaining Trust:** Doctors must show respect for patients, treat patients and colleagues fairly and without discrimination and must act with honesty and integrity (General Medical Council, 2014).

These principles are commendable. They certainly go a long way to ensuring that physicians in training attain and maintain high standards of quality, and provide a solid reference base for medical regulation. However, in this author's opinion, they still fall short of the holistic development and attention to the health and well-being of the physician-in-training described in this chapter.

We can no longer ignore the fact that Cartesian dualism had and continues to have a significant, negative influence on our view of human beings in general as well as a negative influence on our approach to managing our patients (Robinson, 2016; Kriel, 1988). The philosophical discussion of a mental state as opposed to a physical state, is moot when one considers the evidence before us. Studies have confirmed that over half the persons on a general medical or surgical ward have significant psychological morbidity. When that morbidity is addressed appropriately, the overall morbidity of the patient improves, mortality decreases, and the rate of readmission goes down. So, while we reflect on these scientific observations let us also remember how much we do not know and, at the same time, remember how important quality of life is for doctor and patient alike in our finite existence.

So, now we get to the point where we should discuss the elephant in the room—the stigmatizing attitude that non-psychiatric colleagues (not all, but far too many) have toward mental illnesses and by extension mental health. Mental health is not given the priority it should have and students, or physicians for that matter, who have a psychiatric disorder or any psychological morbidity are viewed as weak, fragile or disabled. They certainly are not given the same understanding or leeway as a student who develops diabetes or fractures a leg. That is unfortunate, but more importantly, it is unfair and only serves to reinforce and strengthen stigma.

CONCLUSION

We owe it to our undergraduate and postgraduate students to declare to them that their personal growth and development, along with their overall health (body, soul and spirit) and well-being, are our priority focus, hand in hand with the development of their medical knowledge, technical competencies and skills. Recently Se Ri Pak, a well-known and very successful female golfer from South Korea retired. She is sure to be included in the Hall of Fame for women's golf when eligible. She was said to reflect on her life at the time of retiring in this way: 'I am an incomplete person.... I took care of my golf, I didn't take care of myself' (Mell, 2016, para. 2), a sad but true reflection that, after having put all her best into her profession, she neglected her personal growth and development.

To test the effectiveness of these interventions future research should focus on measuring the distress levels of medical students, the quality of life of the physicians so trained, and the experience of the patients. Too often, we develop and maintain a paternalistic view toward the patients we serve which coincides with the whole concept of compliance. Today we speak more about adherence to the treatment regime, which involves helping the patient to understand what the treatment is all about, and why it is important to continue the therapy as prescribed, rather than to do so because the doctor says it must be done. Anecdotally, personal coaches assigned to postgraduate doctors in training has been shown to dramatically reduce the stress levels while increasing quality of life and productivity of those doctors.

Perhaps the readers of this chapter will choose to reflect on their own personal growth and development and may even take time out to do some introspection. It is never too late to start the process of improvement in any area of life. Let us pass that message on to the ones we are responsible for training and developing by making their well-being, personal growth and holistic development our priorities.

REFERENCES

Beilock, S. L., & Carr, T. H. (2005). When high-powered people fail: Working memory and choking under pressure in math. *Psychological Science*, *16*(2), 101–105. doi:10.1111/j.0956-7976.2005.00789.x PMID:15686575

Bendapudi, N. M., Berry, L. L., Frey, K. A., Parish, J. T., & Rayburn, W. L. (2006, March). Patients perspectives on ideal physician behaviors. *Mayo Clinic Proceedings*, *81*(3), 338–344. doi:10.4065/81.3.338 PMID:16529138

Billingsley, M. (2015). More than 80% of medical students with mental health issues feel under-supported, says Student BMJ survey. *Student BMJ*, *23*. https://doi.org/10.1136/sbmj.h4521

Blair, S. N., Morris, J. N. (2009). *Annals of epidemiology*. Elsevier.

Brackett, M. A., Rivers, S. E., & Salovey, P. (2011). Emotional intelligence: Implications for personal, social, academic, and workplace success. *Social and Personality Psychology Compass*, *5*(1), 88–103. doi:10.1111/j.1751-9004.2010.00334.x

Brooks, S. K., Chalder, T., & Gerada, C. (2011). Doctors vulnerable to psychological distress and addictions: Treatment from the Practitioner Health Programme. *Journal of Mental Health (Abingdon, England)*, *20*(2), 157–164. doi:10.3109/09638237.2011.556168 PMID:21542716

Castells, M. (2014). The impact of the internet on society: a global perspective. In *Change: 19 key essays on how internet is changing our lives*. Retrieved from https://www.bbvaopenmind.com/wp-content/uploads/2014/03/BBVA-OpenMind-Technology-Innovation-Internet-Francisco-Gonzalez-Knowledge-Banking-for-a-Hyperconnected-Society.pdf

Conlon, A. (2012). *Problems faced by undergraduate medical students*. Retrieved from the Royal Medical Benevolent Fund website: http://www.rmbf.org/pages/problems-faced-by-undergraduate-medical-students-.html

Covey, S. R. (2015). *Primary greatness: The 12 levers of success*. New York, NY: Simon & Schuster.

Dyer, W. W. (2006). *Being in balance: 9 principles for creating habits to match your desires*. Carlsbad, CA: Hay House.

Engelberg, E., & Sjöberg, L. (2004). Internet use, social skills, and adjustment. *Cyberpsychology & Behavior, 7*(1), 41–47. doi:10.1089/109493104322820101 PMID:15006168

General Medical Council. (2014). *The meaning of fitness to practice*. London, England: Author. Retrieved from http://www.gmc-uk.org/the_meaning_of_fitness_to_practise.pdf_25416562.pdf

Goleman, D. (2006). *Emotional intelligence: Why it can matter more than IQ*. New York, NY: Bantam Books.

Grant, A. M. (2007). Enhancing coaching skills and emotional intelligence through training. *Industrial and Commercial Training, 39*(5), 257-266. https://doi.org/10.1108/00197850710761945

Hettler, W. (1976). Six dimensions of wellness model. St. Paul, MN: National Wellness Institute. Retrieved from http://c.ymcdn.com/sites/www.nationalwellness.org/resource/resmgr/docs/sixdimensionsfactsheet.pdf

Kriel, J. R. (1988). Removing medicine's Cartesian mask: The problem of humanising medical education part 1. *Journal of Biblical Ethics in Medicine, 3*(2), 18–22. Retrieved from http://w.biblicalworldview21.org/bmei/jbem/volume3/num2/kriel_removing_medicines_cartesian_mask.pdf

Maxwell, J. C. (2012). *The 15 invaluable laws of growth: Live them and reach your potential*. New York, NY: Center Street.

Mell, R. (2016, December 23). *My 2016 moment: Pak's retirement*. Retrieved from http://www.golfchannel.com/news/golf-central-blog/my-2016-moment-paks-retirement/

Miller, L. (2009). Doctors, their mental health and capacity for work. *Occupational Medicine, 59*(1), 53–55. doi:10.1093/occmed/kqn111 PMID:18796700

National Academy of Sciences. (1997). *Advisor, teacher, role model, friend: On being a mentor to students in science and engineering*. Washington, DC: National Academy Press. https://doi.org/10.17226/5789

National Wellness Institute. (2017). *Definition of wellness*. Retrieved from http://www.nationalwellness.org/?page=AboutWellness

Qual, T. N. S. +. (2011, September). *Well-being: Aggregrate report*. European Commission. Retrieved from http://ec.europa.eu/public_opinion/archives/quali/wellbeing_final_en.pdf

Robinson, H. (2016). Dualism. In Stanford Encyclopedia of Philosophy. Stanford, CA: Stanford University. Retrieved from https://plato.stanford.edu/entries/dualism/

Wang, S., Lee, S., & Wahid, Z. T. (2013). *University student mental health: The Australian context*. Barton, ACT: Australian Medical Students' Association Student Mental Health and Wellbeing Committee. Retrieved from http://www.amsa.org.au/wp-content/uploads/2013/09/AMSA-SMHW-The-Australian-Context-of-Student-Mental-Health-Report.pdf

World Health Organization. (1948). *WHO definition of health*. Retrieved from http://www.who.int/about/definition/en/print.html

KEY TERMS AND DEFINITIONS

Academics: Relating to school or study; acquisition of education.

Cartesian Dualism: The division of mind and body as separate entities.

Darwinian Way: Survival of the fittest or strongest.

Hippocratic Oath: Oath historically taken by physicians when graduating.

Morbidity: Degree of illness or sickness.

Mortality: Ability to cause death.

Social Skills: Tools necessary for communicating and interacting with others effectively.

Spirituality: The relationship one has with God or a higher power; one's beliefs.

Stressor: An event that triggers the stress response.

Yerkes-Dodson Law: Relationship between arousal (stress) and performance where performance increases with mental or physical arousal up to a point and then declines.

Conclusion

Exploring the Pressures of Medical Education From a Mental Health and Wellness Perspective is a reference book written to offer a centralised view of the global crisis of the invisible mental health problems experienced by medical students on their quest for medical training that can last for more than a decade. The subject of medical students' mental ill health has been taboo in the culture of medical school and the profession and continues to prevent students from seeking the help they need to successfully navigate the pressures associated with medical school.

This book aims to condense in one useful format an overview of the lived experiences of many medical students who share common stressors unique to medical education. Many medical articles in recent times have described the problems of mental ill health in medical schools amongst its students, as have newspaper stories, student blogs, and organisations responsible for the policies that govern medical education. However, there is not a singular source that offers an overview of the extent of the problem with solutions and suggestions aimed at medical educators, medical students, prospective medical students, their families and friends, and the myriad people connected with the training of medical students. This book is intended to provide readers with an understanding of what the formidable journey called medical school involves and how, after students enter medical training, documented evidence of serious mental health issues, including the burnout and suicide ideation unique to medical students, has reached a level of international crisis. Solutions and recommendations from practitioners working in medical education and higher education represent the positive steps being taken to address the global mental health and well-being crisis at the international and national levels and within medical education. When doctors are healthy, all of us benefit from an improved quality of care.

HOW THIS BOOK CONTRIBUTES TO THE SUBJECT MATTER

This book seeks to provide an overview of the subject matter in broad terms: Who are medical students? What are their characteristics? How does becoming a physician produce pride, power, and prestige in the view of students, their families, and society at large? Discussions on perfectionism and burnout in students, residents, and medical faculty are included to provide awareness of these hot-button issues. An in-depth chapter on the cultural influences of stigma on help-seeking behaviour of medical students is tackled by medical school administrators and adds to the understanding missing on the topic of stigma and the ingrained problems associated with diminishing its impact on medical school culture. Other topics in the book, including how higher education students are experiencing a crisis similar to students of the general ages of medical students, are useful in gaining information on how to use data from lessons learnt to design student services that prevent, not react to, students with mental health problems. Finally, the notion that medical education curricula must be drastically restructured from its intense academic format to one based upon adult learning theories and strategies is useful in creating healthy cultures where self-care amongst students, staff, and faculty is the norm.

The subject matter of medical students' mental health crises related to the stressors of prolonged and difficult routines is addressed in the solutions and recommendations by the book's authors and represents a powerful tool for readers to draw upon information useful in creating good practice in medical schools in the support of students with mental health concerns.

Ultimately, this book provides prospective medical students, current medical students, their families and friends, educators, and health professionals with resources to better understand the pressures associated with becoming a physician.

Medical education is known for its rigorous process in which a structured academic curriculum is offered to students in various stages of learning and over a period of years. In addition to the formal curriculum, medical students are exposed to the hidden beliefs and expectations of what is required through an informal curriculum whereby the habits of faculty, staff, and others in the environment seem to honour and respect students who do not complain. Additionally, myths abound about how medical school is supposed to be and how fortunate students should feel for being accepted into a medical programme. Chapter 1, 'Medical Students' Quest Towards the Long White Coat: Impact Upon Mental Health and Well-Being', offered a context for the problems, issues, and controversies impacting the general society and students within the higher education system as a perspective for considering the pressures associated with medical education, which leads to a serious decline in the mental health of many medical students. The author, Dr. Ramirez-Smith, has worked for more than 30 years with student populations in the K–12 and higher education systems in the United States and the Bahamas and serves as a consultant to companies around the world in the development of human resources to fill jobs in education, business, and healthcare-related fields. Thus, this chapter seeks to make meaning of the big picture of global mental health concerns affecting millions of people in the general society and noticeably in the college and university age group in order to better examine the context for understanding how certain types of pressures affect the mental health of medical students. This chapter's broad perspective about the problems of mental health drives home the importance of stakeholders changing the type of training currently used in educating future professionals, in this instance, medical students. Ramirez-Smith notes that research documenting the problems, issues, and controversies associated with mental health and well-being provides governments, higher education institutions, medical schools and their related helping professionals, and all stakeholders concerned about the welfare of future doctors to use the information available and to move beyond the stage of reporting on the crisis to taking bold steps to change the culture of shame that prohibits many from seeking help. Finally, the chapter renders solutions and recommendations suitable for faculty, staff, and administrators in the medical education environment as well as stakeholders concerned with policy, planning, and administration of medical education.

Chapter 2, 'Medical Students' Perceptions of Stigma When Seeking Medical Care for Chronic or Mental Issues: Specific Examination of Cultural Factors', describes the negative impact stigma plays within the culture of medical school, which is compounded by the fact that, in our society, stigma associated with mental ill health is highly pervasive. Furthermore, there is much misinformation about the cultural aspects of understanding how students from diverse cultures, ethnicities, and backgrounds manifest behaviours when under duress. The authors recognise that working towards a preventative approach in helping students highlights the importance of accessible and visible opportunities for peer and social support. Awareness of the type of issues medical students confront is necessary in working towards a stigma-free learning culture. The fact that the stigma around mental health is a powerful barrier to students seeking help, and the understanding of problems and mental health issues by faculty, staff, family, friends, and others, is conducive to developing an inclusive environment where all students feel accepted.

Chapter 3, 'Perfectionism: Managing High Expectations', discusses the evidence that shows that medical students will push themselves because of character traits such as perfectionism and will ignore illness and feelings of distress. Medical students differ widely in the personality traits, self-perceptions, and values that may have an impact on their well-being. This chapter, written by a current medical student and a student affairs practitioner, discusses the types of perfectionism seen in medical students and the stress-related illness that results due to some personality traits, such as a driven personality or type A personality, that are useful in meeting the heavy workloads and long hours of study required of medical students. However, these same traits can be detrimental to students' well-being in times of distress. When combined with a deep feeling of professional obligation to excel, a tradition of self-sacrifice can ensue, leaving these highly motivated medical students adrift. This chapter offers a rare insight into the voice of a medical student who has found strategies to manage her perfectionistic behaviours. The chapter concludes with solutions and recommendations based on the authours' experiences and is an excellent chapter for prospective and current medical students. Stakeholders involved in the day-to-day training of medical students will find the chapter compelling in addition to being useful. The chapter concludes with tips for students to address perfectionistic behaviours and for faculty and administrators to recognise signs of distress in medical students that may be a result of perfectionism.

Sobering information is presented in Chapters 4 and 5, where the two most prevalent problems in medical education today are discussed: burnout and suicide. In Chapter 4, 'Medical Student Burnout: A Social Cognitive Learning Perspective on Medical Student Mental Health and Wellness', Drs. Hamlin and Lubin brilliantly discuss how burnout manifests in the medical school learning environment. This chapter is particularly useful to medical educators, preceptors, and academic and student affairs officers at the undergraduate medical level and graduate level because of the specific recommendations on how to teach medical students. The pragmatic recommendations in this chapter confirm many of the problems with traditionally organised medical school formal curriculum. For example, the authors note 'that many medical school educational innovations are instituted to address a specific gap in the curriculum but are not designed or implemented in a systematic way'. To address burnout, the authors agree with findings from leading medical educators warning that efforts to remedy burnout require specific courses or programmes that must go beyond addressing the symptoms of a stressful learning environment. In fact, the authors call for curricula to address the deep roots of the problems of burnout. Without a systematic and transformational change in the curriculum that owns up to the problems associated with the pressures in the learning environment, courses and seminars will continue to be 'Band-Aids' and miss the opportunities to fix the problem. In an effort to create depth and breadth in a curriculum designed to attack medical student burnout, the authors provide a framework for medical educators and others connected with curriculum development to follow: the curricular changes must be based upon best practices in the field and should be derived from research in the learning sciences. Using theory to guide the development of the medical learning environment promotes the explicit and appropriate professional attributes in medical students. Accompanying the creation of theory-based learning instruction, the authors recommend that the needs and learning styles of medical students must be accessed and that teaching of humanistic medical care is necessary, in addition to the basic science models found in most medical schools. Ultimately, this chapter proposes teaching and learning components of medical education from a cognitive apprenticeship model. Communities of practice where practitioner reflection and strong role model relationships between students and faculty are in place are more likely to help shape the future of medical students. When students perceive strong mentoring-type relationships, medical students' motivation and achievement can be strengthened. There are many implications for faculty development and curricular innovations in this chapter. Awareness of and specific knowledge about what aspects of medical training produces extraordinary pressures will enhance what, when, why, and how medical students' tasks are assigned and in turn will improve students' ability to cope.

Chapter 5, 'Deliberate Self-Harm and Suicide Ideology in Medical Students: Self-Harm and Suicide Among Medical Students' by Dr. Vinod Gopalan and medical students Erick Chan and Debbie Thao Thanh Ho from the School of Medicine at Griffith University in Australia, tackles the most difficult topic in the book. Being alone with thoughts of suicide is a factor known to increase the risk of self-harm. Like many doctors, medical students learn to self-manage illness early in the process of medical training. The learned behaviours and the hidden curriculum, where ill health is minimised and replaced by expectations of resilience, contribute to students' reluctance to seek help. Additionally, medical students' own perceptions of what it means to be a medical student coupled with the culture of medicine and inappropriate responses to stress and anxiety push some students over the edge. The authors point out that, worldwide, suicide is the second leading cause of death amongst 15- to 29-year-olds and that global statistics show that medical students and doctors are at a higher risk of suicide than the general population. This chapter imparts the facets of suicide that are useful in spotting or recognising symptoms connected to deep distress. Concrete strategies that medical educators could utilise to aide medical students are presented. The authors conclude that medical educators' training requires an awareness of the relationship between deliberate self-harm and suicide ideology in order to create and implement systems of support, which includes screening, assessment, and intervention.

Chapters 6 and 7 stress the importance of gaining an understanding of the transition for resident physicians from medical school to doctors. Along the same lines, the negative impact of faculty burnout on preparing medical students warrants further research, as many habits internalised and practised later on may be attributed to the unintended messages transferred to students via the informal curriculum in medical schools, where students' first role models are overwhelmed themselves and struggling with managing their own heavy workloads and expectations. Both chapters provide promising solutions and methods to help medical students and residents manage the pressures of their intensive educational quests.

Chapter 6, 'Medical School and the Transition to Graduate Education: Medical Resident', addresses a critical transitional period in the life of a medical student. The associated pressures with this transition might go unnoticed by medical faculty, family, friends, and even resident graduate education placements (residency). The authors stress the fact that, when medical students graduate from medical school, they are suddenly doctors and not students. Changing roles from medical student to physician is a major life stress because residents who may have been supported financially by family, friends, and student loans for at least 20 years are faced with a new perception of them. Specifically, medical school faculty, residencies, families, and friends see a newly minted physician, and the expectation is for the resident to perform as well as a physician who has been practising for 20 years. The biggest stress, according to the chapter, is the new culture of residency that strangely resembles on some levels the medical education undergraduate experience. Residents who have never held a full-time job before graduating from medical school are shocked at the work hours and the insensitive responses from co-workers or attending physicians to matters of physical illness where calling in sick is not an option. Being late for work is unaccepted and not overlooked. On day one of the residency, the resident is tasked with the full rights and responsibilities of patient care and life-and-death decision making. Graduate medical education, as noted by the authors, has not changed much in recent times, and the transition from medical student to resident is no different. In fact, the authors, Drs. Martin, McDonald and Salzberg reported that the most recent and significant change to graduate medical education in the United States has been the implementation of a restriction on the number of legal work hours for residents. In the past, residents worked holidays, weekends, nights, and continuous shifts of up to 30 hours. In 2002, the Accreditation Council for Graduate Medical Education mandated that intern resident shifts be reduced to a maximum of 80 hours of work per week and up to 16-hour shifts. The RDH (Resident Duty Hours) mandate has met with controversy, as many hospitals are struggling to maintain and implement the RDH as stipulated for many reasons. Those reasons are beyond the scope of the chapter but warrant further research to document the effectiveness of reduced work hours on the well-being of residents. A framework developed by the authors based upon four pillars of prevention is useful when creating a comprehensive strategy to improve residents' well-being: education, screening, treatment, and support. The four recommended domains offer an invaluable source of information to those administrators, such as residency programme directors, who are charged with identifying and preventing mental health problems in the residency.

Chapter 7 offers a beneficial template for use by administrators when designing wellness programmes. Authored by two practicing physicians, this chapter is suitable for prospective students, current medical students and even family members who may use the information to understand the transitions experienced by medical students upon graduation to residency and for administrators to reconsider the roles and responsibilities of medical academic faculty in view of burnout issues.

Chapters 8–10 complete the book with detailed solutions and recommendations for managing the pressures unique to medical students in the twenty-first century. Chapter 8, 'Developing a Comprehensive Wellness Program for Medical Students', is written by Drs. LaTanya Love, a practising paediatrician and medical school administrator, and Dana McDowelle, the current director of admissions at the University of Texas medical system. The chapter presented a thorough description of the undergraduate American medical education 4-year programme. This insightful chapter describes the structure of medical education whereby the pressures and stressors are described from years 1 to 4. The information in this chapter will enlighten prospective students, their families, and especially, high school and college-level counsellors involved with premedical academic advisement. The remainder of the chapter sets forth a dynamic approach to creating a comprehensive wellness programme that goes beyond being reactive and instead is designed to address both the academic and the non-academic sources of stress within the medical learning environment. Five areas emerge as key components of the comprehensive development of a wellness programme: academic support, occupational development, professionalism, self-care, and interpersonal development. The politics of education stemming from how internal dollars are allocated in academic versus student affairs is deemed as important in the successful development of wellness programmes. Medical students, along with high-level administrators (boards of trustees, national- and state-level agencies), must buy into the process of change that will contribute to providing students with a high-quality learning experience in what is one of education's most arduous processes.

Chapter 9, 'Medical School Wellness Initiatives', authored by Dr. Lynda Konecny, professor at America's oldest osteopathic medical school, is replete with information on existing medical education programmes in the United States that can serve as models of innovation and bold movement in developing wellness programmes based upon solid theoretical knowledge in how systemic and real change occurs. The chapter presents sound examples of health education theories and models that support the development, implementation, and evaluation of health promotion programmes. Similar to the recommendations in Chapter 8, Dr. Konecny asserts that a comprehensive wellness model must include a variety of dimensions beyond the physical and psychological aspects of well-being. Superb advice to medical school administrators, faculty, staff, and medical students warns against choosing generic wellness models, since each medical education programme embodies its own culture. The author affirms that one size does not fit all. Therefore, considerations regarding the most appropriate model for each medical education programme must be taken into account in addition to best practices and models of excellence.

Chapter 10, 'Essentials for Physician Training in the 21st Century' is a thought-provoking conclusion to the book authored by licensed chief psychiatrist and leading medical educator in The Bahamas, Dr. Timothy Barrett. The ideas presented in this chapter sum up the key tenets of the previous nine chapters by delineating how medical education can improve the care for all patients by developing and training doctors to be whole people. Dr. Barrett's work in this chapter draws heavily from interpersonal and personal areas of self-development. Dr. Barrett argues that the medical education curriculum fails students when teaching is wholly based on the academic preparation of future doctors. With more than 30 years of practice and leadership within the medical community working with medical students and residents, Dr. Barrett maintains that the most 'beloved and effective doctors', who might be intellectually brilliant, never failed an examination, and are technically excellent, may not turn out to be the best physicians. Through formal and informal observations, Dr. Barrett's experiences confirm his personal belief that those doctors who treat patients with warmth and genuineness and embrace the opportunity to relieve their pain and suffering demonstrate the ideals of being a 'good doctor'. Similar to the discussion in Chapter 4 about the character traits necessary to help medical students learn how to become doctors possessing fundamental character traits such as empathy and compassion, Dr. Barrett's recommended curriculum for the twenty-first century is designed with a patient-first point of view. The question posed is: 'What do patients want from doctors?' In response to the research that addresses this question, the chapter concludes with suggestions for designing innovative courses to expand the academic curriculum offered in medical training. Such courses would require staff development, sensitivity training, mentorships, and additional strategies that include teaching doctors to learn how to communicate with patients; therefore, embracing the skills, competencies, and knowledge embodied in personal and interpersonal development.

There is a strong and mounting awareness globally that a key dimension of life is the possession of sound mental health and well-being. In instances where problems exist, societies, colleges, and universities are obligated to actively develop comprehensive policies and services that address mental health and its related disorders. There is also growing realisation by governments and helping organisations across the globe that physicians are not untouchable, and emphasis on self-care and help-seeking behaviour to improve one's mental health is a sign of strength. In response to the international awareness discussions come the following recommendations:

- Proactively examine existing policies with a view to assessing how these policies negatively impact studies of mental illnesses.
- Recognise that funding for student services extends to the type of student being served in addition to the presenting mental health problem. Students must be treated with diversity in mind. All students will not view seeking help the same way.
- Create a culture and environment whereby self-care is encouraged amongst the faculty, staff, and students, and the profession in general promotes prevention.
- Employ curricular innovations that address and use learning theories to provide foundations for creating learning environments suited to adult learning styles and needs.
- Encourage opportunities for inclusive campus communities where medical students are supported and socially connected through a system that improves well-being by developing intervention strategies based upon empirical testing.

A primary purpose of medical education is to prepare physicians to be compassionate, knowledgeable, competent, and caring towards patients. In order to achieve this ideal, training in medical school necessitates teaching medical students how to prioritise their own mental health and well-being without feelings of guilt or personal weakness. Although the focus of this book is medical student mental health and well-being, the mental health of the faculty and staff working in medical schools, hospitals, the helping professions, and other environments is no less significant. The quality of the connections amongst students, faculty, and staff impacts their mental health. The development of an environment that promotes mental health and well-being will benefit the entire campus community, support learning, and contribute to the welfare and care of all citizens. Efforts to represent a movement towards the promotion of mental health and well-being for all matters to everyone on the planet.

REFERENCES

Benner, P., & Sutphen, M. (2007). Learning across the professions: The clergy, a case in point. *Journal of Nursing Education, 46*(3), 103-8. Retrieved from http://search.proquest.com/docview/203971539?accountid=14376

Berragan, L. (2013). Conceptualising learning through simulation: An expansive approach for professional and personal learning. *Nurse Education in Practice*, *13*(4), 250–255. doi:10.1016/j.nepr.2013.01.004 PMID:23402772

Dyrbye, L. N., Power, D. V., Stanford Massie, F., Eacker, A., Harper, W., Thomas, M. R., & Shanafelt, T. D. (2010). Factors associated with resilience to and recovery from burnout: A prospective, multi-institutional study of US medical students. *Medical Education*, *44*(10), 1016–1026. doi:10.1111/j.1365-2923.2010.03754.x PMID:20880371

Franco, K. (2013). Retrieved from news.com/education/blogs/medical-school-admissions-doctor/2013/10/22/understand-common-reasons-leave-medical-school

Greeno, J. G. (1997). On claims that answer the wrong questions. *Educational Researcher*, *26*, 1, 5–17.

Greeno, J. G., & Van De Sande, C. (2007). Perspectival understanding of conceptions and conceptual growth in interaction. *Educational Psychologist*, *42*(1), 9–23. doi:10.1080/00461520709336915

Hafferty, F. W. (1998). Beyond curriculum reform: Confronting medicines hidden curriculum. *Academic Medicine*, *73*(4), 403–407. doi:10.1097/00001888-199804000-00013 PMID:9580717

Muzafar, Y., Khan, H. H., Ashraf, H., Hussain, W., Sajid, H., Tahir, M., & Ahmad, W. (2015). Burnout and its Associated Factors in Medical Students of Lahore, Pakistan. *Cureus, 7*(11). 10.7759/cureus.390

Noone, J. (2009). Teaching to the three apprenticeships: Designing learning activities for professional practice in an undergraduate curriculum. *The Journal of Nursing Education*, *48*(8), 468–471. doi:10.3928/01484834-20090518-08 PMID:19681538

Rotenstein, L.S., Ramos, M.A., Torre, M., Segal, J.B., Oeluso, M.J., Guille, C., … Mata, D.A. (2016). Prevalence of Depression, depressive symptoms, and suicidal ideation among medical students: A systematic review and meta-analysis. *JAMA, 316*(21), 2214-2236. doi:10.1001/jama.2016.17324

YouGov. (n.d.). *One in four students suffer from mental health problems*. Retrieved from https://yougov.co.uk/news/2016/.../quarter-britains-students-are-afflicted-mental-hea/

Appendix

APPENDIX 1

Mental Health and Well-Being Toolkit

Listed below are some organisations working in the field of mental health, and well-being:

- American College of Mental Health Administration
- Independent professional organisation for mental health administrators from various disciplines.
- American Counseling Association
- Counselling organisation site featuring resources for counsellors and students.
    - Contact: 202-966-7300

Resources useful for:

- Medical Students and Residents
    - This organisation works to relieve and support those living with anxiety disorders by providing information, support and understanding via an extensive range of services, including 1:1 therapy.
- Association of Practicing Psychologists
    - Goal to advance the practice of psychology while promoting human welfare.
- Centre for Disease Control CDC - Burden of Mental Illness - Mental Illness - Mental ...
    - https://www.cdc.gov/mentalhealth/basics/burden.htm
- Centre for Global Mental Health
    - www.centreforglobalmentalhealth.org
- Child Mind Institute
    - Contact: 212-308-3118

        - The Child Mind Institute's Symptom Checker - updated based on the DSM-V
        - Mental Health Guide provides information about diagnostic criteria for various disorders.
- Committee of Interns and Residents (CIR)/SEIU Healthcare
    - Contact: info@cirseiu.org; 800-247-8877
        - The Committee of Interns and Residents (CIR) gives residents, interns, and fellows a voice to improve their salary and working conditions, their education and training, and the quality of care they provide to patients. CIR members and alumni are available to be speakers and/or facilitators at community conversations about mental health as well as provide resources for dialogue speakers and facilitators.
- Community Anti-Drug Coalitions of America (CADCA)
    - Contact: 800-54-CADCA
    - The Community Anti-Drug Coalitions of America (CADCA) is a membership organization representing those working to make their communities safe, healthy and drug-free. CADCA provides expertise in building coalitions to address local conditions including:
        - Underage and binge drinking
        - Youth tobacco use
        - Illicit drug use
        - Abuse of over-the-counter and prescription medicines.
- Families for Depression Awareness is a nonprofit organization working to promote depression awareness by uniquely focusing on the friends, family, and caregivers of those experiencing depression and/or bipolar.
- Medical Education Resources Global Medical Education
    - https://www.gmeded.com/resources
        - Medical Education Resources. Global Medical Education (GME) provides a list of recommended medical education resources below for clinicians and patients.
- Mental Health America (MHA)
    - Contact: 800-969-6642
    - Mental Health America (MHA) is a nonprofit organization dedicated to helping all people live mentally healthier lives. Helpful resources from Mental Health America:
    - Find mental health treatment services
    - Mental Health America's Public Education Programs:
        - MHA's Live Your Life Well provides helpful wellness tools
        - General information about mental health.

- Mental Health Foundation (UK)
    - Committed to improving the lives of citizens with mental health problems or learning difficulties.
- National Alliance of Multi-Ethnic Behavioural Health Associations. The mission of NAMBHA is to collectively promote the behavioural well-being and full potential of people of color and to eliminate disparities in behavioural health services and treatment through policy reform, culturally appropriate research and evaluation, systems change and transformation, acquisition and distribution of resources, and consumer involvement.
- National Alliance on Mental Illness (NAMI)
    - Contact: info@nami.org; 800-950-6264
    - The National Alliance on Mental Illness is dedicated to building better lives for the millions of Americans affected by mental illness. Contact NAMI to access support, information, and free education programs for families and individuals living with mental health problems. Helpful resources from NAMI:
    - NAMI Walks - mental health awareness raising events
    - Brochures and information about specific mental illnesses and treatment options
    - NMHA, a nonprofit organization addressing all aspects of mental health and mental illness, works to improve the mental health of all Americans, especially the 54 million individuals with mental disorders, through advocacy, education, research and service.
- National Physicians Alliance
  Contact: npa@npalliance.org
        - The National Physicians Alliance supports research and education programs that promote health and foster active engagement of physicians within communities to achieve high quality, affordable health care for all.
        - NPA can identify physicians with mental health expertise who can participate in or speakers at awareness events and community conversations.
        - Connect with NPA's Local Networks for additional ways to collaborate with physicians in local region, state or community.
- Screening for Mental Health
    - Facilitates mental health screening programmes in hospitals, universities, primary care offices and social services agencies.
- The Jed Foundation
    - Contact: 212-647-7544

    - The Jed Foundation provides expertise in promoting emotional and mental health and preventing suicide among teens, young adults, and college students. Helpful resources provided by the Jed Foundation include:
    - Resources for campus professionals that address emotional and mental health systems in college and university campuses and crisis management on college and university campuses.
    - Online communications strategies and resources for supporting the emotional and mental health of college students and young adults
- Time to Change, a U.K.-based campaign run by the mental health charity organizations Mind and Rethink Mental Illness, works with adults, children, and youth to end discriminatory attitudes and behaviour toward those with mental health concerns across England.
- National Federation of Families for Children's Mental Health
    - Contact: 240-403-1901
    - The National Federation of Families for Children's Mental Health is a s a national family-run organization focused on the issues of children and youth with emotional, behavioural, or mental health needs and their families. Helpful Resources provided by the National Federation of Families for Children's Mental Health include:
        - Networks of family members available to participate as speakers at awareness events and community dialogues.
    - See Me, Scotland's response to the stigmatization of mental health concerns, is a national program dedicated to ending the discrimination affecting outcomes for those facing mental and emotional challenges.
- Teenmentalhealth.org, a nonprofit dedicated to providing youth, their families, and educators with reliable, evidence-based mental health information, works to combat stigma through accurate information and greater mental health literacy.
- Working to improve the quality of life for people with mental health problems
- The NoStigmas Network is an organization seeking to unite individuals with a common goal: the elimination of stigma toward mental health concerns.
- The Trevor Project Programs provide life-saving and life-affirming resources for LGBTQ youth and to create safe, accepting and inclusive environments for all young people, regardless of sexual orientation or gender identity.
- Educator and Parent Resources including brochures, books, and films
- Archived webinars focus on how to reduce the risk for suicide, promote resiliency, and incorporate the best practices to create positive environments for all youth and are designed for service providers, educators, and other adults across the country.

World Health Organisation. Provides a plethora of fact sheets and Mental health news from around the world.

- World Federation for Mental Health
    - Global organization which aims to promote the advancement in the mental health field.
    - Mental Health Speakers Bureau provides a directory of Active Minds speakers that can bring the mental health conversation to your community.
    - Contact Active Minds about holding an event on a college campus or for information about involving youth in mental health programming and events.
    - Send Silence Packing is a program to reduce college student suicide and promote a dialogue about mental health issues on college campuses,
    - Awareness activities that address negative attitudes and beliefs about mental illness, stress, eating disorders, and veteran student mental health.
    - Emerging Scholars Fellowship provides an opportunity for students to complete independent research or creative projects devoted to mental health with emphasis on issues relevant to younger communities.

APPENDIX 2

Prospective and Current Medical Student Toolkit

- American Medical Association - AMA
    - https://healthfinder.gov/FindServices/Organizations/Organization...
- Association of American Medical Colleges - Official Site
    - https://www.aamc.org
- American Osteopathic Association - Official Site
    - www.osteopathic.org
- American Association of Colleges of Osteopathic Medicine
    - www.aacom.org
- Doctors' health and well-being
    - https://www.rsm.ac.uk/events/events-listing/2013-2014/sections/
- The Health and Wellbeing of Doctors and Medical Students
    - https://ama.com.au/position-statement/health-and-wellbeing-doctors
- Improving mental health and well-being - Living Well
    - https://www.livingwell.org.au/

- Medical Student Well-Being
  - amsa.org
- Mental Health of Students
  - https://www.nasn.org/
- University Student Mental Health
  - mentalhealth.amsa.org.au/

APPENDIX 3

Administrators, Counsellors, Student Affairs and Medical Academic Faculty Toolkit of useful Assessments

- **Dreem Measure:** The Dundee Ready Educational Environment Measure (DREEM). The DREEM's Social Self-Perception subscale measures the way a student perceives their learning and development.
- **Dreem Sub-Scale:** The Academic Self-Perception sub-scale indicates how students feel about the learning environment
- **Jefferson Scale of Empathy–Student Version**: Used to measure self-reported levels of empathy.
- **Maslach's Burnout Inventory (MBI):** This inventory is a leading measure of burnout and defines the three dimensions of burnout: Emotional Exhaustion, Depersonalisation and Personal Accomplishment.
- **Oldenburg Burnout Inventory (OLBI-S):** The Oldenburg Burnout Inventory for college students. This inventory was adapted to measure academic burnout.
- **Patient Health Questionnaire (PHQ-9):** An anonymous screening system used to identify affective disorders and suicide in medical students.
- **Psychological or Psychosocial Interventions:** Include problem-solving therapy, cognitive behavioural therapy (CBT) and psychodynamic interpersonal therapy. These methods are effective in reducing the number of recurrent Deliberate Self-Harm (DSH) events.
- **The Columbia –Suicide Severity Rating Scale (C-SSRS):** This scale is utilised to assess suicide ideation, lethality and severity of suicide attempt.
- **The Depression Anxiety Stress Scale (DASS):** The DASS is a 42-itemself report instrument designed to measure the three -related negative emotional states of depression, anxiety, tension/stress.
- **The Healer Education Assessment and Referral (HEAR) Programme:** A two-tiered screening and referral system used to identify affective disorders and suicide in medical students.

- **The Mindful Attention Awareness Scale (MAAS):** The MAAS is a 15-item scale designed to assess a core characteristic of dispositional mindfulness.
- **The Spectrum of Stress Tool:** Useful to measure distress, chronic stress, burnout and mental illness in Residents.

APPENDIX 4

Toolkit: Acronyms

AACOM: American Association of Colleges of Osteopathic Medicine
AAHC: Association of Academic Health Centres
AAHE: American Association for Health Education
AAMA: American Academy of Medical Administrators
AAMC: American Association of Medical Colleges
ACGME: Accreditation Council on Graduate Medical Education
AMA: American Medical Association
AMA: The Australian Medical Association
BMA: The British Medical Association
CMA: The Canadian Medical Association
CAMC: The Caribbean Association of Medical Councils
CMA: Chinese Medical Association
CDC: Centre for Diseases Control
CEC: Continuing Education Credits
CEU: Continuing Education Units
CAMA: Chinese American Medical Association
GMC: General Medical Council
GME: Graduate Medical Education
LCME: The Liaison Committee on Medical Education
MET: Medical Education and Training
RSM: The Royal Society of Medicine
WHO: World Health Organisation
UKMSA: The United Kingdom Medical Students Association

Glossary

Academy of Medical Educators (AME): The Academy of Medical Educators is the professional organisation for all those involved in medical education—the education and training of students and practitioners in medicine, dentistry and veterinary science. Established in 2006 and gaining charitable status in 2009, the Academy exists to provide leadership, promote standards and support all those involved in the Academic discipline of medical education.

Academics: Relating to school or study; acquisition of education.

Adaptive Perfectionist: Hold themselves to high personal standards, while not engaging in overly self-critical behaviours and thinking when they do not meet high standards.

Adult Learning: Different from children, adults prefer to create their own goals for learning, they like to take advantage of their already established competencies and favour problem solving educational techniques in which they actively participate in and share the responsibility for the learning outcomes.

Allopathic Medical School: Relating to or being a system of medicine that aims to combat disease by using remedies (as drugs or surgery) that produce effects that are different from or incompatible with those of the disease being treated.

Alternative Medicine: An approach to healthcare that does not have its roots in conventional (Western) medicine. The term is often used inter-changeably with complementary medicine in terms of the range of treatments used (Complementary and Alternative Medicine CAM), the word 'alternative' signifying its use instead of, rather than alongside, conventional medicine. Examples of alternative/complementary medicine include: homeopathy, acupuncture, osteopathy, chiropractic and herbalism.

American Medical Association (AMA): According to its mission statement, this professional association represents the voice of the American medical profession and constitutes the partnership of physicians and their professional associations dedicated to promoting the art and science of medicine and the betterment of public health. The AMA serves physicians and their patients by establishing and promoting ethical, educational, and clinical standards for the medical profession and by advocating the highest principle of all: the integrity of the physician/patient relationship. http://www.ama-assn.org/.

Apprenticeship Learning: Is learning for practise.

Association for Medical Education in Europe (AMEE): A worldwide association concerned with education in the medical and health professions, including teachers, curriculum developers, deans, administrators, researchers and students. AMEE works across the continuum of education to promote its quality, facilitate and develop high quality research, and serve as a source of advice on matters relating to medical education. AMEE assists with the development of skills required by medical teachers and facilitates the exchange of information in the rapidly changing world of medical education. AMEE's activities include: annual conferences; publications including the peer-reviewed journal Medical Teacher; courses such as Essential Skills in Medical Education (ESME); Best Evidence Medical Education (BEME) Collaboration; and the MedEdWorld website. www.amee.org/index.asp www.mededworld.org.

Association of American Medical Colleges (AAMC): A non-profit association of the 141 accredited United States medical schools, the 17 accredited Canadian medical schools, more than 400 major teaching hospitals and health systems, and 90 academic and scientific societies representing faculty members, medical students and resident physicians. www.aamc.org.

Association of Faculties of Medical Education Canada (AFMC): The Association of Faculties of Medicine of Canada (AFMC) represents Canada's 17 faculties of medicine. AFMC has 3 standing committees which provide guidance on continuing, postgraduate, and undergraduate medical education, and a fourth standing committee on research and graduate studies. It also has eleven resource groups that provide national engagement on a wide range of issues relating to their social accountability mandate such as diversity in our medical schools, global health, professionalism, and student affairs. Representatives from the AFMC and CMA, along with students and public representatives are members of the Committee on Accreditation of Canadian Medical Schools (CACMS) which accredit the MD program in all 17 faculties of medicine in Canada. The accreditation is undertaken jointly between CACMS in Canada and the Liaison Committee on Medical Education in the U.S. Additionally, AFMC, through the Committee on Accreditation of Continuing Medical Education, also participates in the accreditation of the offices of Continuing Medical Education at all Canadian faculties of medicine. Since 2005, AFMC has also served as the secretariat for the Canadian Conference on Medical Education, delivered through a partnership between the AFMC, the Canadian Association for Medical Education, the College of Family Physicians of Canada, the Medical Council of Canada and the Royal College of Physicians and Surgeons of Canada.

American Osteopathic Association (AOA): Organisation that regulates and accredits osteopathic training programmes. This agency is equivalent to the LCME which accredits allopathic medical schools. http://www.am-osteo-assn.org.

Anxiety: An abnormal and overwhelming sense of apprehension and fear often marked by physical signs (such as tension, sweating, and increased pulse rate), by doubt concerning the reality and nature of the threat, and by self-doubt about one's capacity to cope with it.

Articulation: Social learning method used to help students develop the cognitive and metacognitive skills that are the target of cognitive apprenticeship.

Attitude: A settled way of thinking or feeling about someone or something, typically one that is reflected in a person's behaviour.

Attrition: Student attrition is the reduction in numbers of students attending courses as time goes by. Medical students may dropout or may leave medical school for a number of reasons, not all related to educational issues, for example due to the development of health problems.

Assessment: A system of evaluation of professional accomplishments using defined criteria and usually including an attempt at measurement either by grading on a rough scale or by assigning numerical value. The purpose of assessment in an educational context is to make a judgment about the level of skills or knowledge, to measure improvement over time, to evaluate strengths and weaknesses, to rank students for selection or exclusion, or to motivate. Assessment should be as objective and reproducible as possible. A reliable test should produce the same or similar scores on two or more occasions or if given by two or more assessors. The validity of a test is determined by the extent to which it measures whatever it sets out to measure. One can distinguish three types of assessment: 1) Formative assessment is testing that is part of the developmental or on-going teaching/learning process. It should include delivery of feedback to the student. 2) Summative assessment is testing which often occurs at the end of a term or course, used primarily to provide information about how much the student has learned and how well the course was taught. 3) Criterion-referenced assessment refers to testing against an absolute standard such as an individual's performance against a benchmark.

Authentic Assessment: An assessment requiring students to use the same competencies, or combinations of knowledge, skills, and attitudes, that they need to apply in the criterion situation in professional life. The level of authenticity of an assessment is thus defined by its degree of resemblance to the criterion situation.

Authentic Leaders: Are positive people with truthful self-concepts who promote openness.

Authentic Leadership: Is an approach to leadership that emphasises building the leader's legitimacy through honest relationships with followers which value their input and are built on an ethical foundation.

Balance in Dimensions of Wellness: The ability to self-assess or understand dimensions of wellness and how to ensure equality among dimensions.

Basic Medical Education: Undergraduate medical education.

Basic Science Model: Taught as part of the medical curriculum to provide an overview of fundamental scientific theories and concepts for clinical application. Subjects traditionally taught as part of the medical curriculum include anatomy, histology, physiology, biochemistry and pathology. The current teaching model includes genetics, cell and molecular biology, epidemiology, nutrition and energy metabolism, and the science of healthcare delivery and bioinformatics. Following the Flexner model, basic medical sciences were traditionally taught before clinical exposure. However, the dominant teaching model has shifted to a more integrated approach, and either paired with related clinical disciplines are taught in blocks by organ system.

Basic Science Years: A term that usually refers to the initial two years of a medical school's programme. However, in some schools, this may entail more or less than two years. With the introduction of new learning methodologies such as

Problem-Based Learning (PBL) and early exposure to patients, basic science learning has become more integrated with clinical instruction and the division between basic science years and clinical years has eroded.

Best Practice: Professional procedures that are accepted or prescribed as being correct or most effective.

Blog: A personal website or web page on which an individual records opinions and links to other sites, etc. on a regular basis. Blogs can range from personal, diary-like pages to in-depth public affairs analysis. Some provide description of… selected links, others tell about details of a writer's day and some offer personal opinions and commentaries on the news of a day.

Bloom's Taxonomy: Is a classification system used to define and distinguish different levels of human cognition—i.e., thinking, learning, and understanding. Bloom's taxonomy was originally published in 1956 by a team of cognitive psychologists at the University of Chicago. It is named after the committee's chairman, Benjamin Bloom (1913–1999). The original taxonomy was organized into three domains: Cognitive, Affective, and Psychomotor. Educators have primarily focused on the Cognitive model, which includes six different classification levels: Knowledge, Comprehension, Application, Analysis, Synthesis, and Evaluation. The group sought to design a logical framework for teaching and learning goals that would help researchers and educators understand the fundamental ways in which people acquire and develop new knowledge, skills, and understandings. Their initial intention was to help academics avoid duplicative or redundant efforts in developing different tests to measure the same educational objectives. Some users of the taxonomy place more emphasis on the hierarchical nature of the framework, asserting that the first three elements—Knowledge, Comprehension, and Application—represent lower levels of cognition and learning, while Analysis, Synthesis, and Evaluation are considered higher-order skills. For this reason, the taxonomy is often graphically represented as a pyramid with higher-order cognition at the top.

Board Exam: After successfully completing an accredited residency programme, trainees take a national evaluation in their specialty. Typically, passing the board exam is one requirement for board certification.

Burnout: A syndrome of emotional exhaustion, loss of meaning in work, feelings of ineffectiveness, and a tendency to view people as objects rather than human beings.

Canadian Association for Medical Education (CAME): Established in 1987, CAME is a grassroots organisation for the promotion and advancement of excellence in medical education. Their goal is to promote excellence and scholarship in all aspects of medical education by advocating for medical education and medical educators, by supporting faculty and educational development, and by encouraging research in medical education through networking and scientific activities.

Cartesian Dualism: The division of mind and body as separate entities.

Chronic Stress: Prolonged states of arousal and alertness in response to stress.

Clerkships: A rotation around the clinical settings of the medical school. Some clerkships are obligatory (e.g., internal medicine, paediatrics, surgery), while others are elective or selective. In the United States, medical students participate in clerkships in their third and fourth year while in Europe, this typically occurs in the fourth through sixth year of medical school.

Clinical Years: This typically refers to the third and fourth year of medical school when students spend their time gaining basic clinical competencies in clerkships. In the past, it was often not until that time that students had contact with patients. However, in recent years, medical education has become more integrated and students often experience clinical settings already in the first year of medical school.

Coaching: Social learning method used to help students develop the cognitive and metacognitive skills that are the target of cognitive apprenticeship.

Cognitive Apprenticeship: The application of apprentice learning to the teaching of cognitive skills in applied settings.

Collaborative Learning: In collaborative learning students learn from each other without the assignment of specific roles of tutor and tutee. Students work together as members of a group or team to solve a problem, complete a task or create a product.

Comlex: The Comprehensive Osteopathic Medical Licensing Examination of the United States (COMLEX-USA or the Boards) is a series of three osteopathic medical licensing examinations administered by the National Board of Osteopathic Medical Examiners (NBOME) similar to the United States Medical Licensing Examination(USMLE).

Compassion: Awareness of and feeling for the pain and suffering of others; sympathy.

Competence: Possession of a satisfactory level of relevant knowledge and acquisition of a range of relevant skills that include interpersonal and technical components at a certain point in the educational process. Such knowledge and skills are necessary to perform the tasks that reflect the scope of professional practises. Competence may differ from "performance", which denotes actions taken in a real-life situation. Competence is therefore not the same as "knowing" on the contrary, it may well be about recognizing one's own limits. The more experienced the professional being tested, the more difficult it is to create a tool to assess their actual understandings and the complex skills of the tasks they undertake. A holistic integration of understandings, abilities and professional judgments, i.e., a "generic" model, is one where competence is not necessarily directly observable, but rather can be inferred from performance.

Contextualisation: Practical reasoning and requires that the practitioner select the elements of professional knowledge most relevant to the given context.

Continuing Medical Education (CME): A continuous process of acquiring new knowledge and skills throughout one's professional life. As undergraduate and postgraduate education is insufficient to ensure lifelong physicians' competencies, it is essential to maintain the competencies of physicians, to remedy gaps in skills, and to enable professionals to respond to the challenges of rapidly growing knowledge and technologies, changing health needs and the social, political and economic factors of the practise of medicine. Continuing medical education depends highly upon learner motivation and self-directed learning skills. See also Life-Long Learning; Continuing Professional Development (CPD); Faculty Development.

Crisis: Is generally described as situations or events that exceed ones' capabilities and/or resources and leave one feeling void of coping mechanisms.

Critical Reflection: Involves a critique of the presuppositions on which our beliefs have been built which transforms learning into a new experience.

Critical Thinking: Is the ability to apply higher-order cognitive skills (conceptualisation, analysis, evaluation) and the disposition to be deliberate about thinking (being open-minded or intellectually honest) that lead to action that is logical and appropriate. Papp et al. have developed a model of five stages of critical thinking:

(1) Unreflective thinker; (2) Beginning critical thinker; (3) Practising critical thinker; (4) Advanced critical thinker; and (5) Accomplished critical thinker.

Culture: The collective programming of the mind that distinguishes the members of one group or category of people from another.

Curriculum: Is a sophisticated blend of educational strategies, course content, learning outcomes, educational experiences, assessment, the educational environment and the individual students' learning style, personal timetable and the programme of work.

Darwinian Way: Survival of the fittest or strongest.

Deferment: The act or an instance of delaying or putting off student loan repayments.

Deliberate Self-Harm: Direct behaviour that causes minor to moderate physical injury, that is undertaken without conscious suicidal intent and that occurs in the absence of psychoses and/or organic intellectual impairment.

Depersonalisation: Depersonalisation is described as feeling callousness towards others. Using internal attributes for academic success such as doing well academically because of good studying techniques could explain the strong correlation with depersonalisation.

Distress: A sense of real or implied threat that activates involuntary mechanisms.

Doctor of Medicine: A practitioner of the healing arts, as one graduated from a college of medicine, osteopathy, chiropractic, optometry, podiatry, dentistry, or veterinary medicine, and licensed to practice.

Doctor of Osteopathic Medicine (D.O. or DO): Is a professional degree for physicians and surgeons offered by medical schools in the United States. Holders of the D.O. degree are known as osteopathic physicians and have the same rights, privileges, and responsibilities as physicians with a Doctor of Medicine degree (M.D.). D.O. physicians are licensed to practice the full scope of medicine and surgery in sixty countries, including all 50 states in the US, and make up 7 percent of the total U.S. physician population. As of 2012, there were more than 82,500 D.O. physicians in the United States.

Dysphoric: An emotional state characterized by anxiety, depression, or unease.

Educational Climate: The way in which students perceive their educational environment and teaching practices.

Efficacy: The ability to produce the necessary or desired result.

Emotional Intelligence: Intelligence regarding the emotions, especially in the ability to monitor one's own or others' emotions.

Empathy: Empathy is a predominantly cognitive (rather than emotional) attribute that involves an understanding (rather than feeling) of experiences, concerns and perspectives of the patients, combined with a capacity to communicate this understanding.

Ethnicity: People who share a common culture or nationality.

Exploration: Social learning method used to help students develop the cognitive and metacognitive skills that are the target of cognitive apprenticeship. Exploration is the last technique in cognitive apprentice instruction and is an attempt to move the student to independently execute expert problem solving and to seek out and define new problems that can be solved with the newly acquired skills and strategies.

Evaluation: A process that attempts to systematically and objectively determine relevance, effectiveness, and impact of activities in relation to specified objectives. Evaluation can be related to structure, process, or outcome. One can distinguish these various types: 1) Formative individual evaluation provides feedback to an individual (usually a learner) in order to improve that individual's performance. This type of evaluation identifies areas for improvement and provides specific suggestions for improvement serving as an educational tool. 2) Summative individual evaluation measures whether specific objectives were accomplished by an individual in order to place a value on the performance of that individual. It may certify competency or lack of competency in performance in a particular area. 3) Formative programme evaluation provides information in order to improve a programme's performance. It usually takes the form of surveys of learners to obtain feedback about and suggestions for improving a curriculum. Quantitative information such as ratings of various aspects of the curriculum can help identify areas that need revision. Qualitative information, such as responses to open-ended questions about programme strengths and weaknesses, as well as suggestions for change, provide feedback in areas that may not have been anticipated and provide ideas for improvement. Information can also be obtained from faculty or other observers, such as nurses and patients. 4) Summative programme evaluation measures the success of a curriculum in achieving learner objectives for all targeted learners, its success in achieving its process objectives, and/or its success in engaging, motivating, and pleasing its learners and faculty. In addition to quantitative data, summative programme evaluation may include qualitative information about unintended barriers or unanticipated effects encountered in programme implementation. 5) Formative evaluations generally require the least amount of rigor, whereas summative individual and summative programme evaluation for external use (e.g., certification of competence) requires the greatest amount of rigor. When a high degree of methodological rigor is required, the measurement instrument must be appropriate in terms of content, reliability, validity, and practicality.

Extracurricular Activities: Are those performed by students that fall outside the realm of the normal curriculum of school or university education. Such activities may form an important part of integrating students into university life and offer opportunities for developing key life and social skills. Examples may include: sports, drama, languages, politics, debating, journalism, events organising, choir, music, amongst many others.

Flexner Report: This report, written and published by Abraham Flexner (1866-1959) in 1910 for the Carnegie Foundation and entitled "Medical Education in the United States and Canada" is known today as the Flexner Report. It triggered much-needed reforms in the standards, organisation, and curriculum of North American medical schools. At the time of the Flexner Report, many medical schools were proprietary schools operated more for profit than for education. Flexner proposed that medical schools operate instead in the German tradition of combining strong biomedical sciences with hands-on clinical training. The report caused many medical schools to close down. It remains one of the most important publications on medical education in the 20th century. Abraham Flexner was not a doctor, but a secondary school teacher and principal for 19 years in Louisville, Kentucky. He did graduate work at Harvard University and the University of Berlin and joined the research staff of the Carnegie Foundation for the Advancement of Teaching. In 1930, Flexner founded the Institute for Advanced Study at Princeton University and served as its first director. Flexner was one of the great educators of the 20th century. Modern medical education and medicine in North America owes a large debt to this educator.

Forbearance: The temporary suspension of loan repayments. Interest continues to accrue during forbearance and may result in extending the repayment period or cause payments to increase once they are resumed. A borrower must apply to the lender to be considered for forbearance.

Formation: A pedagogy that produces habits of mind or what some have labelled habitus which is the ability to think in context and perform like a member of the profession.

General Medical Council (GMC): The General Medical Council (GMC) is the independent regulator for medical doctors in the United Kingdom. The purpose of the GMC is to protect, promote and maintain the health and safety of the public by ensuring proper standards in the practice of medicine. www.gmc-uk.org/.

Goal: A general aim, object, or end-effect which one strives to achieve.

Graduate Medical Education (GME): In the United States, this term typically refers to residency training and fellowships; the education physicians receive after finishing medical school. In many other countries' it is called specialty training or postgraduate education.

Graduate Training or Internship: The phase of acquiring widening clinical experience through the practise of basic clinical skills and judgment. This is normally used to designate the period of hospital clerkship. The periods of undergraduate education and graduate training together comprise the doctor's basic medical education.

Habitus of Practice: Habitus or habits of practice are an interactive process whereby a new identity is formed so that students begin to see themselves as members of the profession rather than just acting the part.

Health: In accordance with the Constitution of the World Health Organisation (1948) health is "a state of complete physical, mental and social well-being and not merely the absence of disease and infirmity". Health is defined as a positive concept, emphasising social and personal resources as well as physical capabilities.

Health and Well-Being: In accordance with the Constitution of the World Health Organisation (1948) health is "a state of complete physical, mental and social well-being and not merely the absence of disease and infirmity". Health is defined as a positive concept, emphasising social and personal resources as well as physical capabilities.

Health Care: Services provided to individuals or communities by a health care system or by professionals to promote, maintain, monitor, or restore health. Health care contains a broad spectrum of services and activities delivered by a team of health personnel. This contrasts with medical care, which concentrates on diagnostic and therapeutic actions performed by or under the supervision of an individual physician.

Health Education: To develop and provide learning opportunities focused on improving health and wellness for individuals and communities.

Health Education Models: Models that provide guidance for the planning, implementing, and assessing health promotion programmes.

Health Education Theories: Theories that provide guidance in explaining how and why changes occur.

Health Promotion: The process of enabling individuals to increase control over and improve their health. It involves the population as a whole in the context of their everyday lives, rather than focusing on people at risk for specific diseases, and is directed toward action on the determinants or causes of health.

Healthy Behaviour: The combination of knowledge, practices and attitudes that together contribute to motivate actions we take regarding our own health. Healthy behaviour may promote and preserve good health. On the other hand, behaviours harmful to health such as tobacco smoking, alcohol drinking, drug abuse and lack of physical exercise may be determinants of disease.

Helicopter Parents: Parents likened to a military or police helicopter hovering overhead. These parents are overly involved in a student's life.

Hidden Curriculum: Unwritten expectation of medical students to push through stressors and not complain or seek assistance.

Higher Education: Education beyond high school and provided by colleges, graduate and professional schools.

Hippocratic Oath: An affirmation usually taken by physicians about to enter the practice of medicine. It is attributed to Greek physician, Hippocrates of Cos, who is called the "Father of Medicine" (circa 460-377 B.C.). Its content reflects the ethical code of the physicians' attitudes and behaviour and obligations towards patients, colleagues and society.

Humanistic Medical Care: Includes attitudes and actions that demonstrate interest and respect for a patient and related to issues of psychological, social and spiritual concerns.

Impaired Physician Programmes: Every state has an agency that helps physicians who are impaired (e.g., due to drugs or alcohol) to overcome their problems and return to the health care system.

Informal Curriculum: Refers to lessons that are not explicitly taught. In medicine, for example, there are skills and behaviours medical students and doctors learn that are rarely recorded in textbooks or overtly discussed during rounds or lectures.

Information Overload: This is a problem particularly acute in medicine. New articles, Web sites, drugs, and treatments are arriving daily and it takes special skills in information management to maximise their usefulness without drowning in information.

Institute for International Medical Education (IIME): A non-profit medical Institute established in 1999 by a grant from the China Medical Board of New York, which began its own operations in 1914 as a division of The Rockefeller Foundation. The IIME has been entrusted with the development of 'Global Minimum Essential (Core) Requirements' which include knowledge, clinical skills, professional ethical values and fundamental competencies to the practise of health care worldwide. These essential requirements represent only a portion of the educational experience, since each country and even each medical school has unique needs that the educational curriculum should address. Three committees composed of medical experts from around the globe supervise the work of IIME: The Core Committee, the Steering Committee and the Advisory Committee. The Institute is located just outside of New York City in suburban White Plains, New York. http://www.iime.org.

Intern: First year medical resident.

Internship: A first postgraduate training year in which graduates practice medicine under supervision. In some countries, this is a requirement for licensure. In many countries and for many specialties such as internal medicine, paediatrics and surgery, this is the first year of residency. However, as there are some specialties that are too narrow to provide a broad medical practice experience, those residents may have to attend a transitional year in one of the above specialties or a rotating internship.

Interpersonal Skills: Are the skills a person uses to communicate and interact with others. These skills usually include active listening, delegation, persuasion and leadership.

Intolerance of Uncertainty: A perception of ambiguous situations as a threat.

Jefferson Scale of Empathy: The Jefferson Scale of Empathy (JSE, 20 items) was specifically developed for measuring empathy in the context of medical education and patient care, relying on the conceptualisation of empathy as a predominantly cognitive (as opposed to affective or emotional) attribute that involves an understanding (as opposed to feeling) of patients' pain, experiences, concerns, and perspectives, combined with a capacity to communicate this understanding, and an intention to help.

Learning Communities: Is a group of people who share common emotions, values or beliefs, are actively engaged in learning together from each other and by habituation.

Learning Environment: The physical or virtual setting in which learning takes place.

Liaison Committee on Medical Education (LCME): A group organised under the sponsorship of the American Medical Association (AMA) and American Association of Medical Colleges (AAMC) to accredit educational programmes leading to the M.D. degree in the US and Canada. www.lcme.org.

Long White Coat: Most senior doctors, called attending physicians, wear long coats.

Maladaptive Perfectionist: Hold themselves to high standards, but differ in how they respond to falling short of those high standards. Maladaptive perfectionists experience higher levels of self-critical behaviours and thinking in response to failure.

Medical Education: The process of teaching, learning and training of students with an on-going integration of knowledge, experience, skills, qualities, responsibility and values which qualify an individual to practise medicine. It is divided into undergraduate, postgraduate and continuing medical education, but increasingly there is a focus on the "lifelong" nature of medical education. Undergraduate education or basic medical education refers to the period beginning when a student enters medical school and ends with the final examination for basic medical qualification.

This period of education comprises a pre-clinical and a clinical period. It can result in granting a license to practise, which may be provisional and subject to conditions as to supervision; or permitting the start of postgraduate education. In the United States, however, undergraduate education refers to pre-medical college education, which results in a Bachelor's degree and is the training most students receive before entering medical school. Postgraduate education, graduate medical education or specialty training is used to designate the more or less continuous period of post-basic training which, when it occurs, normally directly follows undergraduate training and is designed to lead to competence in a chosen branch of medical practise.

Medical Educator: A professional who focuses on the educational process necessary to transform students into physicians. Some medical educators are physicians, but an increasing number have backgrounds in education, behavioural or other health sciences.

Medical Resident: A physician in graduate medical education who practises

Medical School: A higher education or university level institution offering a prescribed course of medicine. The following are examples of the names that such institutions may bear and which vary from one country to another or even within countries: Medical College; College of Surgeons; Medical Institute; Institute of Medicine and Pharmacy; Institute of Medicine and Surgery; Faculty of Medicine; Faculty of Medical Sciences; Faculty of Medicine and Surgery; Academy of Medicine or Medical Academy; University Centre for Health Sciences; Medical University; Faculty of Medicine and Pharmacy.

Medical School Culture: Customs, rules, and ethics which medical schools place on the management of the institution, being on structure or student's well-being.

Medium Length White Coat: Staff-length (below the hips) is generally worn by residents.

Mental Health: A person's condition with regard to their psychological and emotional well-being.

Mental Health Literacy: The understanding of mental health in regards to awareness, presenting symptoms, and how to seek help.

Mental Health Sequelae: A morbid condition following or occurring as a consequence of another condition or event.

Mental Ill-Health: Covers a very wide spectrum, from the worries and grief we all experience as part of everyday life to the most bleak, suicidal depression or complete loss of touch with everyday reality.

Mental Illness: A wide range of mental health conditions that adversely affect moods, cognitions, and behaviours.

Mentor: Someone who gives advice to a mentee.

Mentor Role: A mentoring role involves a two-way relationship between a mentor and a mentee. A mentor is usually a person with greater experience in the same field than the mentee, who can offer advice, information and critically, support in times of need.

Mindfulness: A mental state achieved by directing one's awareness on the present moment, while acknowledging and accepting one's feelings, thoughts and sensations; it is often used as a therapeutic technique.

Modelling: Social learning method used to help students develop the cognitive and metacognitive skills that are the target of cognitive apprenticeship.

Morbidity: Degree of illness or sickness.

Mortality: Ability to cause death.

Night Float System: One or more residents are assigned to work all or part of the night in order to provide a rest period for the remaining trainees. This scheduling system was designed in response to the limitation on resident work hours. Among the benefits one can find a decrease in fatigue and an increase in morale; on the negative side, residents lose some continuity in providing patient care and may have less opportunity to attend lecture and conference programmes while on night rotation.

Obeah: A form of folk magic and belief among some black cultures, especially African and West Indian. It is used to ward off misfortune or to cause harm, and also, to prescribed herbal medicine.

Occupational Development: The process of developing towards a career.

On-Call Duties: In order to provide coverage for patient care around the clock, medical trainees and practicing physicians have selected evenings, nights, and weekends when they have to be available to manage admissions, medical emergencies and generally provide continuity in diagnostic and treatment activities in in- and out-patient settings.

Osteopathic Medical School: Four years in total length, the first two years of medical school focus on the biomedical and clinical sciences, followed by two years of core clinical training in the clinical specialties. One notable difference in the education at D.O.-granting medical schools is the inclusion of 300 – 500 additional hours in the study of hands-on manual medicine and the body's musculoskeletal system. This training, referred to as osteopathic manipulative medicine, absent in the M.D. curricula.

Osteopathy: A system of medical practice based on a theory that diseases are due chiefly to loss of structural integrity, which can be restored by manipulation of the parts supplemented by therapeutic measures (as use of drugs or surgery).

Pan-American Federation of Associations of Medicals Schools (PAFAMS): A non-governmental, academic and educational organization that gathers information on medical schools in the Western Hemisphere from Canada to Argentina. Founded in 1962 in Chile, PAFAMS is striving through collaboration toward the improvement and development of innovative medical education. The constituency is integrated by 13 national Associations of Medical Schools, and comprises over 500 Medical schools. The mission is: "The promotion and advancement of medical education and the biomedical sciences in the Americas and the Caribbean." www.fepafempafams.org.

Passionate Engagement: Refers to a type of professional practice that includes the practitioner's ability to situate their learning and practices within their own experience and world view, a contextual awareness of the critical elements of the situation and the knowledge of best practices in the profession.

Pedagogy: The art or profession of teaching.

Peer Assessment: Concerns the active participation of students in assessing their peers. Such assessment can be in the form of formative feedback in the course of study, but may also be part of summative assessment and contribute to the final score, particularly in a team-based or group-work situation. It is important that guidance is provided on learning outcomes, marking criteria and rating scales.

Peer Mentoring: Concerns a more equal relationship between people at the same stage of experience in a mutually supportive relationship.

Peer Teaching: Involves students taking an active role in presenting and discussing themes and issues and learning from each other in ways that supplement the teaching of academic staff. Examples may include a student taking responsibility, perhaps within a small group, to investigate one aspect of a topic and give a short summary to the group, leading or facilitating discussions.

Peer-Assisted Learning (PAL): People from similar social groupings who are not professional teachers helping each other to learn and learning themselves by teaching. Those persons helping their peers to learn are from similar social groupings to the learners (although not necessarily from the same course or year of study) and are not themselves professional teachers or 'experts' in the subject. PAL tutors therefore typically have less expansive knowledge of subject matter, less developed teaching skills and less authority than 'expert' tutors. Other terms used: Peer appraisal, Peer assessment, Peer tutoring, Peer teaching, Student teaching/tutoring/mentoring, Peer assisted writing, Study advisory schemes, Peer supported learning.

Perceptions: Is the process of recognising and interpreting sensory stimuli.

Perfectionism: A subjective state in which a person pursues an extremely high standard of performance and, in many cases, demands the same standards of others. Failure to attain the goals may lead to feelings of defeat and other adverse psychological consequences.

Performance: Denotes what an individual actually does in a real-life situation. In medicine, it denotes what a student or doctor actually does in an encounter with a patient when applying learned knowledge and skills, mediated by clinical judgment and the use of interpersonal communication skills. From this standpoint, competence implies professional maturity and ease in making difficult decisions. Although these elements are inherent in good practise, it is not easy to demonstrate them. Assessment of clinical performance is of the greatest importance but is often difficult to measure.

Pharmacological: Relating to pharmacology or to the composition, properties, and actions of drugs.

Physician: A professional, qualified by education and authorised by law to practice medicine. The essence of being a professional is an ability to find solutions to difficult problems for which there are no easily discovered answers and to effectively handle medical situations where no two patients are identical even if they have the same condition. This differentiates the professional, who must deal with complex problems that tend not to have unambiguous, clear-cut solutions, from the technician.

Population Health: Organised efforts focused on the health of defined populations in order to promote and maintain or restore health, to reduce the amount of disease, premature death and disease-produced discomfort and disability. programmes, services and institutions here emphasise the prevention of disease and the health needs of the population as a whole. Among a broad scope of disciplines, various knowledge and skills are utilised such as biostatistics, epidemiology, planning, organization, management, financing and evaluation of health programmes, environmental health, application of social and behavioural factors in health and disease, health promotion, health education and nutrition.

Positive Psychology: A field focused on emphasising the meaningful and optimistic aspects of life. A change from the focus on reaction to dysfunction, to the promotion of enhancing personal fulfillment.

Post-Graduate Year (PGY): This nomenclature designates the years after graduating from medical school. Lately the abbreviation PGY has been replaced with R (for resident), thus one refers to someone who is in the second year of postgraduate training as an R-2 rather than a PGY-2.

Preceptor: Faculty member who is usually in a non-academic practice setting.

Preceptorships: An appointment as a preceptor.

Pre-Med Student: Pre-medical (often referred to as pre-med) is an educational track that undergraduate students pursue prior to entering medical school.

Pressures: Gives us energy, helps with performance and inspires confidence. But excessive pressure can lead to stress.

Prevention: The goals of medicine are to promote health, to preserve health, to restore health when it is impaired, and to minimise suffering and distress. These goals are embodied in the word prevention, which is easiest to define in the context of levels, customarily called primary, secondary and tertiary prevention: Primary prevention refers to the protection of health by personal and community wide effects, such as preserving good nutritional status, physical fitness, and emotional well-being, immunising against infectious diseases, and making the environment safe; Secondary prevention can be defined as the measures available to individuals and populations for the early detection and prompt and effective intervention to correct departures from good health; Tertiary prevention consists of the measures available to reduce or eliminate long-term impairments and disabilities, minimise suffering caused by existing departures from good health, and to promote the patient's adjustment to irremediable conditions. This extends the concept of prevention into the field of rehabilitation. There are no precise boundaries between these levels.

Preventive Medicine: A specialised field of medical practise composed of distinct disciplines that focus on the health of defined populations in order to promote and maintain health and well-being and prevent disease, disability and premature death. It aims at the application of preventive measures within all areas of clinical medicine. In addition to the knowledge of basic and clinical sciences and the skills common to all physicians, practitioners of preventive medicine possess knowledge of and competence in other disciplines. Among a broad scope of such disciplines are: bio-statistics, epidemiology, planning, organization, management, financing, and evaluation of health programmes, environmental health, application of social and behavioural factors in health and disease, health promotion, health education and nutrition.

Primary Health Care: The World Health Organisation defines primary health care as the principal vehicle for the delivery of health care at the most local level of a country's health system. It is essential health care made accessible at a cost the country and community can afford with methods that are practical, scientifically sound and socially acceptable. Everyone in the community should have access to it, and everyone should be involved in it. Beside an appropriate treatment of common diseases and injuries, provision of essential drugs, maternal and child health, and prevention and control locally endemic diseases and immunisation, it should also include at least education of the community on prevalent health problems and methods of preventing them, promotion of proper nutrition, safe water and sanitation.

Primary Prevention: Invention or action that aims to prevent disease or injury before it ever occurs.

Problem-Based Learning (PBL): In this approach, students learn in small groups supported by a tutor. They initially explore a predetermined problem. The problem contains triggers designed to evoke objectives or concepts which are used to set the agenda for individual or group investigation and learning after the initial session. Subsequent group meetings permit students to monitor their achievements and to set further learning goals as required. The tutor's role is to offer support for learning and to help reach the expected outcomes. PBL enables students to develop the ability to translate knowledge into practice at an early stage, encourages individual participation in learning and also allows the development of teamwork skills. Students in PBL courses have been found to place more emphasis on "meaning" (understanding) than "reproduction" (memorisation). Students must engage in a significant amount of self-directed learning; lectures are kept to a minimum. PBL originated at McMaster University in Canada, and then at Maastricht University, and is now widely adopted in medical schools in many countries. Each school makes its own adjustments to the basic model. It does require a heavy investment in resources (library books, IT, tutorial rooms) as well as requiring education and training for tutors.

Professionalism: Adherence to a set of values comprising both a formally agreed-upon code of conduct and the informal expectations of colleagues, clients and society. The key values include acting in a patient's interest, responsiveness to the health needs of society, maintaining the highest standards of excellence on the practise of medicine and in the generation and dissemination of knowledge. In addition to medical knowledge and skills, medical professionals should present psychosocial and humanistic qualities such as caring, empathy, humility and compassion, as well as social responsibility and sensitivity to people's cultures and beliefs. All these qualities are expected of members of highly trained professions. The American Board of Internal Medicine's Project Professionalism indicates the most important elements of professionalism to be: altruism, accountability, duty, excellence, honour and integrity, and respect for others. Professional Altruism: constitutes the essence of professionalism and is based on the rule that the best interest of patients and not self-interest is the professional obligation. Professional Accountability is an important element of professionalism which is required of physicians at several levels: to their patients for fulfilling the implied contract governing the patient/physician relationship, to society for addressing the health needs of the public, and to their profession for adhering to medicine's time-honoured ethical precepts. Professional Duty can be expressed by the free acceptance of a commitment to service, availability and responsiveness when "on call," accepting inconvenience to meet the needs of one's patients, enduring unavoidable risks to oneself when a patient's welfare is at stake, and advocating the best possible care regardless of the patient's ability to pay. It is willingness to seek an active role in professional organisations and volunteering one's skills and expertise for the welfare of the community. Professional Excellence entails a conscientious effort to exceed ordinary expectations. Commitment to excellence is an acknowledged goal for all physicians and includes a commitment to life-long learning. Professional Honour and Integrity implies being fair, being truthful, keeping one's word, meeting commitments, and being straightforward. It also requires recognition of the possibility of conflict of interest and avoiding any situation in which the interest of the physician is placed above that of the patient or allowing personal gain to supersede the best interest of the patient. It constitutes an integral part of professionalism. The importance of professionalism in the patient/physician relationship cannot be overstated. Professional Respect for Others is reflected in the respect towards the patients and their families, other physicians and professional colleagues such as nurses, medical students, and residents. It is the essence of humanism, and humanism is both central to professionalism and fundamental to enhancing collegiality among physicians.

Psychoeducational Intervention: A broad range of activities, combining education, counselling and support interventions. These may be delivered individually or in groups, may be tailored or standardised.

Psychosocial Disability: This term is used to describe students who have a mental illness that periodically interferes with their ability to function and may require accommodation in an academic setting. Counsellors may use the term psychosocial instead of more commonly used terms such as mental impairment or disorder. Its use is preferred as the stigma attached to mental illness may cause further distress to a student labelled mentally ill.

Psychosocial Rounds: Some institutions hold special rounds which include medical and mental health personnel to jointly address patients' psychosocial and psychiatric needs (e.g., depression, compliance, family matters).

Quality of Care: A level of performance or accomplishment that characterises health care. Ultimately, measures of the quality of care always depend upon clinical outcomes or value judgments, but there are ingredients and determinants of quality that can be measured objectively, such as structure, process or procedures, and outcomes.

Reflection: Has been defined as intellectual and affective activities in which individuals engage to explore their experiences in order to lead to new understandings and appreciation. Reflection is a social learning method used to help students develop the cognitive and metacognitive skills that are the target of cognitive apprenticeship.

Reflective Learning Process: An important model of learning that is based on the principle of gaining from the learner's own experience; this is significantly different from the traditional model of undergraduate medical education. It has very clear links with the model of self-directed learning based on a portfolio which gives evidence of activity, reflection and the outcomes of learning. Students use their knowledge, skills and attitudes to solve problems in the workplace. However, many problems are ambiguous and create surprises. Recognition of these surprises causes the student to review problems and create alternative hypotheses, which is termed "Reflection in Action". This leads to a search for more information, seeking help from colleagues or experts, reading texts or searching on-line to solve the problem. In order to turn the new information into new learning, a further step is required, which takes place after the problem has been solved: "Reflecting on Action" involves looking back critically over the initial 'surprise' and the resolution of the problem. The process of reviewing and evaluating information leads to learning and this in turn adds to expertise. The process of learning itself tends to generate new questions and motivates the professional to undertake further inquiry, which results in the learning process being determined more by the learner than by the person who designed the activity. This process of reflection provides a stimulus for learning and helps learners to derive maximum benefit from their own experiences.

Reflective Practitioners: Knowledge and skills are blended in a complex, network of skilled practise.

Research: Scientific inquiry or an organised quest for new knowledge and better understanding, such as of the natural world or determinants of health and disease. Research can take several forms: empiric (observational), analytic, experimental, theoretical and applied.

Residency: The period of training in a specific medical specialty. It occurs after graduation from medical school and its length varies from three to seven years, depending upon the specialty.

Resident or Resident Physician: An individual at any level in a Graduate Medical Education programme, including subspecialty programmes. Other terms used to refer to these individuals include interns, house officers, house staff, trainees, or fellows. The term "intern" is often used to denote physicians in their first year of training. The term "fellow" is frequently used to denote physicians in subspecialty programmes (versus residents in specialty programmes) or in Graduate Medical Education programmes that are beyond the eligibility requirements for first board certification in the discipline.

Resilience: A concept that proposes a recurrent human need to weather periods of stress and change successfully throughout life. The ability to weather each period of disruption and reintegration leaves the person better able to deal with the next change.

Scaffolding: Social learning method used to help students develop the cognitive and metacognitive skills that are the target of cognitive apprenticeship.

Secondary Prevention: Intervention or action that aims to reduce the impact of a disease or injury that has already occurred through screening, early detection or halting.

Self-Assessment: The process of evaluating one's own deficiencies, achievements, behaviour or professional performance and competencies. Self-assessment is an important part of self-directed and lifelong learning because it creates a need for improvement while it justifies confidence in one's competence.

Short White Coat: Most medical students, who are sometimes called "short white coats," wear hip-length coats that are bestowed upon them in a solemn ceremony when they begin medical school.

Situated Learning Theory: Sociocultural perspective focus on the social nature of learning and thinking and many make the claim that all learning and thinking is situated in and tied to social contexts.

Skill: The ability to perform a task well, usually gained by training or experience; a systematic and coordinated pattern of mental and/or physical activity.

Snow Plough Parent: The 'snow plough' parent is defined as a person who constantly forces obstacles out of their kids' paths.

Social Skills: Tools necessary for communicating and interacting with others effectively.

Socialisation: The process of learning, and acting in accord with, societal norms, cultural customs, or professional or organisational roles.

Spirituality: The relationship one has with God or a higher power; one's beliefs.

Stakeholders: A person with an interest or concern in something.

Step 1&2: United States Medical Licensing Examination (USMLE): A 3-step examination procedure that provides a common evaluation system for United States medical licensure applicants. Results of the USMLE are reported to State Medical Boards granting the initial license to practice medicine. Each medical licensing authority requires, as part of its licensing procedure, a successful completion of an examination or other certifications demonstrating qualification for licensure.

Stigma: A set of negative and often unfair beliefs that a society or group of people have about something.

Stress: A state of mental or emotional strain or tension resulting from adverse or demanding circumstances.

Stress Management: Methods to cope with one's stressors.

Stressor: An event that triggers the stress response.

Sub-Internship: In the United States this is a rotation in the fourth year of medical school that serves as an introduction to the first post-graduate year.

Suicide: The act of deliberately killing oneself.

Suicide Ideology: Concerns, thoughts about or unusual preoccupation with suicide. Also known as suicide ideation.

Team-Based Learning (TBL): Is a learner-centred, instructor-directed strategy that incorporates class-based teamwork and assessment to enhance active learning and critical thinking. Originally developed by Larry Michaelsen in a business school environment to promote the benefits of small-group teaching in a large group setting, it has since been increasingly used within medical education. It can be used with large or small classes, and involves dividing a class into multiple small groups of between 5-7 students in a single classroom. One content-expert can instruct 20 or more teams, and grading, peer evaluation and feedback are used to promote individual and team accountability and learning. It is recommended that teams are created by the instructor with members selected on the basis of diversity of skills and other characteristics, and that members should work together in the same teams for as long as possible. The approach is characterised by three key components: 1) Individual student preparation in advance of the class. Students receive a list of learning activities and a set of learning goals to be completed before the class. 2) Individual (iRATs) and Team readiness assurance tests (tRATs). A set of 10-20 multiple choice questions (MCQs) focussing on the concepts the students need to master in order to complete the next stage. This is completed individually, and then again as a team through consensus-building discussion, and is followed by a clarification review by the instructor. 3) In class team application (tAPP) assignments. Students are presented with a significant problem, authentic to the type they will encounter in the workplace, which they must interpret and as a team select a specific response from a range of answers that they should also be able to explain and defend. All teams have the same problem and must make a simultaneous report of their answer. A backward design, outcomes-based approach is recommended to ensure the focus remains on what learners should be able to do. As such, instructors should establish the situational factors and learning goals before the team application, readiness assurance tests and advance assignments. Students are graded on all stages of the work. Teams can appeal a question in the readiness assurance tests and team application if they think it is poorly written or have an alternative answer by providing an alternative question and a written, referenced argument to support their case.

Tertiary: Education at a college or university.

Tertiary Prevention: Intervention, action or treatment for disease or injury that prevents complication and/or progression.

Undergraduate Medical Education (UGME): In the United States of America medical education is a term that refers to medical school. More generally, however, undergraduate refers to college education which results in a Bachelor's degree. It is the training most students have before entering medical school.

United States Medical Licensing Examination (USMLE): A 3-step examination procedure that provides a common evaluation system for United States medical licensure applicants. Results of the USMLE are reported to State Medical Boards granting the initial license to practice medicine. Each medical licensing authority requires, as part of its licensing procedure, a successful completion of an examination or other certifications demonstrating qualification for licensure.

Well-Being: A state of health, happiness and prosperity, which is affected by various factors, including: a balanced diet, regular exercise, supportive relationships, adequate financial resources, stimulating work, education and leisure activity, health monitoring, preventive services (i.e., screening and vaccinations), and risk management to protect individuals and promote personal safety.

Wellness Dimensions: A specific aspect of a wellness model such as spiritual, physical fitness, physical health, emotional, environmental, intellectual, occupational and social.

Wellness Programmes: Structured initiatives designed to educate and promote balance in dimensions of wellness.

Western Psychotherapy: The different theoretical approaches to counselling which focuses on psychological symptoms and is used to strengthen the self in order to improve functioning, facilitate healthy regulation of emotions, and increase ability to cope with both internal and external stressors.

Witchcraft: The act of magic, sorcery or supernatural powers used to protect from harm or cause harm. Witchcraft is embedded in the African and West Indian Cultures.

World Federation for Medical Education (WFME): A non-governmental organization with ties to WHO and UNESCO, the WFME is concerned with global education and training of medical doctors and umbrella organization for six regional associations for medical education. The WFME's general objective is to strive for the highest scientific and ethical standards in medical education and to take initiatives with respect to new methods, tools and management of medical education. The central office has been located at the University of Copenhagen, Denmark since 1996, in collaboration with Lund University in Sweden. www.wfme.org.

Yerkes-Dobson Law: The relationship between stress and performance has been known for about a century in psychology. This is a different way of thinking about how the brain operates to help or hurt performance, whether at work, in learning, in a sport, in any domain of ability. There are three primary states described in the Yerkes-Dodson Law: disengagement, frazzle, and flow. Each of these states has powerful impacts on a person's ability to perform at their best: disengagement and frazzle torpedo our efforts, while flow eases our efforts and lets them soar.

Compilation of References

Abbiati, M., Baroffio, A., & Gerbase, M. W. (2016). Personal profile of medical students selected through a knowledge-based exam only: Are we missing suitable students. *Med Educ Online, 21*(29705). doi:.v21.2970510.3402/meo

Abuhusain, H., Chotirmall, S. H., Hamid, N., & O'Neill, S. J. (2009). Prepared for internship?. *Irish Medical Journal, 102*(3), 82–84. PMID:19489196

Accreditation Council for Graduate Medical Education (ACGME). (n.d.). *Resident Survey – Duty Hours FAQ*. Chicago: USA. Retrieved on January 19, 2017 from https://www.acgme.org/Portals/0/dhfaqsresidents.pdf

Adlaf, E. M., Begin, P., & Sawka, E. (2005). *Canadian Addiction Survey (CAS): A national survey of Canadians' use of alcohol and other drugs: Prevalence of use and related harms: Detailed report*. Ottawa, Canada: Canadian Centre on Substance Abuse.

Adsett, C. A. (1968). Psychological health of medical students in relation to the medical education process. *Journal of Medical Education, 43*(6).

Agarwall, G., & Lakel, M. (2016). Personal transition to the profession: A novel longitudinal professional development and wellness medical student curriculum. *Academic Psychiatry, 40*(1), 105–108. doi:10.1007/s40596-015-0463-1 PMID:26742500

Age of Anxiety. (n.d.). In *The Concise Oxford Dictionary of Music*. Retrieved March 02, 2017 from Encyclopedia.com: http://www.encyclopedia.com/arts/dictionaries-thesauruses-pictures-and-press-releases/age-anxiety

Ahmed, H., Rhydderch, M., & Cohen, D. (2012). Prevalence of common mental health disorders in medical students: A systematic review and meta-analysis. *From Awareness to Action*. Retrieved from http://www.cma.ca/multimedia/PhysicianHealth/ICPH/ ICPH2012_PrelProg_EN.pdf

Ajdacic-Gross, V. (2008). Methods of suicide: International suicide patters derived from the WHO mortality database. *Bulletin of the World Health Organization, 86*(9), 726–732. doi:10.2471/BLT.07.043489 PMID:18797649

AlFaris, E., Irfan, F., Qureshi, R., Naeem, N., Alshomrani, A., Ponnamperuma, G., … van der Vleuten, C. (2016). Health professions' students have an alarming prevalence of depressive symptoms: exploration of the associated factors. BMC Medical Education, 16(279).

Alladin, W. J. (2002). Ethnic Matching in Counselling: How Important is it to Ethnically Match Clients and Counsellors? In S. Palmer (Ed.), *Multicultural Counselling: A Reader*. New York: SAGE.

Allen, A. A. (1988). West Indians. In *Clinical Guidelines in Cross-cultural Mental Health*. Oxford, UK: John Wiley & Sons.

Alshehri, S. A., Alshehri, A. F., & Erwin, T. D. (2012). Measuring the medical school educational environment: Validating an approach from Saudi Arabia. *Health Education Journal*, *71*(5), 553–564. doi:10.1177/0017896912450875

Altindag, A., Yanik, M., Ucok, A., Alptekin, K., & Ozkan, M. (2006). Effects of an Antistigma Programme on Medical Students Attitudes Towards People with Schizophrenia. *Psychiatry and Clinical Neurosciences*, *60*(3), 283–288. doi:10.1111/j.1440-1819.2006.01503.x PMID:16732743

Amarasuriya, S., Jorm, A., & Reavley, N. (2015). Perceptions and intentions relating to seeking help for depression among medical undergraduates in Sri Lanka: A cross-sectional comparison with non-medical undergraduates. *BMC Medical Education*, *15*(1), 162. doi:10.1186/s12909-015-0453-8 PMID:26419827

American Association of Medical Colleges. (1984). *Physicians for the Twenty-First Century*. The GPEP Report: Report of the Panel on the General Professional Education of the Physician and College Preparation for Medicine. ERIC Number: ED252102.

American Association of Medical Colleges. (2016). *Creating a Culture of Wellbeing and Resilience in Academic Medicine*. AAMC's Leadership Forum, Washington, DC. Retrieved 27 February http://www. aamc.org.AAMCacrnm1

American Medical Association (AMA). (2014). *Education*. Retrieved from http://www.ama-assn.org/ama

Amiri, L., Voracek, M., Yousef, S., Galadari, A., Yammahi, S., Sadeghi, M., & Dervic, K. et al. (2013). Suicidal Behavior and Attitudes Among Medical Students in the United Arab Emirates. *Crisis*, *34*(2), 116–123. doi:10.1027/0227-5910/a000170 PMID:23195458

Anfosi & Numico. (2014). Empathy in the Doctor-Patient Relationship. *Journal of Clinical Oncology*, *22*, 12258–12259. Retrieved from http://jco.ascopubs.org/content/22/11/2258.1.short PMID:15169824

Anxiety and Depression Association of America (ADAA). (2016). *Master's Level Videos*. Retrieved from http://www.adaa.org

Arboleda-Flórez, J., & Stuart, H. (2012). From Sin to Science: Fighting the Stigmatisation of Mental Illnesses. *Canadian Journal of Psychiatry*, *57*(8), 457–463. doi:10.1177/070674371205700803 PMID:22854027

Armstrong, E. (1997). Rehabilitating troubled doctors. *BMJ (Clinical Research Ed.)*, 7095.

Arnett, J. (2000). Emerging Adulthood: A theory of development from the late teens to the late twenties. *The American Psychologist*, *55*(5), 469–480. doi:10.1037/0003-066X.55.5.469 PMID:10842426

Association of American Medical Colleges (AAMC). (1984). *Physicians for the Twenty-First Century*. AAMC.

Astrom, S., Nilsson, M., Norberg, A., Sandman, P., & Winblad, B. (1991). Staff burnout in dementia care relations to empathy and attitudes. *International Journal of Nursing Studies*, *28*(1), 65–75. doi:10.1016/0020-7489(91)90051-4 PMID:1856035

Australia Medical Students' Association Student Mental Health and Wellbeing Committee. (2013). *Student Based Mental Health Interventions: Australian Medical Schools*. Canberra: AMSA. Retrieved from http://mentalhealth.amsa.org.au/wp-content/uploads/2015/09/AMSA-SMHW-Australian-Medical-Student-Report-2013.pdf

Ayalon, L., & Young, M. (2005). Racial Group Differences in Help-Seeking Behaviours. *The Journal of Social Psychology*, *145*(4), 391–403. doi:10.3200/SOCP.145.4.391-404 PMID:16050338

Back, A., & Arnold, R. (2013). "Isn't there anything more you can do?": When empathic statements work, and when they don't. *Journal of Palliative Medicine*, *16*, 1429–1432. doi:10.1089/jpm.2013.0193

Bahora, M., Hanafi, S., Chien, V. H., & Compton, M. T. (2008). Preliminary Evidence of Effects of Crisis Intervention Team Training on Self-Efficacy and Social Distance. *Administration and Policy in Mental Health*, *35*(3), 159–167. doi:10.1007/s10488-007-0153-8 PMID:18040771

Barry, M. M., & Jenkins, R. (2007). *Implementing Mental Health Promotion*. Oxford, UK: Churchill Livingstone, Elsevier.

Bateman, A. (2014). *Self-Harm. Royal College of Psychiatrists*. Retrieved 1 October 2016, from http://www.rcpsych.ac.uk/healthadvice/problemsdisorders/self-harm.aspx

Baxter, A. (2013). Global prevalence of anxiety disorders: A systematic review and meta-regression. *Psychological*, *43*, 897–910.

Beating burnout: Confidential access to health services for trainees. (n.d.). Retrieved from https://wire.ama-assn.org/life-career/beating-burnout-confidential-access-health-services-trainees?utm_source=Selligent&%3Butm_medium=email&%3Butm_term=%25m%25d%25y&%3Butm_content=Med%2BEd_addr1_12-14-16&%3Butm_campaign=Med%2BEd&%3Butm_uid=8710492&%3Butm_effort

Beckman, T. J., Reed, D. A., Shanafelt, T. D., & West, C. P. (2012). Resident physician well-being and assessments of their knowledge and clinical performance. *Journal of General Internal Medicine*, *27*(3), 325–330. doi:10.1007/s11606-011-1891-6 PMID:21948207

Beilock, S. L., & Carr, T. H. (2005). When high-powered people fail: Working memory and choking under pressure in math. *Psychological Science*, *16*(2), 101–105. doi:10.1111/j.0956-7976.2005.00789.x PMID:15686575

Bell Curve. (2012). Retrieved from www.SciTechDaily.com

Beltran, R. O., Scanlan, J. N., Hancock, N., & Luckett, T. (2006). The Effect of First Year Mental Health Fieldwork on Attitudes of Occupational Therapy Students Towards People with Mental Illness. *Australian Occupational Therapy Journal*, 42–48.

Benbassat, J. (2014). Changes in wellbeing and professional values among medical undergraduate students: A narrative review of the literature. *Advances in Health Sciences Education: Theory and Practice*, *19*(4), 597–610. doi:10.1007/s10459-014-9500-1 PMID:24615278

Benbassat, J., Baumal, R., Chan, S., & Nirel, N. (2011). Sources of distress during medical training and clinical practice: Suggestions for reducing their impact. *Medical Teacher*, *33*(6), 486–490. doi:10.3109/0142159X.2010.531156 PMID:21609178

Bendapudi, N. M., Berry, L. L., Frey, K. A., Parish, J. T., & Rayburn, W. L. (2006, March). Patients perspectives on ideal physician behaviors. *Mayo Clinic Proceedings*, *81*(3), 338–344. doi:10.4065/81.3.338 PMID:16529138

Benner, P., & Sutphen, M. (2007). Learning across the professions: The clergy, a case in point. *Journal of Nursing Education, 46*(3), 103-8. Retrieved from http://search.proquest.com/docview/203971539?accountid=14376

Benner, P. (1984). *From Novice to Expert: Excellence and Power in Clinical Nursing Practice*. Menlo Park, CA: Addison-Wesley Publishing Company.

Benner, P., & Sutphen, M. (2007). Learning across the professions: The clergy, a case in point. *The Journal of Nursing Education*, *46*, 103–108. Retrieved from http://search.proquest.com/docview/203971539?accountid=14376 PMID:17396548

Benson, E. (2003). The many faces of perfectionism. *Monitor on Psychology*, *34*(10), 18.

Berk, R. A. (2010). Where's the Chemistry in Mentor-Mentee Academic Relationships? Try Speed Mentoring!. *The International Journal of Mentoring and Coaching*, 85-92.

Berragan, L. (2013). Conceptualising learning through simulation: An expansive approach for professional and personal learning. *Nurse Education in Practice*, *13*(4), 250–255. doi:10.1016/j.nepr.2013.01.004 PMID:23402772

Bhatia, T. (2016, May 24). *Use of bell curve in performance appraisals- Good or bad?* [Weblog post]. Employee Appraisals, HR Best Practices, Human Resources, Performance Management.

Bieling, P. J., Israeli, A. L., & Antony, M. M. (2004). Is perfectionism good, bad, or both? Examining models of the perfectionism construct. *Personality and Individual Differences*, *36*(6), 1373–1385. doi:10.1016/S0191-8869(03)00235-6

Billingsley, M. (2015). More than 80% of medical students with mental health issues feel under-supported, says Student BMJ survey. *Student BMJ, 23*. https://doi.org/10.1136/sbmj.h4521

Billings, M. E., Lazarus, M. E., Wenrich, M., Curtis, J. R., & Engelberg, R. A. (2011). The effect of the hidden curriculum on resident burnout and cynicism. *Journal of Graduate Medical Education, 3*(4), 503–510. doi:10.4300/JGME-D-11-00044.1 PMID:23205199

Blair, S. N., Morris, J. N. (2009). *Annals of epidemiology*. Elsevier.

Blasi, Z. D., Harkness, E., Ernst, E., Georgiou, A., & Kleijnen, J. (2001). Influence of context effects on health outcomes: A systematic review. *Lancet, 357*(9258), 757–762. doi:10.1016/S0140-6736(00)04169-6 PMID:11253970

Bloom, B. S. (Ed.). (1956). Taxonomy of Educational Objectives. In Handbook I: The Cognitive Domain. New York: David McKay Co Inc.

Bolster, L., & Rourke, L. (2015). The effect of restricting residents duty hours on patient safety, resident well-being, and resident education: An updated systematic review. *Journal of Graduate Medical Education, 7*(3), 349–363. doi:10.4300/JGME-D-14-00612.1 PMID:26457139

Bond, K. S., Jorm, A. F., Kitchener, B. A., & Reavley, N. J. (2015). *Mental health first aid training for Australian medical and nursing students: An evaluation study. BMC Psychology.*

Bourdieu, P. (1990). Structures, habitus, practices. *The Logic of Practice*, 52-65.

Bowler, D. L., & Pettit, W. G. (2001). The Albuquerque Police Department's Crisis Intervention Team: A Report Card. *FBI Law Enforcement Bulletin*, 1-6.

Brackett, M. A., Rivers, S. E., & Salovey, P. (2011). Emotional intelligence: Implications for personal, social, academic, and workplace success. *Social and Personality Psychology Compass, 5*(1), 88–103. doi:10.1111/j.1751-9004.2010.00334.x

Bradburn, N. M. (1969). *The structure of psychological well-being*. Chicago: Aldine.

Brazeau, C. M. (2010). The Surest Way to Prevent Burnout in Medical School and Beyond. *Academic Medicine, 85*(4), 569–570. doi:10.1097/ACM.0b013e3181d2d643 PMID:20354360

Brazeau, C. M., Schroeder, R., Rovi, S., & Boyd, L. (2010). Relationships between medical student burnout, empathy, and professionalism climate. *Academic Medicine, 85*, S33–S36. doi:10.1097/ACM.0b013e3181ed4c47 PMID:20881699

Brice-Baker, J. (1994). West Indian Women: The Jamaican Woman. In *Women of Colour: Integrating Ethnic and Gender Identities in Psychotherapy* (pp. 139–160). New York: Gilford Press.

Brooks, S. K., Chalder, T., & Gerada, C. (2011). Doctors vulnerable to psychological distress and addictions: Treatment from the Practitioner Health Programme. *Journal of Mental Health (Abingdon, England), 20*(2), 157–164. doi:10.3109/09638237.2011.556168 PMID:21542716

Brown, B. (2013). *Overcoming perfectionism*. Retrieved from http://www.huffingtonpost.com/2013/06/29/brene-brown-daring-greatly-perfectionism-oprah_n_3468501.html

Bryde, J. F., & Milburn, C. M. (1990). Helping to make the transition from school to college. In R. L. Emans (Ed.), *Understanding undergraduate education* (pp. 203–213). Vermillion, SD: University of South Dakota Press.

Burns, D. D. (1980). The perfectionist's script for self-defeat. *Psychology Today*, *14*, 34–52.

Carnegie Foundation for the Advancement of Teaching. (2007). *Preparation for the Professions Program*. Retrieved January 3, 2015, from http://www.carnegiefoundation.org/publications/new-agenda-higher-education-shaping-life-mind-practice

Carr, S. E., & Johnson, P. H. (2013). Does self-reflection and insight correlate with academic performance in medical students?. *BMC Medical Education, 13*, 113. doi:10.1186/1472-6920-13-113

Carter, R., Golant, S. K., & Cade, K. E. (2010). Within Our Reach: Ending the Mental Health Crisis. Rodale Press, Inc.

Carter, G., Page, A., Large, M., Hetrick, S., Milner, A., Bendit, N., & Christensen, H. et al. (2016). Royal Australian and New Zealand College of Psychiatrists clinical practice guideline for the management of deliberate self-harm. *The Australian and New Zealand Journal of Psychiatry*, *50*(10), 939–1000. doi:10.1177/0004867416661039 PMID:27650687

Castells, M. (2014). The impact of the internet on society: a global perspective. In *Change: 19 key essays on how internet is changing our lives*. Retrieved from https://www.bbvaopenmind.com/wp-content/uploads/2014/03/BBVA-OpenMind-Technology-Innovation-Internet-Francisco-Gonzalez-Knowledge-Banking-for-a-Hyperconnected-Society.pdf

Cedfeldt, A. S., Bower, E., Flores, C., Brunett, P., Choi, D., & Girard, D. E. (2015). Promoting resident wellness: Evaluation of a time-off policy to increase residents utilization of health care services. *Academic Medicine: Journal of the Association of American Medical Colleges*, *90*(5), 678–683. doi:10.1097/ACM.0000000000000541 PMID:25354073

Celluci, T., Krogh, J., & Vik, P. (2006). Help seeking for alcohol problems in a college population. *The Journal of General Psychology*, *133*(4), 421–433. doi:10.3200/GENP.133.4.421-433 PMID:17128960

Center for Collegiate Mental Health. (2015, January). *2010 Annual Report* (Publication No. STA 15-30). Author.

Chambers, R. (1993). What should doctors do if they become sick? *Family Practice*, *10*(4), 416–423. doi:10.1093/fampra/10.4.416 PMID:8168678

Chang, D., & Berk, A. (2009). Making cross-racial therapy work: A phenomenological study of clients experiences of cross-racial therapy. *Journal of Counseling Psychology*, *56*(4), 521–536. doi:10.1037/a0016905 PMID:20414342

Chang, E., Eddins-Folensbee, F., & Coverdale, J. (2012). Survey of the prevalence of burnout, stress, depression, and the use of supports by medical students at one school. *Academic Psychiatry*, *36*(3), 177–182. doi:10.1176/appi.ap.11040079 PMID:22751817

Chan, W., Batterham, P., Christensen, H., & Galletly, C. (2014). Suicide literacy, suicide stigma and help-seeking intentions in Australian medical students. *Australasian Psychiatry*, *22*(2), 132–139. doi:10.1177/1039856214522528 PMID:24526795

Chemers, M. M., Hu, L., & Garcia, B. F. (2001). Academic self-efficacy and first-year college student performance and adjustment. *Journal of Educational Psychology*, *93*(1), 55–64. doi:10.1037/0022-0663.93.1.55

Chew-Graham, C., Rogers, A., & Yassin, N. (2003). I wouldn't want it on my CV or their records: Medical students experiences of help-seeking for mental health problems. *Medical Education*, *37*(10), 873–880. doi:10.1046/j.1365-2923.2003.01627.x PMID:12974841

Choy, G., & McInerney, V. (2007). Multi-dimensions of perfectionism and self- concept in school Aged Children. *Paper presented at Australian international education conference*, School of Psychology, Self- Research Centre, University of Western Sydney, Australia.

Christopher, J. C. (2001). Culture and Psychotherapy: Towards a Hermeneutic Approach. *Psychotherapy (Chicago, Ill.)*, *38*(2), 115–128. doi:10.1037/0033-3204.38.2.115

Chun, K. H., Park, Y. S., Lee, Y. H., & Kim, S. Y. (2014). Academic burnout and selection-optimization- compensation strategy in medical students. *Korean Journal of Medical Education*, *26*(4), 299–308. doi:10.3946/kjme.2014.26.4.299 PMID:25800237

Coates, W. C., Spector, T. S., & Uijtdehaage, S. (2012). Transition to life-A sendoff to the real world for graduating medical students. *Teaching and Learning in Medicine*, *24*(1), 36–41. doi: 10.1080/10401334.2012.641485 PMID:22250934

Cohen, D., & Rhydderch, M. (2013). *Support for tomorrow's doctors: getting it right, meeting their needs.* Retrieved from occmed.oxfordjournals.org/content/63/1/2.full

Cohen, M. J. M., Kay, A., Youakim, J. M., & Balacius, J. M. (2009). Identity transformation in medical students. *American Journal of Psychoanalysis*, *69*, 43-52. doi:10.1057/ajp.2008.38

Colbert, J. A., & Chokshi, D. A. (n.d.). Technology in Medical Education-Osler Meets Watson. *Journal of General Internal Medicine*, *12*, 29.

Collins, A., Brown, J. S., & Holum, A. (1991). *Cognitive Apprenticeship: Making Thinking Visible.* Retrieved from: http://elc.fhda.edu/transform/resources/collins_brown_holum_1991.pdf

Collins, A., Brown, J. S., & Newman, S. E. (1987). *Cognitive Apprenticeship: Teaching the craft of reading, writing and mathematics.* Center for the Study of Reading, Technical report No. 403. University of Illinois. Retrieved from: http://files.eric.ed.gov/fulltext/ED284181.pdf

Columbia School of Physicians and Surgeons (CSPS). (2017). *The white coat ceremony.* Retrieved from http://psclub.columbia.edu/orientation/whitecoatceremony

Compton, M., Esterberg, M., McGee, R., Kotwicki, R., & Oliva, J. (2006). Brief Reports: Crisis Intervention Team Training: Changes in Knowledge, Attitudes, and Stigma Related to Schizophrenia. *Psychiatric Services (Washington, D.C.)*, *57*(8), 1199–1202. doi:10.1176/ps.2006.57.8.1199 PMID:16870973

Conlon, A. (2012). *Problems faced by undergraduate medical students*. Retrieved from the Royal Medical Benevolent Fund website: http://www.rmbf.org/pages/problems-faced-by-undergraduate-medical-students-.html

Corrigan, P. W. (2004). How stigma interferes with mental health care. *The American Psychologist*, *59*(7), 614–625. doi:10.1037/0003-066X.59.7.614 PMID:15491256

Costa, P. T., & McCrae, R. (1992). *Revised NEO Personality Inventory (NEO-PI-R) and NEO Five Factor Model (NEO-FFI) Professional manual*. Odessa, FL: Psychological Assessment Center.

Coulehan, J. L., Platt, F. W., Egener, B., Frankel, R., Lin, C., Lown, B., & Salazar, W. H. (2001). Let Me See If I Have This Right…: Words That Help Build Empathy. *Annals of Internal Medicine*, *135*(3), 221–227. doi:10.7326/0003-4819-135-3-200108070-00022 PMID:11487497

Coulter, M. A., & Abney, P. C. (2009). A study of burnout in international and country of origin teachers. *International Review of Education*, *55*(1), 105–121. doi:10.1007/s11159-008-9116-x

Covey, S. R. (2015). *Primary greatness: The 12 levers of success*. New York, NY: Simon & Schuster.

Crandall, J. S., Volk, R. J., & Loemker, V. (1993). Medical Students Attitudes Toward Providing Care for the Underserved: Are We Training Socially Responsible Physicians? *JAMA*, *269*(19), 2519–2523. doi:10.1001/jama.1993.03500190063036 PMID:8487415

Cruce, S., Pashak, T., Handal, P., Munz, D., & Gfeller, J. (2012). Conscientious perfectionism, self-evaluative perfectionism, and the five-factor model of personality traits. *Personality and Individual Differences*, *53*(3), 268–273. doi:10.1016/j.paid.2012.03.013

Crum, A. J., Salovey, P., & Achor, S. (2013). Rethinking stress: The role of mindsets in determining the stress response. *Journal of Personality and Social Psychology*, *104*(4), 716–733. doi:10.1037/a0031201 PMID:23437923

Dabrow, S., Russell, S., Ackley, K., Anderson, E., & Fabri, P. J. (2006). Combating the stress of residency: One schools approach. *Academic Medicine: Journal of the Association of American Medical Colleges*, *81*(5), 436–439. doi:10.1097/01.ACM.0000222261.47643.d2 PMID:16639197

Dahlin, M., & Runeson, B. (2007). Burnout and psychiatric morbidity among medical students entering clinical training: A three year prospective questionnaire and interview-based study. *BMC Medical Education*, *7*(1), 6. doi:10.1186/1472-6920-7-6 PMID:17430583

Dankoski, M. E., Palmer, M. M., Laird, T. F. N., Ribera, A. K., & Bogdewic, S. P. (2012). An expanded model of faculty vitality in academic medicine. *Advances in Health Sciences Education : Theory and Practice*, *17*(5), 633–649. doi:10.1007/s10459-011-9339-7 PMID:22134490

Davies-Black, Mata, D. A., Ramos, M. A., Kim, M. M., Guille, C., & Sen, S. (2016). In their own words: An analysis of the experiences of medical interns participating in a prospective cohort study of depression. *Academic Medicine*, *91*(9), 1244–1250. doi:10.1097/ACM.0000000000001227

de Oliveira, G. S. Jr, Chang, R., Fitzgerald, P. C., Almeida, M. D., Castro-Alves, L. S., Ahmad, S., & McCarthy, R. J. (2013). The prevalence of burnout and depression and their association with adherence to safety and practice standards: A survey of united states anesthesiology trainees. *Anesthesia and Analgesia*, *117*(1), 182–193. doi:10.1213/ANE.0b013e3182917da9 PMID:23687232

Deci, E.L., & Ryan, R.M. (2008). Hedonia, Eudaimonia, and wellbeing. *Journal of Happiness Studies*, *9*(1). doi:10.1007/s10902-006-9018-1

Deosthalee, P. G. (2002). Job satisfaction of teachers in comparison with non-teachers. *Pakistan Journal of Psychological Research*, 17.

Department of Experimental and Clinical Medicine. (n.d.). *Frontiers in Psychology* [2016, 7:1682]. Retrieved from www.europepmc.org.mg alt=”Cover image” src=”http://ars.els-cdn.com/content/image/1-s2.0-S0272735813X00078-cov150h.gif”class=”toprightlogo

Derksen, F., Bensing, J., & Largo-Janssen, A. (2013). Effectiveness of empathy in general practice: A systematic review. *The British journal of general practice. The Journal of the Royal College of General Practitioners*, *63*(606), 76–84. doi:10.3399/bjgp13X660814

Diagnostic and statistical manual of mental disorders. (2013). Washington, DC: Academic Press.

Diamond, G. M. (2005). Counseling and Therapy with Minority Group Counselors /Therapists. In D. W. Sue & D. Sue (Eds.), *Counseling the Culturally Diverse: Theory and Practice* (pp. 317–344). Hoboken, NJ: Wiley.

Diener, E. (2009). Assessing well-being: the collected works of Ed Diener. New York: Springer.

Diener, E., Lucas, R. E., & Scollon, C. N. (2006). Beyond the hedonic treadmill: Revising the adaptation theory of well-being. *The American Psychologist*, *61*(4), 305–314. doi:10.1037/0003-066X.61.4.305 PMID:16719675

Dieserud, G., Roysamb, E., Ekeberg, O., & Kraft, P. (2001). Toward an Integrative Model of Suicide Attempt: A Cognitive Psychological Approach. *Suicide & Life-Threatening Behavior*, *31*(2), 153–168. doi:10.1521/suli.31.2.153.21511 PMID:11459248

DiLalla, L. F., Hull, S. K., & Dorsey, J. K. (2004). Effect of Gender, Age, and Relevant Course Work on Attitudes Toward Empathy, Patient Spirituality, and Physician Wellness. *Teaching and Learning in Medicine: An International Journal*, *16*, 165-170. Retrieved from: http://www.tandfonline.com/doi/abs/10.1207/s15328015tlm1602_8

DiMaggio, G., Lysaker, P. H., Calarco, T., Pedone, R., Marsigli, N., Riccardi, I., & Paviglianiti, A. et al. (2015). Perfectionism and personality disorders as predictors of symptoms and interpersonal problems. *American Journal of Psychotherapy*, *69*(3), 317–330. PMID:26414312

DiPrima, A. J., Ashby, J. S., Gnilka, P. B., & Noble, C. L. (2011). Family relationships and perfectionism in middle-school students. *Psychology in the Schools*, *48*(8), 815–827. doi:10.1002/pits.20594

Doherty, E. M., & Nugent, E. (2011). Personality factors and medical training: A review of the literature. *Med Educ.*, *45*(2), 132-40. doi: . 20.10.1111/j.1365-2923

Doherty, E. M., & Nugent, E. (2011). Personality factors and medical training: A review of the literature. *Medical Education*, *45*(2), 132–140. doi:10.1111/j.1365-2923.2010.03760.x PMID:21208259

Doja, A., Bould, M. D., Clarkin, C., Eady, K., Sutherland, S., & Writer, H. (2016). The hidden and informal curriculum across the continuum of training: A cross-sectional qualitative study. *Medical Teacher*, *38*(4), 410–418. doi:10.3109/0142159X.2015.1073241

Douce, L. A., & Keeling, R. P. (2014). *A strategic primer on college student mental health. American Council on Education (ACE).*

Downs, N., Feng, W., Kirby, B., McGuire, T., Moutier, C., Norcross, W., & Zisook, S. et al. (2014). Listening to Depression and Suicide Risk in Medical Students: The Healer Education Assessment and Referral (HEAR) Program. *Academic Psychiatry*, *38*(5), 547–553. doi:10.1007/s40596-014-0115-x PMID:24705825

Drolet, B. C., & Rodgers, S. (2010). A comprehensive medical student wellness programdesign and implementation at Vanderbilt school of medicine. Academic Medicine. *Journal. Association of American Medical Colleges*, *85*(1), 103–110. doi:10.1097/ACM.0b013e3181c46963

Dunkley, D. M., Sanislow, C. A., Grilo, C. M., & McGlashan, T. H. (2009). Self-criticism versus neuroticism in predicting depression and psychosocial impairment for 4 years in a clinical sample. *Comprehensive Psychiatry, 50,* 335–346. doi:psych.2008.09.00410.1016/j.comp

Dunkley, D. M., Blankstein, K. R., & Flett, G. L. (1997). Specific cognitive-personality vulnerability styles in depression and the five-factor model of personality. *Personality and Individual Differences*, *23*(6), 1041–1053. doi:10.1016/S0191-8869(97)00079-2

Dunkley, D. M., Blankstein, K. R., Zuroff, D. C., Lecce, S., & Hui, D. (2006). Self-critical and personal standards factors of perfectionism located within the five-factor model of personality. *Personality and Individual Differences*, *40*(3), 409–420. doi:10.1016/j.paid.2005.07.020

Dunn, H. L. (1961). *High-level wellness.* Arlington, VA: Beatty Press.

Dunn, H. L. (1973). *High level wellness.* Arlington, VA: R.W. Beatty, Ltd.

Dunn, L. B., Moutier, C., Hammond, K. A. G., Lehrmann, J., & Roberts, L. W. (2008). Personal health care of residents: Preferences for care outside of the training institution. *Academic Psychiatry*, *32*(1), 20–30. doi:10.1176/appi.ap.32.1.20 PMID:18270277

Dunn, L., Iglewicz, A., & Moutier, C. (2008). A Conceptual Model of Medical Student Well-Being: Promoting Resilience and Preventing Burnout. *Academic Psychiatry*, *32*(1), 44–53. doi:10.1176/appi.ap.32.1.44 PMID:18270280

Dyer, W. W. (2006). *Being in balance: 9 principles for creating habits to match your desires.* Carlsbad, CA: Hay House.

Dyrbye, L.N., Thomas, M.R., & Shanafelt, T.D. (2005). Medical student distress: Causes, consequences, and proposed solutions. *Mayo Clinic Proc., 80*(12), 1613-1622.

Dyrbye, L. N., Power, D. V., Stanford Massie, F., Eacker, A., Harper, W., Thomas, M. R., & Shanafelt, T. D. (2010). Factors associated with resilience to and recovery from burnout: A prospective, multi-institutional study of US medical students. *Medical Education*, *44*(10), 1016–1026. doi:10.1111/j.1365-2923.2010.03754.x PMID:20880371

Dyrbye, L. N., & Shanafelt, T. D. (2011). Commentary: medical student distress: a call to action. Academic medicine. *Journal of the Association of American Medical Colleges*, *86*(7), 801–803. doi:10.1097/ACM.0b013e31821da481

Dyrbye, L. N., Thomas, M. R., Harper, W., Massie, F. S. Jr, Power, D. V., Eacker, A., & Shanafelt, T. D. et al. (2009). The learning environment and medical student burnout: A multicentre study. *Medical Education*, *43*(3), 274–282. doi:10.1111/j.1365-2923.2008.03282.x PMID:19250355

Dyrbye, L. N., Thomas, M. R., Massie, F. S., Power, D. V., Eacker, A., Harper, W., & Shanafelt, T. D. et al. (2008). Burnout and suicidal ideation among U.S. medical students. *Annals of Internal Medicine*, *149*(5), 334–341. doi:10.7326/0003-4819-149-5-200809020-00008 PMID:18765703

Dyrbye, L. N., Thomas, M. R., & Shanafelt, T. D. (2005). Medical student distress: Causes, consequences, and proposed solutions. *Mayo Clinic Proceedings*, *80*(12), 1613–1622. doi:10.4065/80.12.1613 PMID:16342655

Dyrbye, L. N., Thomas, M. R., & Shanafelt, T. D. (2006). Systematic review of depression, anxiety, and other indicators of psychological distress among U.S. and Canadian medical students. *Academic Medicine*, *81*(4), 354–373. doi:10.1097/00001888-200604000-00009 PMID:16565188

Dyrbye, L. N., West, C. P., Satele, D., Boone, S., Tan, L., Sloan, J., & Shanafelt, T. D. (2014). Burnout among U.S. medical students, residents, and early career physicians relative to the general U.S. population. Academic Medicine. *Journal. Association of American Medical Colleges*, *89*(3), 443–451. doi:10.1097/ACM.0000000000000134

Dyrbye, L., & Shanafelt, T. (2016). A narrative review on burnout experienced by medical students and residents. *Medical Education*, *50*(1), 132–149. doi:10.1111/medu.12927 PMID:26695473

Eckleberry-Hunt, J., Lick, D., Boura, J., Hunt, R., Balasubramaniam, M., Mulhem, E., & Fisher, C. (2009). An exploratory study of resident burnout and wellness. *Academic Medicine: Journal of the Association of American Medical Colleges*, *84*(2), 269–277. doi:10.1097/ACM.0b013e3181938a45 PMID:19174684

Eckleberry-Hunt, J., Van Dyke, A., Lick, D., & Tucciarone, J. (2009). Changing the Conversation From Burnout to Wellness: Physician Well-being in Residency Training Programs. *Journal of Graduate Medical Education, 1*(2), 225–230. doi:10.4300/JGME-D-09-00026.1 PMID:21975983

Edwards, M. T., & Zimet, C. N. (1976). Problems and concerns among medical students. *Journal of Medical Education, 51*(8).

Egan, J. S. (2008). *An investigation of Positive and Negative Perfectionism.* Retrieved from http://adt.curtin.edu.au

Egan, J. S., Wade, T. D., Shafran, R., & Antony, M. M. (2014). *Cognitive-behavioral treatment of perfectionism.* New York: Guilford Press.

Egan, S. J., Wade, T. D., & Shafran, R. (2011). Perfectionism as a trans diagnostic progress: A clinical review. *Clinical Psychology Review, 31*(2), 203–212. doi:10.1016/j.cpr.2010.04.009 PMID:20488598

Eisenberg, D., Hunt, J., Speer, N., & Zivin, K. (2011). Mental health service utilisation among college students in the United States. *The Journal of Nervous and Menal Disease*, 301-308.

Eisenberg, D., Hunt, J., & Speer, N. (2012). Help Seeking for Mental Health on College Campuses: Review of Evidence and Next Steps for Research and Practice. *Harvard Review of Psychiatry, 20*(4), 222–232. doi:10.3109/10673229.2012.712839 PMID:22894731

Ellis, A. (2002). The role of irrational beliefs in perfectionism. In G.I. Flett & P.L. Hewitt (Eds.), Perfectionism: Theory, Research and Treatment (pp. 217-229). Washington, DC: American Psychological Association. doi:10.1037/10458-009

Elnicki, D. M., Curry, R. H., Fagan, M., Friedman, E., Jacobson, E., Loftus, T., & Linger, B. et al. (2002). Medical students' perspectives on and responses to abuse during the internal medicine clerkship. *Teaching and Learning in Medicine, 14*(2), 92–97. doi:10.1207/S15328015TLM1402_05 PMID:12058552

Engelberg, E., & Sjöberg, L. (2004). Internet use, social skills, and adjustment. *Cyberpsychology & Behavior, 7*(1), 41–47. doi:10.1089/109493104322820101 PMID:15006168

Enns, S. C., Perotta, B., Paro, H.B., Gannam, S., Peleias, M., Mayer, F. B., … Zen, T. P. (2016). Medical Students Perception of Their Educational Environment and Quality of Life: Is There a Positive Association?. Academic Medicine, 91(3), 409-417.

Enns, M. W., & Cox, B. J. (2001). The nature and assessment of perfectionism: A critical analysis. In G. L. Flett & P. L. Hewitt (Eds.), *Perfectionism: Theory research and treatment.* American Psychological Association.

Enns, M. W., Cox, B. J., Sareen, J., & Freeman, P. (2001). Adaptive and maladaptive perfection in medical students: A longitudinal investigation. *Medical Education, 35*(11), 1034–1042. doi:10.1046/j.1365-2923.2001.01044.x PMID:11703639

Epstein, R. (2017). *Attending: Medicine, Mindfulness, and Humanity.* Scribner.

Epstein, R. M., & Krasner, M. S. (2013). Physician Resilience: What It Means, Why It Matters, and How to Promote It. *Academic Medicine*, *88*(3), 301–303. doi:10.1097/ACM.0b013e318280cff0 PMID:23442430

Eskin, M., Voracek, M., Stieger, S., & Altinyazar, V. (2011). A cross-cultural investigation of suicidal behavior and attitudes in Austrian and Turkish medical students. *Social Psychiatry and Psychiatric Epidemiology*, *46*(9), 813–823. doi:10.1007/s00127-010-0254-7 PMID:20563550

Etzersdorfer, E., Vijayakumar, L., Schöny, W., Grausgruber, A., & Sonneck, G. (1998). Attitudes toward suicide among medical students: Comparison between Madras (India) and Vienna (Austria). *Social Psychiatry and Psychiatric Epidemiology*, *33*(3), 104–110. doi:10.1007/s001270050029 PMID:9540384

Eum, K., & Rice, K. G. (2011). Test anxiety, perfectionism, goal orientation, and academic performance. *Anxiety Stress Coping, 24*(2), 167-78. doi: 10.1080/10615806.2010.488723

Ey, S., Moffit, M., Kinzie, J. M., Choi, D., & Girard, D. E. (2013). If you build it, they will come: Attitudes of medical residents and fellows about seeking services in a resident wellness program. *Journal of Graduate Medical Education*, *5*(3), 486–492. doi:10.4300/JGME-D-12-00048.1 PMID:24404315

Fahrenkopf, A. M., Sectish, T. C., Barger, L. K., Sharek, P. J., Lewin, D., Chiang, V. W., & Landrigan, C. P. et al. (2008). Rates of medication errors among depressed and burnt out residents: Prospective cohort study. *BMJ (Clinical Research Ed.)*, *336*(7642), 488–491. doi:10.1136/bmj.39469.763218.BE PMID:18258931

Federal Reserve Bank of San Francisco (FRB). (2003). *What effects do recessions have on college students?*. FRB.

Fenlkenstein, C., Brownstein, A., Scott, C., & Lan, Y. (2007). Anxiety and stress reduction in medical education: An intervention. *Medical Education*, *41*(3), 258–264. doi:10.1111/j.1365-2929.2007.02685.x PMID:17316210

Firth, J. (1986). Levels and sources of stress in medical students. *British Medical Journal (Clinical Research Ed.)*, *292*(6529), 1177–1180. doi:10.1136/bmj.292.6529.1177 PMID:3085772

Flett, G., Heisel, M., & Hewitt, P. (2014). The destructiveness of perfectionism revisited: Implications for the assessment of suicide risk and the prevention of suicide. *Review of General Psychology*, *18*(3), 156–172. doi:10.1037/gpr0000011

Flo, E., Pallesen, S., Magerøy, N., Moen, B. E., Grønli, J., Nordhus, I. H., & Bjorvatn, B. (2012, April). Shift Work Disorder in Nurses – Assessment, Prevalence and Related Health Problems. *PLoS ONE*, *7*(4), 1–9. doi:10.1371/journal.pone.0033981 PMID:22485153

Foster, C. R., Dahill, L. E., Goleman, L., & Tolentino, B. W. (2006). *Educating clergy: Teaching practices and pastoral imagination.* San Francisco, CA: Kossey-Bass.

Franco, K. (2013). Retrieved from news.com/education/blogs/medical-school-admissions-doctor/2013/10/22/understand-common-reasons-leave-medical-school

Franco, K. (2013). *Understand Common Reasons Students Leave Medical School*. Retrieved from news.com/education/blogs/medical-school-admissions-doctor/2013/10/22/understand-common-reasons-leave-medical-school

Frauenfelder, M. (2001, December 9). The Year in Ideas: A to Z.; Social-Norms Marketing. *The New York Times Magazine*.

Frey, B. S., & Stutzer, A. (2002). *Happiness and economics*. Princeton, NJ: Princeton University Press.

Friedman, H. S., Kern, M. L., & Reynolds, C. A. (2010). Personality and health, subjective well-being, and longevity. *Journal of Personality*, *78*(1), 179–216. doi:10.1111/j.1467-6494.2009.00613.x PMID:20433617

Frost, R. O., Marten, P., Lahart, C., & Rosenblat, R. (1990). The dimensions of perfectionism. *Cognitive Therapy and Research*, *14*(5), 449–468. doi:10.1007/BF01172967

Furber, G., Leach, M., Guy, S., & Segal, L. (2016). Developing a broad categorisation scheme to describe risk factors for mental illness, for use in prevention policy and planning. *The Australian and New Zealand Journal of Psychiatry*. doi:0004867416642844

Gaber, R. R., & Martin, D. M. (2002). Still-well osteopathic medical student wellness program. *The Journal of the American Osteopathic Association*, *102*(5), 289–292. PMID:12033759

Gaber, R. R., & Martin, D. M. (2002). Still-Well osteopathic medical student wellness programme. *The Journal of the American Osteopathic Association*, *102*(5), 289–292. Retrieved from http://jaoa.org/article.aspx?articleid=2092752 PMID:12033759

Gaber, R. R., & Martin, D. M., (2002, May). Still-Well osteopathic medical student wellness program. *The Journal of the American Osteopathic Association*, *102*(5), 289–292. PMID:12033759

Galán, F., Sanmartín, A., Polo, J., & Giner, L. (2011). Burnout risk in medical students in Spain using the Maslach Burnout Inventory-Student Survey. *International Archives of Occupational and Environmental Health*, *84*(4), 453–459. doi:10.1007/s00420-011-0623-x PMID:21373879

Gall, T. L., Evans, D. R., & Bellerose, S. (2000). Transition to first-year university: Patterns of change in adjustment scores across life domains and time. *Journal of Social and Clinical Psychology*, *19*(4), 44–67. doi:10.1521/jscp.2000.19.4.544

Gander, P., Briar, C., Garden, A., Purnell, H., & Woodward, A. (2010). A gender-based analysis of work patterns, fatigue, and work/life balance among physicians in postgraduate training. *Academic Medicine*, *85*(9), 1526–1536. doi:10.1097/ACM.0b013e3181eabd06 PMID:20736682

Gelhaus, P. (2012). The desired moral attitude of the physician (I): Empathy. *Medicine, Health Care, and Philosophy*, *15*(2), 103–111. doi:10.1007/s11019-011-9366-4 PMID:22167298

General Medical Council (GMC). (2009). *Tomorrow's Doctors. Outcomes and standards for undergraduate medical education*. Available from: http://www.gmc-uk.org/Tomorrow_s_Doctors_1214.pdf_48905759.pdf

General Medical Council. (2014). *The meaning of fitness to practice*. London, England: Author. Retrieved from http://www.gmc-uk.org/the_meaning_of_fitness_to_practise.pdf_25416562.pdf

George, P., Dumenco, L., & Dollase, R. (2013). Introducing technology into medical education: Two pilot studies. *Patient Education and Counseling*, *12*, 93. PMID:23684367

Ghetti, C., Chang, J., & Gosman, G. (2009). Burnout, psychological skills, and empathy: Balint training in obstetrics and gynecology residents. *Journal of Graduate Medical Education*, *1*(2), 231–235. doi:10.4300/JGME-D-09-00049.1 PMID:21975984

Givens, J., & Tjia, J. (2002). Depressed Medical Students Use of Mental Health Services and Barriers to Use. *Academic Medicine. Journal. Association of American Medical Colleges*, 918–921. doi:10.1097/00001888-200209000-00024

Glasser, W. (1999). *Choice Theory: A New Psychology of Personal Freedom*. New York, NY: Harper Perennial.

Global Burden of Disease (GBD). (2015). Disease and injury incidence and Prevalence Collaborators, and others. Global, regional, and national incidence, prevalence, and years lived with disability for 310 diseases and injuries, 1990–2015: A systematic analysis for the Global Burden of Disease Study 2015. *Lancet*, *388*, 10053.

Global Knowledge Exchange Network (GKEN). (2009). *An overview of educators and training requirements for global healthcare professionals-Physicians, Workforce and Training Task Force*. Author.

GMC. (2013). *Medical students: professional values and fitness to practice*. Available at www.gmc-uk.org/education/undergraduate/professional behaviour.asp

Gnilka, P. B., Ashby, J. S., & Noble, C. M. (2013). Adaptive and Maladaptive Perfectionism as Mediators of Adult Attachment Styles and Depression, Hopelessness, and Life Satisfaction. *Journal of Counseling and Development*, *91*(1), 78–91. doi:10.1002/j.1556-6676.2013.00074.x

Goffman, E. (2009). *Stigma: Notes on the Management of Spoiled Identity*. New York: Simon and Schuster.

Goitein, L. (2014). Physician well-being: Addressing downstream effects, but looking upstream. *JAMA Internal Medicine*, *174*(4), 533–534. doi:10.1001/jamainternmed.2013.13253 PMID:24515255

Goldhagen, B. E., Kingsolver, K., Stinnett, S. S., & Rosdahl, J. A. (2015). Stress and burnout in residents: Impact of mindfulness-based resilience training. *Advances in Medical Education and Practice*, *6*, 525. PMID:26347361

Goldman, M. L., Shah, R. N., & Bernstein, C. A. (2015). Depression and suicide among physician trainees: Recommendations for a national response. *JAMA Psychiatry*, *72*(5), 411–412. doi:10.1001/jamapsychiatry.2014.3050 PMID:25738529

Goldsmith, S. (2002). *Reducing suicide*. Washington, DC: National Academies Press.

Goldston, D. B., Molock, S. D., Whitbeck, L. B., Murakami, J. L., Zayas, L. H., & Hall, G. C. (2008). Cultural considerations in adolescent suicide prevention and psychosocial treatment. *The American Psychologist, 63*(1), 14–31. doi:10.1037/0003-066X.63.1.14 PMID:18193978

Goleman, D. (2006). *Emotional intelligence: Why it can matter more than IQ*. New York, NY: Bantam Books.

Gopaul-McNicol. (2006). Non-Western Approach to Helping. In C. Lago (Ed.), *Race, Culture and Conselling*. Maidenhead, UK: Open University Press.

Gopaul-McNicol, S., & Brice-Baker, J. (1997). Caribbean Americans. In S. Friedman (Ed.), *Cultural Issues in the Treatment of Anxiety* (pp. 65–68). New York: Guilford Press.

Govardhan, L. M., Pinelli, V., & Schnatz, P. F. (2012). Burnout, depression and job satisfaction in obstetrics and gynecology residents. *Connecticut Medicine, 76*(7), 389. PMID:23248861

Goyal, M., Kohli, C., Kishore, J., & Jiloha, R. C. (2013). Effect of an Educational Booklet on Knowledge and Attitude Regarding Major Depressive Disorder in Medical Students in Delhi. *International Journal of Medical Students*, 16-23.

Gracey, C. F., Haidet, P., Branch, W. T., Weissman, P., Kern, D. E., Mitchell, G., & Inui, T. et al. (2005). Precepting humanism: Strategies for fostering the human dimensions of care in ambulatory settings. *Academic Medicine, 80*(1), 21–28. doi:10.1097/00001888-200501000-00007 PMID:15618087

Grant, A. M. (2007). Enhancing coaching skills and emotional intelligence through training. *Industrial and Commercial Training, 39*(5), 257-266. https://doi.org/10.1108/00197850710761945

Gray, A. J. (2002). Stigma in Psychiatry. *Journal of the Royal Society of Medicine, 95*(2), 72–76. doi:10.1258/jrsm.95.2.72 PMID:11823548

Greeno, J. G. (1997). On claims that answer the wrong questions. *Educational Researcher, 26*, 5–17.

Greeno, J. G., & Van De Sande, C. (2007). Perspectival understanding of conceptions and conceptual growth in interaction. *Educational Psychologist, 42*(1), 9–23. doi:10.1080/00461520709336915

Gresalfi, M. S., & Cobb, P. (2011). Negotiating identities for mathematics teaching in the context of professional development. *Journal for Research in Mathematics Education, 42*, 270–304.

Groopman, J. (2007). *How doctors think*. Houghton Mifflin Harcourt.

Gross, J., & Levenson, R. (1997). Hiding feelings: The acute effects of inhibiting negative and positive emotion. *Journal of Abnormal Psychology, 106*(1), 95–103. doi:10.1037/0021-843X.106.1.95 PMID:9103721

Guille, C., Speller, H., Laff, R., Epperson, C. N., & Sen, S. (2010). Utilization and barriers to mental health services among depressed medical interns: A prospective multisite study. *Journal of Graduate Medical Education, 2*(2), 210–214. doi:10.4300/JGME-D-09-00086.1 PMID:21975622

Gunderman, R. (2016b). *What Do High Rates of Medical Student Depression Say About Health System?* Retrieved from www.realclearhealth.com/.../2016/.../what_do_high_rates_of_medical_student_depres

Gunderman, R. (2006a). *Medical Student depression and our health system.* Academic Press.

Guthrie, E., Black, D., Bagalkote, H., Shaw, C., Campbell, M., & Creed, F. (1998). Psychological stress and burnout in medical students: A five-year prospective longitudinal study. *Journal of the Royal Society of Medicine, 91*(5), 237–243. PMID:9764076

Hafferty, F. W. (1998). Beyond curriculum reform: Confronting medicines hidden curriculum. *Academic Medicine, 73*(4), 403–407. doi:10.1097/00001888-199804000-00013 PMID:9580717

Haight, S. J., Chibnall, J. T., Schindler, D. L., & Slavin, S. J. (2012, April). Associations of medical student personality and health/wellness characteristics with their medical school performance across the curriculum. *Academic Medicine, 87*(4), 476–485. doi:10.1097/ACM.0b013e318248e9d0 PMID:22361792

Hall, S. (1992). New Ethnicities. In J. Donald & A. Rattansi (Eds.), *Race, culture and Difference* (pp. 441–449). London: SAGE.

Hamlin, M. D. (2015). Technology in transformative learning environments. In C. Halupa (Ed.), *Transformative Curriculum Design in Health Sciences Education* (pp. 126–140). Hershey, PA: IGI Global. doi:10.4018/978-1-4666-8571-0.ch004

Hanson, R. (2017). *The 12 Pillars of the Path of Well-Being*. Retrieved from https://fwb.rickhanson.net/affiliate/4474

Hassed, C., de Lisle, S., Sullivan, G., & Pier, C. (2009). Enhancing the health of medical students: Outcomes of an integrated mindfulness and lifestyle programme. *Advances in Health Sciences Education : Theory and Practice, 14*(3), 387–398. doi:10.1007/s10459-008-9125-3 PMID:18516694

Healthy Universities. (2010). Retrieved at http://www.healthyuniversities.ac.uk/index.php?s=1

Hellstén, M., & Prescott, A. (2004). Learning at University: The international student experience. *International Education Journal, 5*, 344–351.

Henderson, A., Twentyman, M., Eaton, E., Creedy, D., Stapleton, P., & Lloyd, B. (2010). Creating supportive clinical learning environments: An intervention study. *Journal of Clinical Nursing, 19*(1-2), 177–182. doi:10.1111/j.1365-2702.2009.02841.x PMID:19686319

Henning, K., Ey, S., & Shaw, D. (1998). Perfectionism, the imposter phenomenon and psychological adjustment in medical, dental, nursing and pharmacy students. *Medical Education, 32*(5), 456–464. doi:10.1046/j.1365-2923.1998.00234.x PMID:10211285

Herrman, H. S., Saxena, S., & Moodie, R. (2005). Promoting Mental Health: Concepts, Emerging Evidence, Practice. A WHO Report in collaboration with the Victoria health Promotion Foundation and the University of Melbourne. Geneva: World Health Organization; Retrieved from http://www.who.int/mental_health/evidence/MH_Promotion_Book.pdf

Hetter, H. M. G. (2011). *No health without mental health: A cross-governmental mental health outcomes strategy for all ages*. 10.1016/j.socscimed.2014.11.027

Hettler, W. (1976). Six dimensions of wellness model. St. Paul, MN: National Wellness Institute. Retrieved from http://c.ymcdn.com/sites/www.nationalwellness.org/resource/resmgr/docs/sixdimensionsfactsheet.pdf

Hewitt, P. L., & Flett, G. L. (1990). Perfectionism and depression: A multidimensional analysis. *Journal of Social Behavior and Personality*, *5*, 423–438.

Hewitt, P. L., & Flett, G. L. (1991). Perfectionism in the self and social contexts: Conceptualization, assessment, and association with psychopathology. *Journal of Personality and Social Psychology*, *60*(3), 456–470. doi:10.1037/0022-3514.60.3.456 PMID:2027080

Hewson, M. G., & Little, M. L. (1998). Giving Feedback in medical education: Verification of recommended techniques. *Journal of General Internal Medicine*, *13*(2), 111–116. doi:10.1046/j.1525-1497.1998.00027.x PMID:9502371

Hill, R. W., Huelsmann, T. J., Furr, R. M., Kibler, J., Vicente, B. B., & Kennedy, C. (2004). A new measure of perfectionism: The Perfectionism Inventory. *Journal of Personality Assessment*, *82*(1), 80–91. doi:10.1207/s15327752jpa8201_13 PMID:14979837

Hirsch, E. M. (2007). The role of empathy in medicine: A medical student's perspective. *The Virtual Mentor*, *9*, 423. Retrieved from: http://journalofethics.ama-assn.org/2007/06/pdf/medu1-0706.pdf

Hirschfeld, R., & Russell, J. (1997). Assessment and Treatment of Suicidal Patients. *The New England Journal of Medicine*, *337*(13), 910–915. doi:10.1056/NEJM199709253371307 PMID:9302306

Hobson, K. (2013, March 21). New medical school programmes help students battle burnout. *U.S. News & World Report.* Retrieved from http://www.usnews.com/education/best-graduate-schools/top-medical-schools/articles/2013/03/21/new-medical-school-programs-help-students-battle-burnout

Hobson, K. (2013, March 21). New Medical School Programmes Help Students Battle Burnout. *US News*.

Hogan, R. (2005). In defense of personality measurement: New wine for older whiners. *Human Performance*, *18*(4), 331–341. doi:10.1207/s15327043hup1804_1

Hogan, R., & Hogan, J. (2001). Assessing leadership: A view from the dark side. *International Journal of Selection and Assessment*, *9*(1&2), 40–51. doi:10.1111/1468-2389.00162

Hojat, M. (2009). Ten Approaches for Enhancing Empathy in Health and Human Services Cultures. *Journal of Health and Human Services Administration*, *31*, 412–450. Retrieved from http://search.proquest.com/docview/199974037?accountid=14376 PMID:19385420

Hojat, M., Mangione, S., Nasca, T. J., Rattner, S., Erdmann, J. B., Gonnella, J. S., & Magee, M. (2004). An empirical study of decline in empathy in medical school. *Medical Education*, *38*(9), 934–941. doi:10.1111/j.1365-2929.2004.01911.x PMID:15327674

Hollender, M. H. (1978). Perfectionism: A neglected personality trait. *The Journal of Clinical Psychiatry*, *39*, 384. PMID:641018

Hopper, S. (1981). Diabetes as a Stigmatised Condition: The Case of Low-Income Clinic Patients in the United States. *Social Science and Medicine. Medical Anthropology*, *15*(1), 11–19. doi:10.1016/0160-7987(81)90004-1 PMID:7209601

Hughes, P. H., Conard, S. E., Baldwin, D. C., Storr, C. L., & Sheehan, D. V. (1991). Resident physician substance use in the united states. *Journal of the American Medical Association*, *265*(16), 2069–2073. doi:10.1001/jama.1991.03460160047027 PMID:2013925

Hughes, P., Kent, A., & Bowman, D. (2008). Medical students and mental health: The UK perspective. *The Clinical Teacher*, *5*(2), 83–87. doi:10.1111/j.1743-498X.2007.00196.x

Humphris, & Kaney, S. (1998). The encouragement of perfect health professionals. *Medical Education, 32*(5), 452-455.

Humphris, G., & Kaney, S. (1998). The encouragement of perfect health professionals. *Medical Education*, *32*(5), 452–455. doi:10.1046/j.1365-2923.1998.00304.x PMID:10211284

Hunt, J., & Eisenberg, D. (2010). Mental health problems and help-seeking behaviour among college students. *The Journal of Adolescent Health*, *46*(1), 3–10. doi:10.1016/j.jadohealth.2009.08.008 PMID:20123251

Hutchins, E. B. (1964). The AAMC longitudinal study: Implications for medical education. *Journal of Medical Education*, *39*, 265–267. PMID:14130655

IsHak, W., Nikravesh, R., Lederer, S., Perry, R., Ogunyemi, D., & Bernstein, C.. (2013). Burnout in medical students: A systematic review. *The Clinical Teacher*, *10*(4), 242–245. doi:10.1111/tct.12014 PMID:23834570

Jackman, S., Ellis, J., Quince, T., Wilkinson, P., Davies, R., & Thiemann, P. (2016). *Improving barriers to medical student mental health help-seeking*. University of Cambridge.

Jackson, E. R., Shanafelt, T. D., Hasan, O., Satele, D. V., & Dyrbye, L. N. (2016). Burnout and Alcohol Abuse/Dependence Among U.S. Medical Students. *Academic Medicine*, *91*(9), 1251–1256. doi:10.1097/ACM.0000000000001138 PMID:26934693

Jenkins, R., Bhugra, D., Bebbington, P., Brugha, T., Farrell, M., Coid, J., & Meltzer, H. et al. (2008). Debt, income, and mental disorder in the general population. *Psychological Medicine*, *38*(10), 1485–1493. doi:10.1017/S0033291707002516 PMID:18184442

Jerant, A., Griffin, E., Rainwater, J., Henderson, M., Sousa, F., Bertakis, K. D., & Franks, P. et al. (2012). Does applicant personality influence multiple mini-interview performance and medical school acceptance offer? *Academic Medicine*, *87*(9), 1250–1259. doi:10.1097/ACM.0b013e31826102ad PMID:22836836

Jorm, A. F., Korten, A. E., Jacomb, P. A., Christensen, H., Rodgers, B., & Pollitt, P. (1997). "Mental health literacy": A survey of the public's ability to recognise mental disorders and their beliefs about the effectiveness of treatment. *The Medical Journal of Australia*, 182–186. PMID:9066546

Kadison, R., & Digeronimo, T. F. (2004). *College of the overwhelmed: The campus mental health crisis and what to do about it.* San Francisco, CA: Jossey-Bass.

Kagawa-Singer, M., & R. C. Y., C. (2002). Towards a new paradigm: A cultural systems approach. In K. Kurasaki, S. Okazaki, & S. Sue (Eds.), *Asian American Mental Health* (pp. 47-66). New York: Kluwer Academic.

Kapinos, K. A., Fitzgerald, P., Greer, N., & Rutks, I. (2012). *The effect of working conditions on patient care: A systematic review.* Academic Press.

Kashani, J. H., Canfield, L. A., Borduin, C. M., Soltys, S. M., & Reid, J. C. (1994). Perceived family and social support: Impact on children. *Journal of the American Academy of Child and Adolescent Psychiatry*, *33*, 819-823. PMID:8083138

Kavan, M. G., & Brumback, R. A. (2009). The White Coat Ceremony: A tribute to the humanism of Arnold P. *Gold. Journal of Child Neurology*, *24*(8), 1051–1052. doi:10.1177/0883073809336133 PMID:19448139

Keller, A., Litzelman, K., Wisk, L. E., Maddox, T., Cheng, E. R., Creswell, P. D., & Witt, W. P. (2012). Does the perception that stress affects health matter? the association with health and mortality. *Health Psychology*, *31*(5), 677–684. doi:10.1037/a0026743 PMID:22201278

Kim, B. S. (2007). Adherence to Asian and European American Cultural Values and Attitudes Toward Seeking Professional Psychological Help Among Asian American College Students. *Journal of Counseling Psychology*, *54*(4), 474–480. doi:10.1037/0022-0167.54.4.474

Kim, S. J., & Lee, S. Y. (2014). The relationship between socially-prescribed perfectionism and anger suppression in college students: Self-silencing as a mediator. *Korean Journal of Counseling*, *15*(2), 729–751. doi:10.15703/kjc.15.2.201404.729

Kirmayer, L. J. (2006). Beyond the New Cross-cultural Psychiatry: Cultural Biology, Discursive Psychology and the Ironies of Globalization. *Transcultural Psychiatry*, *43*(1), 126–144. doi:10.1177/1363461506061761 PMID:16671396

Kligler, B., Linde, B., & Katz, N. T. (2013, April). Becoming a Doctor: A Qualitative Evaluation of Challenges and Opportunities in Medical Student Wellness During the Third Year. *Academic Medicine*, *88*(4), 535–540. doi:10.1097/ACM.0b013e3182860e6d PMID:23425993

Klonsky, E., May, A., & Glenn, C. (2013). The relationship between nonsuicidal self-injury and attempted suicide: Converging evidence from four samples. *Journal of Abnormal Psychology*, *122*(1), 231–237. doi:10.1037/a0030278 PMID:23067259

Koenig, T.W., Parrish, S.K., Terregino, C.A., Williams, J.P., Dunleavy, D.M., & Volsch, J.M. (2013). Core personal competencies important to entering students' success in medical school: what are they and how could they be assessed early in the admission process?. *Acad Med, 88*(5), 603-13. doi: 10.1097/ACM.0b013e31828b3389

Koparan, Ş., Şahin, E., & Kuter, F. (2010). A comparison on of self-efficacy perception and social physical anxiety levels of teacher candidates at physical education department. *Procedia: Social and Behavioral Sciences*, *2*(2), 3932–3937. doi:10.1016/j.sbspro.2010.03.619

Kosky, R., & Hardy, J. (1992). Mental health: Is early intervention the key? *The Medical Journal of Australia*, *3*, 47–58. PMID:1545713

Kötter, T., Tautphäus, Y., Obst, K. U., Voltmer, E., & Scherer, M. (2016). Health-promoting factors in the freshman year of medical school: A longitudinal study. *Medical Education*, *50*(6), 646–656. doi:10.1111/medu.12987 PMID:27170083

Krasner, M. S., Epstein, R. M., Beckman, H., Suchman, A. L., Chapman, B., Mooney, C. J., & Quill, T. E. (2009). Association of an educational program in mindful communication with burnout, empathy, and attitudes among primary care physicians. *Journal of the American Medical Association*, *302*(12), 1284–1293. doi:10.1001/jama.2009.1384 PMID:19773563

Kriel, J. R. (1988). Removing medicine's Cartesian mask: The problem of humanising medical education part 1. *Journal of Biblical Ethics in Medicine*, *3*(2), 18–22. Retrieved from http://w.biblicalworldview21.org/bmei/jbem/volume3/num2/kriel_removing_medicines_cartesian_mask.pdf

Kushner, M. G., & Sher, K. J. (1989). Fear of psychological treatment and its relation to mental health service avoidance. *Professional Psychology, Research and Practice*, *20*(4), 251–257. doi:10.1037/0735-7028.20.4.251

Kushner, R. F., Kessler, S., & McGaghie, W. C. (2011). Using behaviour change plans to improve medical student self-care. *Academic Medicine*, *86*(7), 901–906. doi:10.1097/ACM.0b013e31821da193 PMID:21617509

Kutcher, S., Wei, Y., McLuckie, A., & Bullock, L. (2013). Educator Mental Health Literacy: A Programme Evaluation of the Teacher Training Education on the Mental Health & High School Curriculum Guide. *Advances in School Mental Health Promotion*, 83-93.

Larson, E. B., & Yao, X. Y. (2005). Clinical empathy as emotional labor in the patient-physician relationship. *Journal of the American Medical Association*, *293*(9), 1100–1106. doi:10.1001/jama.293.9.1100 PMID:15741532

Lave, J. (1988). *Cognition in practice: Mind, mathematics, and culture in everyday life*. Cambridge, UK: Cambridge University Press. doi:10.1017/CBO9780511609268

Lave, J., & Wenger, E. (1991). *Situated Learning: Legitimate Peripheral Participation*. Cambridge, UK: Cambridge University Press.

Lazin, R., & Nuemann, L. (1991). Student Characteristics as predicators of drop-out from medical school: Admissions to Beer-Sheva over a decade. *Med Educ., 25*(5), 396-404.

LCME. (2003). *The Changing Face of Medical Education Accreditation*. Retrieved from www.flbog.edu/documents_meetings/0017_0088_0736_9.pdf

LCME. (2016). *Functions and Structure of a Medical School Standards for Accreditation of Medical Education Programs Leading to the MD Degree*. Accessed http://med.virginia.edu/ume-curriculum/wp-content/uploads/sits/216/2016/2017-18_Functions-and-Structure_2016-03-24.pdf

Lee, M. H. (2001). *The positive and negative function of perfectionism: in relations, with achievement goal, stress, psychological well-being and depression* (Unpublished master's thesis). Hanyang University, Seoul, South Korea.

Lee, H. A., & Jo, H. I. (2013). The relation among perfectionism, academic engagement and academic burnout: The mediating effects of motives and goal processes. *Korean Journal of Counseling and Psychotherapy, 25*, 575–601.

Lee, S. H., & Jeon, W. T. (2015). The relationship between academic self-efficacy and academic burnout in medical students. *Korean Journal of Medical Education, 27*(1), 27–35. doi:10.3946/kjme.2015.27.1.27 PMID:25800259

LeFevre, M. (2014). Screening for Suicide Risk in Adolescents, Adults, and Older Adults in Primary Care: U.S. Preventive Services Task Force Recommendation Statement. *Annals of Internal Medicine, 160*(10), 719. doi:10.7326/M14-0589 PMID:24842417

Legassie, J., Zibrowski, E. M., & Goldszmidt, M. A. (2008, July). Measuring Resident Well-Being: Impostorism and Burnout Syndrome in Residency. *Journal of General Internal Medicine, 23*(7), 1090–1094. doi:10.1007/s11606-008-0536-x PMID:18612750

Lempe, H., & Seale, C. (2004). The hidden curriculum in undergraduate medical education: Qualitative study of medical students perceptions of teaching. *British Medical Journal, 329*(7469), 770–773. doi:10.1136/bmj.329.7469.770 PMID:15459051

Leong, F. T., & Lau, A. S. (2001). Barriers to Providing Effective Mental Health Services to Asian Americans. *Mental Health Services Research, 3*(4), 201–214. doi:10.1023/A:1013177014788 PMID:11859966

Leong, F. T., Wagner, N. S., & Kim, H. H. (1995). Group counseling expectations among Asian American students: The role of culture-specific factors. *Journal of Counseling Psychology, 42*(2), 217–222. doi:10.1037/0022-0167.42.2.217

Liaison Committee on Medical Education. (2014). *Accreditation Standards*. Retrieved from: http://www.lcme.org/publications.htm#standards-section

Lievens, F., Coetsier, P., De Fruyt, F., & De Maeseneer, J. (2002). Medical students personality characteristics and academic performance: A five-factor model perspective. *Medical Education, 36*(11), 1050–1056. doi:10.1046/j.1365-2923.2002.01328.x PMID:12406265

Lilley, R., Owens, D., Horrocks, J., House, A., Noble, R., Bergen, H., & Kapur, N. et al. (2008). Hospital care and repetition following self-harm: Multicentre comparison of self-poisoning and self-injury. *The British Journal of Psychiatry, 192*(6), 440–445. doi:10.1192/bjp.bp.107.043380 PMID:18515895

Lin, H., Lin, E., Auditore, S., & Fanning, J. (2016). A narrative review of high-quality literature on the effects of resident duty hours reforms. Academic Medicine. *Journal. Association of American Medical Colleges, 91*(1), 140–150. doi:10.1097/ACM.0000000000000937

Linzer, M., Levine, R., Meltzer, D., Poplau, S., Warde, C., & West, C. P. (2014). 10 bold steps to prevent burnout in general internal medicine. *Journal of General Internal Medicine, 29*(1), 18–20. doi:10.1007/s11606-013-2597-8 PMID:24002633

Lippman, J. (2016). *What does a doctor's white coat really mean?*. Retrieved from www.kevinmd.com/blog/2016/12/doctors-white-coat-really-mean.html

Lipsenthal, L. (2005). The physician personality: Confronting our perfectionism and social isolation. *Holistic Primary Care: News for Health and Healing., 6*, 3.

Lockwood, P., Jordan, C. H., & Kunda, Z. (2002). Motivation by positive or negative role models: Regulatory focus determines who will best inspire us. *Journal of Personality and Social Psychology, 83*(4), 854–864. doi:10.1037/0022-3514.83.4.854 PMID:12374440

Lorgren, R., Karpf, M., Perman, J., & Higdon, C. M. (2006). The U.S. health care system is in crisis: Implications for academic medical centers and their missions. *Academic Medicine, 81*(8), 713–720. doi:10.1097/00001888-200608000-00007 PMID:16868424

Ludwig, A. B., Burton, W., Weingarten, J., Milan, F., Myers, D. C., & Kligler, B. (2015, August 27). Depression and stress amongst undergraduate medical students. *BMC Medical Education, 15*(141). PMID:26311538

Lupo, M. K., & Strous, R. D. (2011). Religiosity, anxiety and depression among Israeli medical students. *The Israel Medical Association Journal, 13*, 613-618. Retrieved from: http://touro.summon.serialssolutions.com/search?s.q=religiosity%2C+anxiety+and+depression+among+Israeli+medical#!/search?q=religiosity,%20anxiety%20and%20depression%20among%20Israeli%20medical

Lutsky, I., Abram, S. E., Jacobson, G. R., Hopwood, M., & Kampine, J. (1991). Substance abuse by anesthesiology residents. *Academic Medicine, 66*(3), 164–166. doi:10.1097/00001888-199103000-00009 PMID:1997028

Lygo-Baker, S., Kokotailo, P., & Young, K. (2015). Developing confidence in uncertainty: Conflicting roles of trainees as they become educators in veterinary and human medicine. *Journal of Veterinary Medical Education, 42*(4), 364–372. doi:10.3138/jvme.1114-107R PMID:26315215

Lykken, D., & Tellegen, A. (1996). Happiness is a stochastic phenomenon. *Psychological Science*, *7*(3), 186–189. doi:10.1111/j.1467-9280.1996.tb00355.x

Lyss-Lerman, P., Teherani, A., Aagaard, E., Loeser, H., Cooke, M., & Harper, G. M. (2009). What training is needed in the fourth year of medical school? views of residency programme directors. Academic Medicine. *Journal. Association of American Medical Colleges*, *84*(7), 823–829. doi:10.1097/ACM.0b013e3181a82426

Lyubomirsky, S., King, L., & Diener, E. (2005). The benefits of frequent positive affect: Does happiness lead to success? *Psychological Bulletin*, *131*(6), 803–855. doi:10.1037/0033-2909.131.6.803 PMID:16351326

Mackean, G. (2011). *Mental health and well-being in post-secondary education settings: A literature and environmental scan to support planning and action in Canada. Canadian Association of College and University Student Services*. CACUSS.

MacLean, L., Booza, J., & Balon, R. (2016). The impact of medical school on student mental health. *Academic Psychiatry*, *40*(1), 89–91. doi:10.1007/s40596-015-0301-5 PMID:25749920

Maher, B. M., Sweeney, C., Khashan, A. S., ORouke, M., Doran, K., Harris, A., & OFlynn, S. (2013). Medical School Attrition-Beyond the Statistics A Ten Year Retrospective Study. *BMC Medical Education*, *13*(1), 13. doi:10.1186/1472-6920-13-13 PMID:23363547

Mahon, K.E, Henderson, M.K., & Kirch, D.G. (2013). Selecting tomorrow's physicians: the key to the future health care workforce. *Acad Med, 88*, 1806.

Mangnall, J., & Yurkovich, E. (2008). A Literature Review of Deliberate Self-Harm. *Perspectives in Psychiatric Care*, *44*(3), 175–184. doi:10.1111/j.1744-6163.2008.00172.x PMID:18577123

Mascaskill, A. (2012). *University student mental health in crisis: A United Kingdom perspective*. Retrieved from https://pdfs.semanticscholar.org/1f78/2c0eb86b7f3d32bc067bfdf8fcbc3b276ae0.pdf

Maslach, C., Jackson, S. E., & Leiter, M. P. (1996). Maslach burnout inventory manual. Mountain View, CA: CPP. Inc.

Maslach, Schaufeli, & Leiter. (n.d.). Job Burnout. *Annual Review of Psychology, 52*, 397–422. Retrieved from: http://www.annualreviews.org/doi/pdf/10.1146/annurev.psych.52.1.397

Maslach, C. (2003). Job burnout new directions in research and intervention. *Current Directions in Psychological Science*, *12*(5), 189–192. doi:10.1111/1467-8721.01258

Matthews, D. A., Suchman, A. L., & Branch, W. T. (1993). Making Connexions: Enhancing the Therapeutic Potential of Patient Clinician Relationships. *Annals of Internal Medicine*, *118*(12), 973–977. doi:10.7326/0003-4819-118-12-199306150-00010 PMID:8489112

Maulana, R., & Opdenakker, C. (2012). Teacher–student interpersonal relationships and academic motivation within one school year: developmental changes and linkage. *School Effectiveness and School Improvement: An International Journal of Research, Policy and Practice, 23.* Retrieved from: http://www.tandfonline.com/doi/abs/10.1080/09243453.2011.619198

Maunder, R. E., Gingham, J., & Rogers, J. (2010). Transition in higher education: Exploring the experiences of first and second year psychology undergraduate students. *Psychology of Education Review*, *34*(1), 50–54.

Maxwell, J. C. (2012). *The 15 invaluable laws of growth: Live them and reach your potential.* New York, NY: Center Street.

Mayer, F. B., Itamar, S. S., Paulo, S. P., Silveira, M. H., Itaqui, L., Souza, A. R., & Tempski, P. et al. (2016). Factors associated to depression and anxiety in medical students: A multicentre study. *BMC Medical Education*, *16*, 1. PMID:26727954

Mayo Clinic. (2005). *Medical Student distress: Causes, consequences and proposed solutions.* Mayo Clinic proceedings.com

McBeth, B. D., Ankel, F. K., Ling, L. J., Asplin, B. R., Mason, E. J., Flottemesch, T. J., & McNamara, R. M. (2008). Substance use in emergency medicine training programs. *Academic Emergency Medicine*, *15*(1), 45–53. doi:10.1111/j.1553-2712.2007.00008.x PMID:18211313

McCue, J. D., & Sachs, C. L. (1991). A stress management workshop improves residents coping skills. *Archives of Internal Medicine*, *151*(11), 2273–2277. doi:10.1001/archinte.1991.00400110117023 PMID:1953233

McEwen, B. S. (2003). Mood disorders and allostatic load. *Biological Psychiatry*, *54*(3), 200–207. doi:10.1016/S0006-3223(03)00177-X PMID:12893096

McEwen, B. S. (2004). Protection and damage from acute and chronic stress: Allostasis and allostatic overload and relevance to the pathophysiology of psychiatric disorders. *Annals of the New York Academy of Sciences*, *1032*(1), 1–7. doi:10.1196/annals.1314.001 PMID:15677391

McGrady, A., Brennan, J., Lynch, D., & Whearty, K. (2012). A wellness programme for first year medical students. *Applied Psychophysiology and Biofeedback*, *37*(4), 253–260. doi:10.1007/s10484-012-9198-x PMID:22699926

McGuire, F. L. (1966). Psycho-social studies of medical students: A critical review. *Journal of Medical Education*, *41*, 728–734. PMID:5328333

McKenna, K. M., Hashimoto, D. A., Maguire, M. S., & Bynum, W. E. IV. (2016). The missing link: Connection is the key to resilience in medical education. *Academic Medicine*, *91*(9), 1197–1199. doi:10.1097/ACM.0000000000001311 PMID:27438155

McKenzie, J. F., Neiger, B. L., & Thackeray, R. (2013). *Planning, implementing, and evaluating health promotion programmes: a primer* (6th ed.). San Francisco: Pearson/Benjamin Cummings.

McKevitt, C., Morgan, M., Dundas, R., & Holland, W. (1997). Sickness absence and working through illness: A comparison of two professional groups. *Journal of Public Health, 19*(3), 295–300. doi:10.1093/oxfordjournals.pubmed.a024633

McManus, I., Woolf, K., Dacre, J., Paice, E., & Dewberry, C. (2009). The academic backbone: Longitudinal continuities in educational achievement from secondary school and medical school to MRCP(UK) and the specialist register in UK medical students and doctors. *BMC Med., 11*(242).

McManus, S., Meltzer, H., Brugha, T., Bebbington, P., & Jenkins, R. (2009). Adult psychiatric morbidity in England, 2007: Results of a household survey. London: National Centre for Social Research.

Mell, R. (2016, December 23). *My 2016 moment: Pak's retirement.* Retrieved from http://www.golfchannel.com/news/golf-central-blog/my-2016-moment-paks-retirement/

Melrose, S. (2011). Perfectionism and depression: Vulnerabilities nurses need to understand. *Nursing Research and Practice, 2011*, 1–7. doi:10.1155/2011/858497 PMID:21994842

Mezirow, J. (2003). Transformative learning as discourse. *Journal of Transformative Education, 1*(1), 58–63. doi:10.1177/1541344603252172

Miletic, V., Lukovic, J., Ratkovic, N., Aleksic, D., & Grgurevic, A. (2014). Demographic risk factors for suicide and depression among Serbian medical school students. *Social Psychiatry and Psychiatric Epidemiology, 50*(4), 633–638. doi:10.1007/s00127-014-0950-9 PMID:25205334

Miller, G. D., Kemmelmeier, M., & Dupey, P. (2013). Gender differences in worry during medical school. *Medical Education, 47*(9), 932.

Miller, L. (2009). Doctors, their mental health and capacity for work. *Occupational Medicine, 59*(1), 53–55. doi:10.1093/occmed/kqn111 PMID:18796700

Mino, Y., Yasuda, N., Tsuda, T., & Shimodera, S. (2001). Effects of a One-Hour Educational Programme on Medical Students Attitudes to Mental Illness. *Psychiatry and Clinical Neurosciences, 55*(5), 501–507. doi:10.1046/j.1440-1819.2001.00896.x PMID:11555346

Miville, M. L., & Constantine, M. G. (2007). Cultural Values, Counselling Stigma, and Intentions to Seek Counseling Among Asian American College Women. *Counseling and Values, 52*(1), 2–11. doi:10.1002/j.2161-007X.2007.tb00083.x

Moate, R. M., Gnilka, P. B., West, E. M., & Bruns, K. L. (2016). *Stress and burnout among* counselor educators: Differences between adaptive perfectionists, maladaptive perfectionists, and nonperfectionists. *Journal of Counseling and Development, 94*(2), 161–171. doi:10.1002/jcad.12073

Modood, T., Berthoud, R., Lakey, J., Nazroo, J., Smith, P., Virdee, S., & Beishon, S. (1997). *The Fourth National Survey of Ethnic Minorities: Ethnic Minorities in Britain.* London: Policy Studies Institute.

Mojtabai, R., Olfson, M., Sampson, N. A., Jin, R., Druss, B., Wang, P. S., & Kessler, R. C. (2011). Barriers to mental health treatment: Results from the National Comorbidity Survey Replication. *Psychological Medicine, 41*(08), 1751–1761. doi:10.1017/S0033291710002291 PMID:21134315

Monroe, A., Quinn, E., Samuelson, W., Dunleavy, D. M., & Dowd, K. W. (2013). An overview of the medical school admission process and use of applicant data in decision making: What has changed since the 1980s?. *Acad Med, 88*, 672-81.

Monrouxe, L. V. (2010). Identity, identification and medical education: Why should we care? *Medical Education, 44*(1), 40–49. doi:10.1111/j.1365-2923.2009.03440.x PMID:20078755

Monrouxe, L. V., Rees, C. E., & Hu, W. (2011). Differences in medical students explicit discourses of professionalism. *Medical Education, 45*(6), 585–602. doi:10.1111/j.1365-2923.2010.03878.x PMID:21564198

Montgomery, M. M., & Côté, J. E. (2003). College as a transition to adulthood. In G. R. Adams & M. D. Berzonsky (Eds.), *Blackwell handbook of adolescence* (pp. 149–172). New York: Blackwell Publishing.

Morra, D. J., Regehr, G., & Ginsburg, S. (2009). Anticipated debt and financial stress in medical. *Medical Education, 41*(2), 105.

Mosby's Medical Dictionary. (2009). Elsevier.

Mousa, O. Y., Dhamoon, M. S., Lander, S., & Dhamoon, A. S. (2016). The MD blues: Under-recognised depression and anxiety in medical trainees. *Plos*. Retrieved from nim.nih.gov

Moutier, C., Cornette, M., Lehrmann, J., Geppert, C., Tsao, C., DeBoard, M. R., & Roberts, L. W. et al. (2009). When residents need health care: Stigma of the patient role. *Academic Psychiatry, 33*(6), 431–441. doi:10.1176/appi.ap.33.6.431 PMID:19933883

Moutier, C., Norcross, W., Jong, P., Norman, M., Kirby, B., McGuire, T., & Zisook, S. (2012). The suicide prevention and depression awareness program at the university of california, san diego school of medicine. *Academic Medicine: Journal of the Association of American Medical Colleges, 87*(3), 320–326. doi:10.1097/ACM.0b013e31824451ad PMID:22373625

Mucci, N., Giorgi, G., De Pasquale, C. S., Fiz-Perez, J., Mucci, F., & Arcangeli, G. (2016). Anxiety, Stress-Related Factors, and Blood Pressure in Young Adults. Academic Press.

Muehlenkamp, J., Walsh, B., & McDade, M. (2009). Preventing Non-Suicidal Self-Injury in Adolescents: The Signs of Self-Injury Program. *Journal of Youth and Adolescence, 39*(3), 306–314. doi:10.1007/s10964-009-9450-8 PMID:19756992

Murinson, B. B., Klick, B., Haythornthwaite, J. A., Shochet, R., Levine, R. B., & Wright, S. M. (2010). Formative experiences of emerging physicians: Gauging the impact of events that occur during medical school. *Academic Medicne, 85*, 1331-1337. Retrieved from: http://journals.lww.com/academicmedicine/Abstract/2010/08000/Formative_Experiences_of_Emerging_Physicians_.18.aspx

Muzafar, Y., Khan, H. H., Ashraf, H., Hussain, W., Sajid, H., Tahir, M., Ahmad, W. (2015). Burnout and its Associated Factors in Medical Students of Lahore, Pakistan. *Cureus,* 7. 10.7759/cureus.390

National Academy of Sciences. (1997). *Advisor, teacher, role model, friend: On being a mentor to students in science and engineering.* Washington, DC: National Academy Press. https://doi.org/10.17226/5789

National Alliance on Mental Illness (NAMI). (2017). *Fact sheets.* Retrieved from http:// www.nami.org

National Institute of Health. (2017). *Transforming the understanding and treatment of mental illnesses.* Author.

National Research Council. (2013). *Subjective Well-Being: Measuring Happiness, Suffering, and Other Dimensions of Experience* (A. Stone & C. Mackie, Eds.). Washington, DC: National Academies Press.

National Wellness Institute. (2017). *Definition of wellness.* Retrieved from http://www.nationalwellness.org/?page=AboutWellness

Nedrow, A., Steckler, N. A., & Hardman, J. (2013). Physician resilience and burnout: Can you make the switch? *Family Practice Management, 20,* 25. Retrieved from https://www.ncbi.nlm.nih.gov/pubmed/23418835 PMID:23418835

Neki, J., Joinet, B., Ndose, N., Kilonzo, G. J. H., & Duvinage, G. (1986). Witchcraft and Psychotherapy. *British Journal of Psychotherapy,* 145–155. PMID:3535977

Neumann, M., Edelhauser, F., Tauschel, D., Fischer, M. R., Wirtz, M., Woopen, C., & Scheffer, C. et al. (2011). Empathy decline and its reasons: A systematic review of studies with medical students and residents. *Academic Medicine, 86*(8), 996–1009. doi:10.1097/ACM.0b013e318221e615 PMID:21670661

No health without mental health: A cross-governmental health outcomes strategy for people of all ages: The mental health strategy for England-GOV.UK. (2011). Retrieved from https://www.gov.uk/government/publications/the-mental-health-strategy-for-england

Noone, J. (2009). Teaching to the three apprenticeships: Designing learning activities for professional practice in an undergraduate curriculum. *The Journal of Nursing Education, 48,* 468–471. Retrieved from http://search.proquest.com/docview/203967665?accountid=14376

Noori, S., Blood, A., Meleca, J., Kennedy, V., & Sengupta, D. (n.d.). *Current directions in medical student wellbeing: A primer for students.* Retrieved February 2017 from https://www.aamc.org/download/450164/data/medstudentwellbeing.pdf

Noori, S., Blood, A., Meleca, J., Kennedy, V., & Sengupta, D. (2017, March 6). Current directions in medical student well-being. *Col Med Rev., 1*(2), 10–19.

O'Connor, M. C., & Paunonen, S. V. (2007). Big five personality predictors of post-secondary academic performance. *Pers Indiv Diff., 43,* 313-315. 10.1080/01421590801953000

OConnor, E., Gaynes, B., Burda, B., Soh, C., & Whitlock, E. (2013). Screening for and Treatment of Suicide Risk Relevant to Primary Care: A Systematic Review for the U.S. Preventive Services Task Force. *Annals of Internal Medicine*, *158*(10), 741. doi:10.7326/0003-4819-158-10-201305210-00642 PMID:23609101

OReilly, C. L., Bell, J. S., Kelly, P. J., & Chen, T. F. (2011). Impact of Mental Health First aid Training on Pharmacy Students Knowledge, Attitudes and Self-Reported Behaviour: A Controlled Trial. *The Australian and New Zealand Journal of Psychiatry*, *45*(7), 549–557. doi:10.3109/00048674.2011.585454 PMID:21718124

Osama, M., Islam, M., Hussain, S., Masroor, S., Burney, M., Masood, M., & Rehman, R. et al. (2014). Suicidal ideation among medical students of Pakistan: A cross-sectional study. *Journal of Forensic and Legal Medicine*, *27*, 65–68. doi:10.1016/j.jflm.2014.08.006 PMID:25287803

Ospina-Kammerer, V., & Figley, C. R. (2003). An evaluation of the respiratory one method (ROM) in reducing emotional exhaustion among family physician residents. *International Journal of Emergency Mental Health*, *5*(1), 29–32. PMID:12722487

Papish, A., Kassam, A., Modgill, G., Vaz, G., Zanussi, L., & Patten, S. (2013). Reducing the stigma of mental illness in undergraduate medical education: A randomised controlled trial. *BMC Medical Education*, 1–10. PMID:24156397

Parkernson, G. R., Broadhead, W. E., & Tse, C. J. (1990). The Health Status and Life Satisfaction of First-year Medical Students. *Academic Medicine*, *65*(9), 586–587. doi:10.1097/00001888-199009000-00009 PMID:2400477

Pasupuleti, R. V. (2013). *Cultural Factors, Stigma, Stress, and Help-seeking Attitudes Among College Students*. University of Rhode Island.

Perfectionism. (2013). Retrieved from http://www.goodtherapy.org/learn-about-therapy/issues/perfectionism

Perfectionism. (n.d.). In *University of Illinois Counseling Center*. Retrieved from http://www.counselingcenter.illinois.edu/?page_id=113

Peters, M. & King, J. (2012). Perfectionism in doctors. *British Medical Journal, 344*, e1674.

Philibert, I., Friedmann, P., & Williams, W. T. (2002). New requirements for resident duty hours. *Journal of the American Medical Association*, *288*(9), 1112–1114. doi:10.1001/jama.288.9.1112 PMID:12204081

Phillips, J. P., Petterson, S. M., Bazemore, A. W., & Phillips, R. L. (2014). A Retrospective Analysis of the Relationship Between Medical Student Debt and Primary Care Practice in the United States. *Annals of Family Medicine*, *12*(6), 542–549. doi:10.1370/afm.1697 PMID:25384816

Pinfold, V., Huxley, P., Thornicroft, G., Farmer, P., Toulmin, H., & Graham, T. (2003). Reducing psychiatric stigma and discrimination - Evaluating an educational intervention with the police force in England. *Social Psychiatry and Psychiatric Epidemiology*, *38*(6), 337–344. doi:10.1007/s00127-003-0641-4 PMID:12799785

Pitt, E., Rosenthal, M. M., Gay, T. L., & Lewton, E. (2004). Mental health services for residents: More important than ever. *Academic Medicine*, *79*(9), 840–844. doi:10.1097/00001888-200409000-00005 PMID:15326006

Plaisant, O., Courtois, R., Toussaint, P. J., Mendelsohn, G. A., John, O. P., Delmas, V., & Moxham, B. J. (2011). Medical students' attitudes toward the anatomy dissection room in relation to personality. *Anatomical Sciences Education*, *4*(6), 305–310. doi:10.1002/ase.251 PMID:22065473

Pololi, L. H., Evans, A. T., Civian, J. T., Gibbs, B. K., Coplit, L. D., Gillum, L. H., & Brennan, R. T. (2015). Faculty vitality-surviving the challenges facing academic health centers: A national survey of medical faculty. *Academic Medicine: Journal of the Association of American Medical Colleges*, *90*(7), 930–936. doi:10.1097/ACM.0000000000000674 PMID:25692560

Population Reference Bureau (PBR). (2015). *Research on Health and Well-Being Aims to Improve Quality of Life in Later Years*. Accessed: http://www.prb.orf

Poulin, M. (2014). Volunteering predicts health among those who value others: Two national studies. *Health Psychology*, *33*(2), 120–129. doi:10.1037/a0031620 PMID:23566179

Poundstone, W. (2014). *Rock Breaks Scissors: A Practical Guide to Outguessing & Outwitting Almost Everybody*. New York: Little, Brown and Company.

Povis, D. (2015). Selecting medical students: An unresolved challenge. *Medical Teacher*, *37*(3), 252–260. doi:10.3109/0142159X.2014.993600 PMID:25532428

Pressman, S. D., & Cohen, S. (2005). Does positive affect influence health? *Psychological Bulletin*, *131*(6), 925–971. doi:10.1037/0033-2909.131.6.925 PMID:16351329

Prinz, P., Hertrich, K., Hirschfelder, U., & de Zwaan, M. (2012). Burnout, depression and depersonalization: Psychological factors and coping strategies in dental and medical students. *GMS Z Med Ausbild*, *29*, Doc10. PMID:22403595

Pscyho, R. C. (2011). *Mental Health of Students in Higher Education*. Retrieved at http://www.rcpsych.ac.uk/files/pdfversion/cr166.pdf

Pullen, D., Lonie, C., Lyle, D., Cam, D., & Doughty, M. (1995). Medical care of doctors. *The Medical Journal of Australia*, 481–484. PMID:7746206

Puthran, R., Zhang, M. W. B., Tam, W. W., & Ho, R. C. (2016). Prevalence of depression amongst medical students: A meta-analysis. *Medical Education*, *50*(4), 456–468. doi:10.1111/medu.12962 PMID:26995484

Puvanendran, R., Park, C., Lee, Y. J., Hong, M., Jung, C.-H., Synn, Y., & Bahn, G. H. et al. (2016). A Multicenter Study Investigating Empathy and Burnout Characteristics in Medical Residents with Various Specialties. *Journal of Korean Medical Science*, *31*, 590–597. doi:10.3346/jkms.2016.31.4.590

Puvanendran, R., Vasanwala, F. F., Kamei, R. K., Hock, L. K., & Lie, D. A. (2012). What do medical students learn when they follow patients from hospital to community? A longitudinal qualitative study. *Medical Education Online*, 17. PMID:22791959

Qual, T. N. S. +. (2011, September). *Well-being: Aggregrate report*. European Commission. Retrieved from http://ec.europa.eu/public_opinion/archives/quali/wellbeing_final_en.pdf

Ramani, S., & Krackov, S. K. (2012). Twelve tips for giving feedback effectively in the clinical environment. *Medical Teacher, 34*(10), 787–791. doi:10.3109/0142159X.2012.684916 PMID:22730899

Ramisetty-Mikler, S. (1993). Asian Indian immigrants in America and sociocultural issues in counseling. *Journal of Multicultural Counseling and Development, 21*(1), 36–49. doi:10.1002/j.2161-1912.1993.tb00581.x

Rapporteur, P. (2016). *Envisioning the Future of Health Professional Education: Workshop Summary*. The National Academic Press. https://doi.org/10.17226/21796

Reavley, N., Ross, A., Killackey, E., & Jorm, A. (2013). Development of guidelines for tertiary education institutions to assist them in supporting students with a mental illness: A Delphi consensus study with Australian professionals and consumers. *Peerj, 1*, e43. doi:10.7717/peerj.43 PMID:23638380

Redmond, B. F. (2014). *Self-Efficacy and Social Cognitive Theories*. Retrieved March 24 2014 from https://wikispaces.psu.edu/display/PSYCH484/7.+Self-Efficacy+and+Social+Cognitive+Theories

Reed, D. A., Shanafelt, T. D., Satele, D. W., Power, D. V., Eacker, A., Harper, W., & Dyrbye, L. N. et al. (2011). Relationship of Pass/Fail Grading and Curriculum Structure with Well-Being Among Preclinical Medical Students: A Multi-Institutional Study. *Academic Medicine, 86*(11), 1367–1373. doi:10.1097/ACM.0b013e3182305d81 PMID:21952063

Rice, K. G., & Ashby, J. S. (2007). An efficient method for classifying perfectionists. *Journal of Counseling Psychology, 54*(1), 72–85. doi:10.1037/0022-0167.54.1.72

Rice, K., & Lopez, F. (2004). Maladaptive perfectionism, adult attachment, and self-esteem in college students. *Journal of College Counseling, 7*(2), 118–128. doi:10.1002/j.2161-1882.2004.tb00243.x

Richardson, M., Abraham, C., & Bond, R. (2012). Psychological correlates of university students' academic performance: A systematic review and meta-analysis. *Psychol Bull, 138*(353), 87.

Richardson, T., Elliott, P., & Roberts, R. (2013). The relationship between personal unsecured debt and mental and physical health: A systematic review and meta-analysis. *Clinical Psychology Review, 33*(8), 1148–1162. doi:10.1016/j.cpr.2013.08.009 PMID:24121465

Ringrose, R., Houterman, S., Koops, W., & Oei, G. (2009). Burnout in medical residents: A questionnaire and interview study. *Psychology Health and Medicine, 14*(4), 476–486. doi:10.1080/13548500903012822 PMID:19697257

Robinson, H. (2016). Dualism. In Stanford Encyclopedia of Philosophy. Stanford, CA: Stanford University. Retrieved from https://plato.stanford.edu/entries/dualism/

Roff, S., McAleer, S., Harden, R. M., & Al-Qahtani, M. (1997). Development and validation of the Dundee ready education environment measure (DREEM). *Medical Teacher, 19*, 295-299. Retrieved from http://search.proquest.com/docview/233249246?accountid=14376

Roger, C. (2012). The "physician personality" and other factors in physician health. *CMAJ, 184*(18). doi:.10.1503/cmaj.109-4329

Rogers, C. R. (1975). Empathic: An unappreciated way of being. *The Counseling Psychologist, 5*(2), 2–10. doi:10.1177/001100007500500202

Roh, M., Jeon, H., Kim, H., Han, S., & Hahm, B. (2010). The prevalence and impact of depression among medical students: A nationwide cross-sectional study in South Korea. *Academic Medicine, 85*(8), 1384–1390. doi:10.1097/ACM.0b013e3181df5e43 PMID:20453812

Rose, G. L., & Rukstalis, M. R. (2008). Imparting medical ethics: the role of mentorship in clinical training. *Mentoring & Tutoring: Partnership in Learning, 16*, 77-89. Retrieved from: http://www.tandfonline.com/doi/pdf/10.1080/13611260701801031

Rosenberg, D. (2014, October 28). *The Secret Dual Lives of People Living With Mental Illness.* Retrieved from Slate Blog: http://www.slate.com/blogs/behold/2014/10/28/liz_obert_dualities_looks_at_the_hidden_and_visible_worlds_of_people_living.html

Rosen, I. M., Gimotty, P. A., Shea, J. A., & Bellini, L. M. (2006). Evolution of sleep quantity, sleep deprivation, mood disturbances, empathy, and burnout among interns. Academic Medicine. *Journal. Association of American Medical Colleges, 81*(1), 82–85. doi:10.1097/00001888-200601000-00020

Rosenthal, O. (2005). White Coat Mood indigo: Depression in Medical school. *NEJM.*

Rosenthal, J. M., & Okie, S. (2005). White coat, mood indigo - depression in medical school. *The New England Journal of Medicine, 353*(11), 1085–1088. doi:10.1056/NEJMp058183 PMID:16162877

Ross, S., Cleland, J., & Macleod, M. J. (2006). Stress, debt and undergraduate medical student performance. *Med Educ, 40*(6), 584–589.

Rotenstein, L. S., Ramos, M. A., Torre, M., Segal, J. B., Peluso, M. J., Guille, C., & Mata, D. A. et al. (2016). Prevalence of Depression, Depressive Symptoms, and Suicidal Ideation Among Medical Students: A Systematic Review and Meta-Analysis. *Journal of the American Medical Association, 316*(21), 2214. doi:10.1001/jama.2016.17324 PMID:27923088

Rubin, R. (2014). Recent suicides highlight need to address depression in medical students and residents. *Journal of the American Medical Association, 312*(17), 1725–1727. doi:10.1001/jama.2014.13505 PMID:25369478

Russo, N. F., & Pirlott, A. (2006). Gender-Based violence: Concepts, methods and findings. *Annals of the New York Academy of Sciences*, *1077*(1), 178–205. doi:10.1196/annals.1385.024 PMID:17189506

Rutter, M. (2012). Resilience as a dynamic concept. *Development and Psychopathology*, *24*(2), 335–344. doi:10.1017/S0954579412000028 PMID:22559117

Salles, A., Liebert, C. A., & Greco, R. S. (2015). Promoting balance in the lives of resident physicians: A call to action. *JAMA Surgery*, *150*(7), 607–608. doi:10.1001/jamasurg.2015.0257 PMID:25992632

Savickas, M. L. (2001). A developmental perspective on vocational behavior: Career patterns, salience, and themes. *International Journal for Educational and Vocational Guidance*, *1*(1/2), 49–57. doi:10.1023/A:1016916713523

Scambler, G. (1998). Stigma and disease: Changing paradigms. *Lancet*, *352*(9133), 1054–1055. doi:10.1016/S0140-6736(98)08068-4 PMID:9759769

Scanlon, L., Rowling, L., & Weber, Z. (2010). You don't have an identity... you are just lost in a crowd: Forming a student identity in the first-year transition to university. *Journal of Youth Studies*, *10*(2), 223–241. doi:10.1080/13676260600983684

Schindler, B. A., Novack, D. H., Cohen, D. G., Yager, J., Wang, D., Shaheen, N. J., & Drossman, D. A. et al. (2006). The impact of the changing health care environment on the health and well-being of faculty at four medical schools. *Academic Medicine*, *81*(1), 27–34. doi:10.1097/00001888-200601000-00008 PMID:16377815

Schneiderman, N., Ironson, G., & Siegel, S. D. (2005). Stress and health: Psychological, behavioral, and biological determinants. *Annual Review of Clinical Psychology*, *1*(1), 607–628. doi:10.1146/annurev.clinpsy.1.102803.144141 PMID:17716101

Schulte, D. L., Skinner, T. A., & Claibom, C. D. (2002). Religious and spiritual issues in counseling psychology training. *The Counseling Psychologist*, *30*(1), 118–134. doi:10.1177/0011000002301009

Schwartz, B. (1987). The Battle for Human Nature: Science, Morality and Modern Life Paperback. W.W. Norton & Company.

Schwenk, T. L., Davis, L., & Wimsatt, L. A. (2010). Depression, stigma, and suicide ideation in medical students. *Journal of the American Medical Association*, *304*(11), 1181–1190. doi:10.1001/jama.2010.1300 PMID:20841531

Scutti, S. (2014). *Perfectionists Are More Likely to Commit Suicide Than The Rest of Us*. Retrieved from http://www.medicaldaily.com/perfectionists-especiallydoctors-architects-and-lawyers-are-higher-risk-suicide-305256

Sen, S., Kranzler, H. R., Krystal, J. H., Speller, H., Chan, G., Gelernter, J., & Guille, C. (2010). A prospective cohort study investigating factors associated with depression during medical internship. *Archives of General Psychiatry*, *67*(6), 557–565. doi:10.1001/archgenpsychiatry.2010.41 PMID:20368500

Seritan, A. L., Rai, G., Servis, M., & Pomeroy, C. (2014, May 20). The Office of Student Wellness: Innovating to Improve Student Mental Health. *Academic Psychiatry*, *39*(1), 80–84. doi:10.1007/s40596-014-0152-5 PMID:24840666

Seritan, A., Hunt, J., Shy, A., Rea, M., & Worley, L. (2012). The state of medical student wellness: A call for culture change. *Academic Psychiatry*, *36*(1), 7–10. doi:10.1176/appi.ap.10030042 PMID:22362429

Serwint, J. R., Bostwick, S., Burke, A. E., Church, A., Gogo, A., Hofkosh, D., & Osta, A. (2016). The AAP Resilience in the Face of Grief and Loss Curriculum. *Pediatrics*, *e20160791*. Retrieved from http://pediatrics.aappublications.org/content/early/2016/10/06/peds.2016-0791 PMID:27940771

Shafran, R., & Mansell, W. A. (2001). Perfectionism and psychopathology: A review of research and treatment. *Clinical Psychology Review*, *21*(6), 879–906. doi:10.1016/S0272-7358(00)00072-6 PMID:11497211

Shanafelt, T. D., Boone, S., Tan, L., Dyrbye, L. N., Sotile, W., Satele, D., & Oreskovich, M. R. et al. (2012). Burnout and satisfaction with work-life balance among US physicians relative to the general US population. *Archives of Internal Medicine*, *172*(18), 1377–1385. doi:10.1001/archinternmed.2012.3199 PMID:22911330

Shanafelt, T. D., Bradley, K. A., Wipf, J. E., & Back, A. L. (2002). Burnout and self-reported patient care in an internal medicine residency program. *Annals of Internal Medicine*, *136*(5), 358–367. doi:10.7326/0003-4819-136-5-200203050-00008 PMID:11874308

Shanafelt, T. D., West, C. P., Sloan, J. A., Novotny, P. J., Poland, G. A., Menaker, R., & Dyrbye, L. N. et al. (2009). Career fit and burnout among academic faculty. *Archives of Internal Medicine*, *169*(10), 990–995. doi:10.1001/archinternmed.2009.70 PMID:19468093

Shanafelt, T., Hasan, O., Dyrbye, L., Sinsky, C., Satele, D., Sloan, J., & West, C. (2015). Changes in burnout and satisfaction with work-life balance in physicians and the general US working population between 2011 and 2014. *Mayo Clinic Proceedings*, *90*(12), 1600–1613. doi:10.1016/j.mayocp.2015.08.023 PMID:26653297

Sherman, E. (2012, January 2). *Are you a perfectionist?*. Retrieved from https://www.psychologytoday.com/blog/couch-meets-world/201201/are-you-perfectionist

Shrank, W. H., Reed, V. A., & Jernstedt, C. (2004). Fostering professionalism in medical education: A call for improved assessment and meaningful incentives. *Journal of General Internal Medicine*, *19*(8), 887–892. doi:10.1111/j.1525-1497.2004.30635.x PMID:15242476

Silver, H. K., & Glicken, A. D. (1990). Medical student abuse. Incidence, severity, and significance. *JAMA, 264*(13), 1657-60.

Simon, G., Rutter, C., Peterson, D., Oliver, M., Whiteside, U., Operskalski, B., & Ludman, E. (2013). Does Response on the PHQ-9 Depression Questionnaire Predict Subsequent Suicide Attempt or Suicide Death? *Psychiatric Services (Washington, D.C.), 64*(12), 1195–1202. doi:10.1176/appi.ps.201200587 PMID:24036589

Simons-Morton, B. G., McLeroy, K. R., & Wendel, M. L. (2012). *Behaviuor theory in health promotion practice and research*. Sudbury, MA: Jones & Bartlett Learning.

Sinha, P. (2014, September 4). Why do doctors commit suicide?. *New York Times*. Retrieved on January 18, 2017 from https://nyti.ms/Wi4ns9

Slavin, S. J. (2016). Medical Student Mental Health Culture, Environment, and the Need for Change. *Retrieved from JAMA., 316*(21), 2195–2196. doi:10.1001/jama.2016.16396 PMID:27923076

Slavin, S. J., & Chibnall, J. T. (2016). Finding the why, changing the how, improving the mental health of medical students, residents, and physicians. *Academic Medicine, 91*(9), 1194–1196. doi:10.1097/ACM.0000000000001226 PMID:27166866

Slavin, S. J., Schindler, D. L., & Chibnall, J. T. (2014). Medical student mental health 3.0: Improving student wellness through curricular changes. *Academic Medicine, 89*(4), 573–577. doi:10.1097/ACM.0000000000000166 PMID:24556765

Smajdor, H. A., & Stöckl, A. (2012). Towards an understanding of resilience and its relevance to medical training. *Med Educ., 46*, 349-356.

Smith, C., Christoffersen, K., Davidson, H., & Herzog, P. (2011). Lost in Transition: The Dark Side of Emerging Adulthood. Oxford University Press, Inc.

Sobral, D. T. (2004). What kind of motivation drives medical students learning quests?. *Medical Education, 38*(9), 950–957. doi:10.1111/j.1365-2929.2004.01913.x PMID:15327676

Social Cognitive Theory. (2014). University of Twente. Retrieved from: http://www.utwente.nl/cw/theorieenoverzicht/Theory%20Clusters/Health%20Communication/Social_cognitive_theory.doc/

Soltani-Kouhbanani, S., & Khosrorad, R. I. (2015). Investigating perfectionism in medicine and architecture majors. *International Journal of Educational Investigation, 2*(2), 128–139.

Sood, A., Prasad, K., Schroeder, D., & Varkey, P. (2011). Stress management and resilience training among department of medicine faculty: A pilot randomized clinical trial. *Journal of General Internal Medicine, 26*(8), 858–861. doi:10.1007/s11606-011-1640-x PMID:21279454

Stalmeijer, R. E., Dolmans, D., Wolfhagen, I., & Scherpbier, A. (2009). Cognitive apprenticeship in clinical practice: Can it stimulate learning in the opinion of students?. *Advances in Health Sciences Education: Theory and Practice, 14*, 535. Retrieved from: http://link.springer.com/article/10.1007/s10459-008-9136-0#page-1

Stanley, B., Sher, L., Wilson, S., Ekman, R., Huang, Y., & Mann, J. (2010). Non-suicidal self-injurious behaviour, endogenous opioids and monoamine neurotransmitters. *Journal of Affective Disorders*, *124*(1-2), 134–140. doi:10.1016/j.jad.2009.10.028 PMID:19942295

Stark, M. A., Hoekstra, T., Lindstrom Hazel, D., & Barton, B. (2012). Caring for self and others: Increasing health care students' healthy behaviors. *Work (Reading, Mass.)*, *42*(3), 393–401. doi:10.3233/WOR-2012-1428 PMID:22523027

Steadman, H. J., Deane, M. W., Borum, R., & Morrissey, J. P. (2000). Comparing Outcomes of Major Models of Police Responses to Mental Health Emergencies. *Psychiatric Services (Washington, D.C.)*, *51*(5), 645–649. doi:10.1176/appi.ps.51.5.645 PMID:10783184

Steel, Z., Marnane, C., Iranpour, C., Jackson, J. W., Patel, V., & Silove, D. (2014). The global prevalence of common mental disorders: A systematics review and meta-analysis 19802013. *International Journal of Epidemiology*, *43*(2), 476–493. doi:10.1093/ije/dyu038 PMID:24648481

Stepien, K. A., & Baernstein, A. (2006). Educating for Empathy. *Journal of General Internal Medicine*, *21*(5), 524–530. doi:10.1111/j.1525-1497.2006.00443.x PMID:16704404

Stoeber, J. (2016). *Comparing Two Short Forms of the Hewitt-Flett Multidimensional Perfectionism Scale Assessment*. Retrieved from https://www.ncbi.nlm.nih.gov/pubmed/?term=multidimensional+of+perfectionsim1073191116659740

Stoeber, J., & Otto, K. (2006). Positive conceptions of perfectionism: Approaches, evidence, challenges. *Personality & Social Psychology*, *10*(4), 295–319. doi:10.1207/s15327957pspr1004_2 PMID:17201590

Stoeber, J., & Rennert, D. (2008). Perfectionism in school teachers: Relations with stress appraisals, coping styles, and burnout. *Anxiety, Stress, and Coping*, *21*(1), 37–53. doi:10.1080/10615800701742461 PMID:18027123

Strecker, E. A., Appel, K. E., Palmer, H. D., & Braceland, F. J. (1936). Psychiatric studies in medical education: Neurotic trends in senior medical students. *The American Journal of Psychiatry*, *92*(4), 937–957. doi:10.1176/ajp.92.4.937

Stumpf, H., & Parker, W. D. (2000). A hierarchical structural analysis of perfectionism and its relation to other personality characteristics. *Personality and Individual Differences*, *28*(5), 837–852. doi:10.1016/S0191-8869(99)00141-5

Suarez, N., & Saunders, K. (2012). Assessment and management of self harm. *Student BMJ, 20*. http://dx.doi.org.libraryproxy.griffith.edu.au/10.1136/sbmj.e511

Suchman, A. L., Williamson, P. R., Litzelman, D. K., Frankel, R. M., Mossbarger, D. L., & Inui, T. S. (2004). Toward an Informal Curriculum that Teaches Professionalism Transforming the Social Environment of a Medical School. *Journal of General Internal Medicine*, *19*(5), 501–504. doi:10.1111/j.1525-1497.2004.30157.x PMID:15109312

Sue, D., & Sue, D. W. (1999). *Counselling the culturally different*. New York: Wiley.

Swift, D. (2017). *The 'Invisible White Coat': Black Women in Medicine*. Medscape Medical News.

Tempski, P., Martins, M. A., & Paro, H. B. (2012). Teaching and learning resilience: a new agenda in medical education. *Med Educ., 46*(4), 345-6. doi: 10.1111/j.1365-2923.2011.04207.x

Tempski, P., Bellodi, P. L., Paro, H., Enns, S. C., Martins, M. A., & Schraiber, B. (2012). What do medical students think about their quality of life? A qualitative study. *BMC Medical Education, 12*(1), 106. doi:10.1186/1472-6920-12-106 PMID:23126332

Tempski, P., Perotta, B., Pose, R. A., & Vieira, J. E. (2009). A questionnaire on the quality of life of medical students. *Medical Education, 43*(11), 1107–1108. doi:10.1111/j.1365-2923.2009.03476.x PMID:19874519

The Gypsy Nesters. (2007-2017). *Boomer Travel, Food, Laugher*. Gypsynester.com.

The Jed Foundation. (2014). *The Comprehensive Approach to Mental Health Promotion and Suicide Prevention on College and University Campuses*. JED Foundation and the Suicide Prevention Resource Center. Retrieved from https://www.jedfoundation.org/what-we-do/

The Lancet. (1980). Stress in medical students. *Lancet, 1*, 129-130.

The Patient Health Questionnaire (PHQ-9). (1999). Centre for Quality Assessment and Improvement in Mental Health. Retrieved 1 October 2016, from http://www.cqaimh.org/pdf/tool_phq9.pdf

The World Health Organisation Mental Health Action Plan 2013 – 2020. (n.d.). Retrieved from http://www.who.int/mental_health/action_plan_2013/en/

Thistlethwaite, J. E., Quirk, F., & Evans, R. (2010). Medical students seeking medical help: A qualitative study. *Medical Teacher, 32*(2), 164–166. doi:10.3109/01421590903434177 PMID:20163234

Thoits, P. A. (2010). Stress and health: Major findings and policy implications. *Journal of Health and Social Behavior, 51*(1), S41–S53. doi:10.1177/0022146510383499 PMID:20943582

Thomas, S., Haney, M., Pelic, C., Shaw, D., & Wong, J. (2011, March 31). Developing a Program to Promote Stress Resilience and Self-Care in First-Year Medical Students. *Canadian Medical Education Journal, 2*(1), E32–E36. PMID:21822458

Thompson, W. T., Cupples, M. E., Sibbett, C. H., Skan, D. I., & Bradley, T. (2001). Challenge of culture, conscience, and contract to general practitioners' care of their own health: Qualitative study. *BMJ (Clinical Research Ed.), 323*(7315), 728–731. doi:10.1136/bmj.323.7315.728 PMID:11576981

Thornicroft, G., Brohan, E., Kassam, A., & Lewis-Holmes, E. (2008). Reducing stigma and discrimination: Candidate interventions. *International Journal of Mental Health Systems*, 3-10.

Thornicroft, G., Mehta, N., Clement, S., Evans-Lacko, S., Doherty, M., Rose, D., & Henderson, C. et al. (2016). Evidence for effective interventions to reduce mental-health-related stigma and discrimination. *Lancet*, *387*(10023), 1123–1132. doi:10.1016/S0140-6736(15)00298-6 PMID:26410341

Tjia, J., Givens, J., & Shea, J. (2005). Factors associated with undertreatment of medical student depression. *Journal of American College Help*, 219-224.

Together for Mental Health: A strategy for mental health and wellbeing in 2010. (n.d.). Retrieved from gov.wales/topics/health/nhswales/mental-health-services/policy/strategy/?lang=en

Tov, W., & Diener, E. (2008). The well-being of nations: Linking together trust, cooperation, and democracy. In B. A. Sullivan, M. Snyder, & J. L. Sullivan (Eds.), *Cooperation: The psychology of effective human interaction* (pp. 323–342). Malden, MA: Blackwell Publishing.

Turiano, N. A., Pitzer, L., Armour, C., Karlamangla, A., Ryff, C. D., & Mroczek, D. K. (2012). Personality trait level and change as predictors of health outcomes: Findings from a national study of Americans (MIDUS). *The Journals of Gerontology. Series B, Psychological Sciences and Social Sciences*, *67*(1), 4–12. doi:10.1093/geronb/gbr072 PMID:21765062

Turner, J. C., & Nolen, S. B. (2015). Introduction: The relevance of the situative perspective in educational psychology. *Educational Psychologist*, *50*(3), 167–172. doi:10.1080/00461520.2015.1075404

Tyssen, R., Vaglum, P., Grønvold, N. T., & Ekeberg, O. (2001). Suicidal ideation among medical students and young physi- cians: A nationwide and prospective study of prevalence and predictors. *Journal of Affective Disorders*, *64*(1), 69–79. doi:10.1016/S0165-0327(00)00205-6 PMID:11292521

U.S.A. Centres for Disease Control Prevention (CDC) Concept Paper. (n.d.). *Wellbeing*. Retrieved 1 March, 2017 www.cdc.gov/hrqol/wellbeing.htm

UNESCO. (2011). *International standard classification of education*. Montréal: UNESCO Institute for Statistics.

University of South Carolina. (2015, January 22). How are student loans affecting the well-being of young adults?. *Science Daily*. Retrieved March 4, 2017 from www.sciencedaily.com/releases/2015/01/150122114430.htm

Utsey, S., Adams, E., & Bolden, M. (2000). Development and initial validation of the Africultural Coping Systems Inventory. *The Journal of Black Psychology*, *26*(2), 194–215. doi:10.1177/0095798400026002005

Vachon, R. (2012). *Foundations of human wellbeing: Social, environmental, economic*. Retrieved from http://www.sustainabledevelopment.un.org

Vaish, A., Grossmann, T., & Woodward, A. (2008). Not all emotions are created equal:the negativity bias in social-emotional development. *Psychological Bulletin*, *134*(3), 383–403. doi:10.1037/0033-2909.134.3.383 PMID:18444702

Vansteenkiste, M., Lens, W., & Deci, E. L. (2006). Intrinsic versus extrinsic goal contents in self-determination theory: Another look at the quality of academic motivation. *Educ Psychol.*, *41*(1), 19–31. doi:10.1207/s15326985ep4101_4

Vaz, F. S., Ferreira, A., Kulkarni, M., Perni, S., Dsouza, D., & Dsouza, L. (2012). Study of health seeking behavior among medical students in Goa, India. *Asian Journal of Medical and Clinical Sciences*, 140-141.

Vessey, J. T., & Howard, K. I. (1993). Who seeks psychotherapy? *Psychotherapy (Chicago, Ill.)*, *30*(4), 546–553. doi:10.1037/0033-3204.30.4.546

Viguera, A., Milano, N., Laurel, R., Thompson, N., Griffith, S., Baldessarini, R., & Katzan, I. (2015). Comparison of Electronic Screening for Suicidal Risk with the Patient Health Questionnaire Item 9 and the Columbia Suicide Severity Rating Scale in an Outpatient Psychiatric Clinic. *Psychosomatics*, *56*(5), 460–469. doi:10.1016/j.psym.2015.04.005 PMID:26278339

Villablanca, , Li, Beckett, & Howell. (2017, February). Evaluating a Medical School's Climate for Women's Success: Outcomes for Faculty Recruitment, Retention, and Promotion. *Journal of Women's Health*. PMID:28170291

Villwock, J. A., Sobin, L. B., Koester, L. A., & Harris, T. (2016). *Impostor syndrome and burnout among American medical students: A pilot study*. Academic Press.

Voltmer, E., Rosta, J., Aasland, O. G., & Spahn, C. (2010). Study-related health and behavior patterns of medical students: A longitudinal study. *Medical Teacher*, *32*(10), e422–e428. doi:10.3109/0142159X.2010.496008 PMID:20854148

Wahl, O. (1999). Mental health consumers experience of stigma. *Schizophrenia Bulletin*, *25*(3), 467–478. doi:10.1093/oxfordjournals.schbul.a033394 PMID:10478782

Walker, E. R., McGee, R. E., & Druss, B. G. (2015). Mortality in mental disorders and global disease burden implications: A systematic review and meta-analysis. *JAMA Psychiatry*, *72*(4), 334–341. doi:10.1001/jamapsychiatry.2014.2502 PMID:25671328

Wallsten, T. S., Pleskac, T. J., & Lejuez, C. W. (2005). Modeling behavior in a clinically diagnostic sequential risk-taking task. *Psychological Review*, *112*(4), 862–880. doi:10.1037/0033-295X.112.4.862 PMID:16262471

Walsemann, K. M., Gee, G. C., & Gentile, D. (2014). Sick of our loans: Student borrowing and the mental health of young adults in the United States. *Social Science & Medicine*, 124.

Wan, Y., Gao, R., Tao, X., Tao, F., & Hu, C. (2012). Relationship between deliberate self-harm and suicidal behaviors in college students. *Zhonghua Liu Xing Bing Xue Za Zhi = Zhonghua Liuxingbingxue Zazhi, 33*(5), 474-477.

Wang, S., Lee, S., & Wahid, Z. T. (2013). *University student mental health: The Australian context.* Barton, ACT: Australian Medical Students' Association Student Mental Health and Wellbeing Committee. Retrieved from http://www.amsa.org.au/wp-content/uploads/2013/09/AMSA-SMHW-The-Australian-Context-of-Student-Mental-Health-Report.pdf

Wang, X., Armstrong, M. E., Cairns, B. J., Key, T. J., & Travis, R. C. (2011, March 25). Shift work and chronic disease: The epidemiological evidence. *Occupational Medicine*, *61*(2), 78–89. doi:10.1093/occmed/kqr001 PMID:21355031

Wasserman, D., Rihmer, Z., Rujescu, D., Sarchiapone, M., Sokolowski, M., Titelman, D., & Carli, V. et al. (2011). The European Psychiatric Association (EPA) guidance on suicide treatment and prevention. *European Psychiatry*, *27*(2), 129–141. doi:10.1016/j.eurpsy.2011.06.003 PMID:22137775

Wasson, L. T. Cusmano, A., Meli, L., Louh, I., Falzon, L., Hampsey, M., … Davidson, K. W. (2016). Association between learning environment interventions and medical student wellbeing: A systematic review. *Journal of the American Medical Association*. doi:10.1001/jama.2016.17573

Watch. (n.d.). *Treating Anxiety Disorders*. Retrieved from https://www.adaa.org/resources-professionals/practice-guidelines-tools

Wayne, S. J., Fortner, S. A., Kitzes, J. A., Timm, C., & Kalishman, S. (2013). Cause or effect? the relationship between student perception of the medical school learning environment and academic performance on USMLE step 1. *Medical Teacher*, *35*(5), 376–380. doi:10.3109/0142159X.2013.769678 PMID:23444883

Wechsler, H., Nelson, T. F., Lee, J. E., Seibring, M., Lewis, C., & Keeling, R. P. (2003). Perception and reality: A national evaluation of social norms marketing interventions to reduce college students heavy alcohol use. *Journal of Studies on Alcohol*, *64*(4), 484–495. doi:10.15288/jsa.2003.64.484 PMID:12921190

Wege, N., Muth, T., Li, J., & Angerer, P. (2016). Mental health among currently enrolled medical students in Germany. *Public Health*, *132*, 92–100. doi:10.1016/j.puhe.2015.12.014 PMID:26880490

Wei, M., Russell, D. W., Young, S., & Hewitt, P. P. (2006). Maladaptive perfectionism and ineffective copping as mediators between attachment and future depression: A prospective analysis. *Journal of Counseling Psychology*, *53*(1), 67–79. doi:10.1037/0022-0167.53.1.67

Weiner, B. (2000). Attributional thoughts about consumer behavior. *The Journal of Consumer Research*, *27*(3), 382–387. doi:10.1086/317592

Weissman, A. N., & Beck, A. T. (1978). *Development and validation of the dysfunctional attitude scale: a preliminary investigation*. Paper presented at the 86th Annual Convention of the American Psychological Association, Toronto, Ontario, Canada.

West, C. P., & Shanafelt, T. D. (2007). The influence of personal and environmental factors on professionalism in medical education. *BMC Medical Education*, *7*, 1. Retrieved from http://bmcmededuc.biomedcentral.com/articles/10.1186/1472-6920-7-29

West, C. P., Dyrbye, L. N., Rabatin, J. T., Call, T. G., Davidson, J. H., Multari, A., & Shanafelt, T. D. et al. (2014). Intervention to promote physician well-being, job satisfaction, and professionalism: A randomized clinical trial. *JAMA Internal Medicine*, *174*(4), 527–533. doi:10.1001/jamainternmed.2013.14387 PMID:24515493

West, C. P., Huschka, M. M., Novotny, P. J., Sloan, J. A., Kolars, J. C., Habermann, T. M., & Shanafelt, T. D. (2006). Association of perceived medical errors with resident distress and empathy: A prospective longitudinal study. *Journal of the American Medical Association*, *296*(9), 1071–1078. doi:10.1001/jama.296.9.1071 PMID:16954486

West, C. P., Tan, A. D., Habermann, T. M., Sloan, J. A., & Shanafelt, T. D. (2009). Association of resident fatigue and distress with perceived medical errors. *Journal of the American Medical Association*, *302*(12), 1294–1300. doi:10.1001/jama.2009.1389 PMID:19773564

Whitley, R., Kirmayer, L. J., & Groleau, D. (2006). Understanding immigrants'reluctance to use mental health services: A qualitative study from Montreal. *Canadian Journal of Psychiatry*, 205–209. PMID:16629344

Whitlock, J., Muehlenkamp, J., Eckenrode, J., Purington, A., Baral Abrams, G., Barreira, P., & Kress, V. (2013). Nonsuicidal Self-Injury as a Gateway to Suicide in Young Adults. *The Journal of Adolescent Health*, *52*(4), 486–492. doi:10.1016/j.jadohealth.2012.09.010 PMID:23298982

WHO Constitution. (n.d.). Retrieved February 2017 http://www.who.int/about/en/

Wilczek-Ruzyczka, E. (2011). Empathy vs. professional burnout in health care professionals. *Journal of US - China Medical Science*, *8*. Retrieved from http://search.proquest.com/docview/1465056775?accountid=14376

Wiles, P. (2015, August 18). Wellness and medical school: Aspiration - or pipe dream?. *Psychiatric Times*. Retrieved from http://www.psychiatrictimes.com/major-depressive-disorder/wellness-and-medical-school-aspiration-or-pipe-dream

William, R. (2005). Towards understanding culture. In C. Lago (Ed.), *Race, Culture and Counseling* (pp. 40–49). Maidenhead, UK: Open University Press.

Williams, D. (2016). Cracking the code on the "hidden curriculum" in medical education pipeline and its contribution to attrition. *Journal of Unschooling & Alternative Learning*, *10*(19), 82–99.

Wolf, T. (1994). M: Stress, coping and health: enhancing well-being during medical school. *Medical Education*, *28*(1), 8–17. doi:10.1111/j.1365-2923.1994.tb02679.x PMID:8208174

Woloschuk, W., & Harasym, P. H. (2004). *Attitude change during medical school: A cohort study*. Retrieved from onlinelibrary.wiley.com/doi/10.1046/j.1365-2929.2004.01820.x/pdf

World Health Organisation (WHO). (2015). Retrieved from http://www.who.int/healthinfo/global_burden_disease/estimates

World Health Organisation (WHO). (2016/2017). *Mental Disorders Fact sheet*. Retrieved from http://www.who.int

World Health Organisation. (1948). *WHO definition of health*. Retrieved from http://www.who.int/about/definition/en/print.html

World Health Organisation. (2003). *Work organization and stress*. Retrieved on January 19, 2017 from http://www.who.int/occupational_health/publications/en/oehstress.pdf

World Health Organisation. (2011). *America's State of Mind Report*. Retrieved from http://apps.who.int/medicinedocs/en/d/Js19032en/

World Health Organisation. (2012). *Health education: Theoretical concepts, effective strategies and core competencies* [pdf file]. Retrieved from http://applications.emro.who.int/dsaf/EMRPUB_2012_ EN_1362.pdf

World Health Organisation. (2012). *Risks to mental health: An overview of vulnerabilities and risk factors*. Retrieved on January 19, 2017 from http://www.who.int/mental_health/mhgap/risks_to_mental_health_EN_27_08_12.pdf

World Health Organization (WHO) & World Federation for Medical Education (WFME). (2005). *WHO/WFME Guidelines for Accreditation of Basic Medical Education*. Available from: http://wfme.org/accreditation/whowfme-policy/28-2-who-wfme-guidelines-for-accreditation-of-basic-medical-education-english/file.www.gken.org

World Health Organization. (1948). *WHO definition of health*. Retrieved from http://www.who.int/about/definition/en/print.html

Wu, D., Rockett, I., Yang, T., Feng, X., Jiang, S., & Yu, L. (2016). Deliberate self-harm among Chinese medical students: A population-based study. *Journal of Affective Disorders*, *202*, 137–144. doi:10.1016/j.jad.2016.05.030 PMID:27262635

Yakunina, E. S., & Weigold, I. K. (2011). Asian International students' intentions to seek counseling: Integrating cognitive and cultural predictors. *Asian American Journal of Psychology*, *2*(3), 219–224. doi:10.1037/a0024821

YouGov. (2014). *One in four students suffer from mental health problems*. Retrieved from https://yougov.co.uk/news/2016/.../quarter-britain-students-are-afflicted-mental-hea/ https:/

YouGov. (n.d.). *One in four students suffer from mental health problems*. Retrieved from https://yougov.co.uk/news/2016/.../quarter-britains-students-are-afflicted-mental-hea/

Yousuf, S., Beh, P., & Wong, P. (2013). Attitudes towards suicide following an undergraduate suicide prevention module: Experience of medical students in Hong Kong. *Hong Kong Medical Journal*, *19*(5), 377–385. doi:10.12809/hkmj133950 PMID:24088587

Yu, J., Chae, S., & Chang, K. (2016). The relationship among self-efficacy, perfectionism and academic burnout in medical school students. *Korean Journal of Medical Education*, *28*(1), 49–55. doi:10.3946/kjme.2016.9 PMID:26838568

Yusoff, M. S. B., Rahim, A. F. A., Baha, A. A., Ismail, S. B., & Pa, M. N. (2013). The impact of medical education on psychological health of students: A cohort study. *Journal of Psychology. Health & Medicine*, *18*(4), 420–430. doi:10.1080/13548506.2012.740162

Zuroff, D. C. (1994). Depressive personality styles and the five-factor model of personality. *Journal of Personality Assessment*, *63*(3), 453–472. doi:10.1207/s15327752jpa6303_5 PMID:7844736

About the Contributors

Christina Ramirez Smith is an Educational Administrator and Professor of Educational and Higher Education Administration, Leadership and Planning. Dr. Ramirez Smith studies higher education with an emphasis upon the preparation of leaders for the global workforce. Her other research interests include the impact of debt on graduate students, organisational development and change, higher education finance and policy, as well as the unique mental health issues experienced by graduate students in addition to medical students. Currently, she is affiliated with University of The Bahamas where she serves in the roles of Advancement fundraiser and Special Assistant to The President.

* * *

Timothy Barrett is a Consultant Liaison Psychiatrist with the Public Hospitals Authority, Bahamas, and Associate Lecturer for the University of the West Indies School of Clinical Medicine and Research, Bahamas. He is a former president of the Medical Association of The Bahamas and former Chair of the Bahamas Medical Council. A veteran medical educator, he is keenly interested in developing people and helping them to maximize their quality of life by using time wisely. He has researched physician stress, factors related to relapse and relapse prevention in polysubstance abuse/dependence and other topics related to the pharmacology of anxiety. He is a noted lecturer and presenter in the area of stress management, conflict resolution and leadership development and has worked throughout the Caribbean in this role. A former Olympic athlete and coach of athletic teams, he uses his broad experience to provide practical strategies for growth and development. A life-long learner, he is committed to developing new strategies to cope with the challenges presented by todays' rapid societal changes. Most importantly, he is committed to a holistic approach understanding the priority of one's spirituality.

Erick Chan is a medical student at Griffith University on the Gold Coast in Australia. He completed his Bachelor of Medical Science in 2013 and is currently the President of the Surgical Interest Association (SURGIA) and the President of the Australasian Students' Surgical Association (ASSA). He writes and presents on student society development, student society leadership and has a keen interest in surgery, medical research and medical education.

Mitchell Dandignac received his MS in Psychological Science from Shippensburg University of Pennsylvania in 2016. In 2015 he was hired as a Learning Specialist at the West Virginia School of Osteopathic Medicine (WVSOM) and is currently the supervisor of the tutoring program at WVSOM. His particular areas of interest include applying the principles of Cognitive Psychology to academic habits, attentional issues, and memory retention. Currently, Mitchell works with medical school students on developing useful studying and test-taking habits and conducts various workshops throughout the year.

Vinod Gopalan is a Senior Lecturer in Medical Education in the School of Medicine at Griffith University, Gold Coast, Australia. Gopalan has over 15 years of experience in teaching/training medical students around the world and primarily focused on promoting self-directed learning and problem based learning among medical students. With a background in medicine and science, Gopalan has published multiple learning and teaching publications and grants in learning and teaching. His primary focuses in education include pathology/histology, pre-clinical, science and work integrated learning.

Michael Hamlin, PhD, has worked and taught in the areas of academic affairs, educational technology and human factors at a number of universities and professional schools including the University of Washington, Pepperdine University, Loyola Marymount University and the Touro College and University System. Starting in Seattle, Washington at the University of Washington Health Sciences and School of Dentistry, he has developed computer-based teaching materials and simulations and also participated in some of the first human factors work in software usability at Microsoft Corporation. Dr. Hamlin is currently Professor of Psychology and Organizational Behavior at Touro University Worldwide where he designed and launched the Professional Doctoral Program in Applied Psychology, a cutting-edge online doctoral program and an innovative online Masters Program in Marriage and Family Therapy.

Debbie Ho is a medical student at Griffith University, Gold Coast Australia. She completed the Bachelor of Medical Science in 2013 and is currently a research assistant at Gold Coast University Hospital. She is a passionate advocate for students and has an interest in emergency, critical care and surgery.

Virginia Joseph is a licensed Psychologist both in St Lucia and the UK. Ms Joseph holds a BSc in psychology, MA in Counselling Psychology and in the process of completing her professional doctorate in Counselling Psychology. Assistant professor at Spartan Health Science University School of Medicine in St Lucia. She also works as a consultant providing seminars and workshops as well operates a private counselling service. Ms Joseph is the founder and director of "Spartan Mental Health Awareness Trust" (SMHAT) a charitable organisation form with medical students. The aim of SMHAT is to bring about more awareness to mental health in St Lucia. Ms Joseph is also an active researcher in the area of culture differences, mindfulness, suicide and mental health.

Lynda Tierney Konecny, DHEd, MCHES, Associate Professor at A.T. Still University, has presented nationally and internationally on wellness, academics, and student services. In addition to her Doctor of Health Education degree, she holds a Master of Science in Counseling/Student Personnel Services, and a Bachelor of Science in Behavioral Psychology. Her passions and experiences include the exploration and evaluation of wellness resources in higher education, innovative teaching methodologies, the practical application of health education theories and models and the educational aspects of health promotion, and examining learning theory in relation to student learning emphasizing behavior modification. In addition to being a Master Certified Health Education Specialist, Dr. Konecny is a nationally certified fitness instructor and personal trainer, and a member of the Editorial Review Board of the Journal of College and Character.

LaTanya Love received her MD from the University of Texas Medical Branch in 2000. She is currently an Associate Professor in Pediatrics and Associate Dean for Admissions and Student Affairs and Diversity and Inclusion at McGovern Medical School at the University of Texas Health Science Center. She oversees student health services and is interested in student wellness and resilience.

Robert Lubin, PsyD, is the Managing Director of the American Medical Program at the Technion School of Medicine in Haifa, Israel. Besides being responsible for overall operations and strategic planning, he provides personal counseling and guidance as well as academic support to the American and Canadian medical students who choose to study medicine in Israel. Dr. Lubin is an Adjunct Faculty Professor of Psychology at Touro College and Touro University Worldwide.

Matt Martin, PhD, LMFT, serves as the Director of Behavioral Medicine at Southern Regional AHEC in Fayetteville, NC where he teaches medical residents and students and manages behavioral health services. His research interests include family-centered care, behavioral medicine curriculum development, and substance use services in primary care. He received graduate degrees from East Carolina University and Brigham Young University. He completed pre-doctoral training at the Dartmouth Family Medicine Residency in Concord, NH and post-doctoral training at the Chicago Center for Family Health in Chicago, IL. He is an AAMFT Clinical Member and Approved Supervisor.

Warren G. McDonald, PhD, is currently Professor and Chair of the Department of Health Care Administration at Methodist University, Fayetteville, NC, and is a noted author and lecturer. He is also Chief Executive Officer of McDonald and Associates, LLC, a consulting firm dedicated to the improvement of healthcare organizations and professionals across the United States and internationally. He holds graduate degrees in Health Care Management (Norwich), Education (East Carolina) and the Doctor of Philosophy in Health Sciences (Touro University), as well as a number of professional certifications. He is a member of the Class of 2005 at the Institute for Management and Leadership in Higher Education at Harvard University, and holds a Graduate Certificate in Health Care Risk Management from the University of Florida. Additional faculty appointments include Contributing Professor in the School of Health Sciences at Walden University where he teaches in the Master of Health Administration program, and mentors doctoral students. He is also serves on the adjunct faculty at Logan University in the Doctor of Health Professions Education program, and the Southern Illinois University Master of Health Administration program. Prior to joining the faculty at Methodist University he held senior-level administrative positions in the University of North Carolina system. He serves on the Board of Trustees of Cape Fear Valley Health Systems, and as chair of the Board of Trustees of the Southern Area Regional Health Education Center.

Dana McDowelle received her PhD from Michigan State University in Environmental Toxicology and Food Science in 1994. She is currently an Assistant Dean of Admissions and Student Affairs at McGovern Medical School. Prior to joining MMS, she served at several institutions, most recently as the Assistant Dean for Diversity and Student Professional Development in the School of Medicine at the University of Texas Health Science Center-San Antonio and prior at Rice University and Xavier University of Louisiana in multiple capacities. At the latter, she was a tenured member of the faculty in the Department of Biology.

Jozelle Miller holds a PhD in health Psychology from the University of Birmingham UK. She also holds a Msc. degree in Applied psychology (specializing in Health), Bsc. (hons), Psychology from the University of the West Indies Mona Campus in Jamaica and is certified as a Qualified Assistant Teacher with special training in Secondary Level Education. Dr Miller is a Health Psychologist with the Ministry of Health, Wellness and the Environment and the Milton Cato Memorial Hospital. With over 10 years working in the area of HIV & AIDS, she is certified as both a trainer and provider of HIV Voluntary Counselling and Testing by JHPIEGO & CHART and completed an Intensive HIV/AIDS course on Strategic Assessments and Responses; Initial Programs for Planning Purposes in the Caribbean Region at the National Institute of Public Health in Mexico. Dr Miller serves also as a Wellness Consultant and is the founder of the VALEO Experience. The VALEO offers Wellness assessments and profiles and a wide range of other services. She is also a weekly columnist in one of the country's leading newspapers; where she provides deep psychological insights to the general public in response to many critical issues affecting their lives. And is also a lecturer at the All Saints College of Medicine.

Fehintola Omidele received her Bachelor of Arts in Biology and a Bachelor of Science in Human Development and Family Sciences at The University of Texas at Austin in 2010. She went on to The University of Texas Medical School at Houston (now McGovern Medical School) to complete her MD in 2014. She is currently pursuing a Master of Public Health from Johns Hopkins Bloomberg School of Public Health, while working as a Health Planner for the City of Houston's Department of Health and Human Services. She writes wellness proposals for medical residency programs and continues to advocate for wellness in her position with the City of Houston.

Emma A. Omoruyi received her Bachelor of Science degree in Biology at Duke University. She subsequently attended Duke University School of Medical School to complete her Medical Degree, and concurrently completed a Master of Public Health from University of North Carolina at Chapel Hill. She finished her pediatric residency at the University of Texas Health Science Center at Houston (UTH) and is currently is a faculty member at McGovern Medical School part of the University of Texas Health Science Center at Houston in the Department of Pediatrics. She enjoys working with medical students and residents. Her research interests include preparing learners to work with diverse patients; serving the underserved; and curriculum design and evaluation.

Lenny Salzberg, M.D., is the Faculty Development Fellowship Director at Southern Regional AHEC in Fayetteville, NC, where he teaches medical residents and students in the Family Medicine Residency. He has served as the Chair of the Society of Teachers of Family Medicine's Group on Faculty Development. Dr. Salzberg graduated from Albany Medical College of Union University, trained at the Duke/FAHEC Family Medicine Residency Program in Fayetteville, N.C., and has completed fellowships in Faculty Development at Duke and at the National Institute of Program Director Development. He also completed the Wildacres Leadership Initiative William C. Friday Fellowship for Human Relations.

Samantha Smith is a medical student at West Virginia School of Osteopathic Medicine. She completed the Bachelor of Arts Degree in English with a minor in Biology from The Boston University, Boston, Massachusetts followed by a Master of Science degree in Medical Science in 2012. She is a certified EMT and presenter on policy matters in the regional AHEC division for West Virginia. She is an avid half-marathon runner and writer. She serves as a mentor for minority and first year students and participates as a WVSOM representative for recruitment of new students. She has an interest in Internal Medicine and Emergency Medicine.

Index

A

Academic Burnout 91
Academic Faculty Wellness 171
Academic Medicine Centres 189
Academic Self-Efficacy 82, 91
Academics 174, 231, 239, 252
Adaptive Perfectionism 73-74, 91
Apprenticeship Learning 105-106, 110, 121

B

Balance 11, 58, 123, 147, 152-155, 175, 180, 192-193, 203, 209, 211-214, 217, 219, 222, 224-226, 228, 239, 241, 245, 247
Balance in Dimensions of Wellness 209, 211-213, 217, 219, 222, 224, 226, 228
Barriers 26, 44, 46, 48-53, 59, 131, 136-137, 176-178, 182, 221, 223-224
Burnout 58, 69-70, 74, 84, 91-93, 95-98, 100-102, 108, 110-112, 121, 123, 145, 147, 151-159, 161-164, 169, 171-173, 175-176, 178-183, 185, 189-191, 194-195, 197, 205, 218-219, 224

C

Cartesian Dualism 249, 252
Chronic Stress 146-147, 151, 155, 157, 163, 169
Clinical Empathy 93-94, 98, 101, 121
Cognitive Apprenticeship 106-107, 110, 112, 121
Competence 69, 80, 91, 100, 108, 111, 150
Conscientiousness 4, 71-72, 82, 91
Contextualization 109-110, 121
Counselling 12, 16, 18, 50, 58, 67, 132, 137, 143, 159, 163, 175-177, 182, 200-201, 204, 210, 217, 239
Culture 1, 8, 18-20, 22-23, 26, 46-53, 59, 67, 69, 102, 105, 130-131, 155, 159-160, 173, 176-177, 182-183, 192, 195-196, 205, 210, 219-220, 226

D

Darwinian Way 247, 252
Deliberate Self-Harm 122-124, 126-129, 131, 134-136, 138, 143
Depression 2, 4, 7, 12-15, 18-19, 45, 47-48, 50, 55, 69-70, 74-75, 84, 91, 93, 123-124, 127, 129-130, 133-134, 145-147, 152-153, 158-159, 163, 173, 176, 178-180, 191-192, 195-196, 200-202, 210-212, 215-217, 219-221, 224, 226, 236, 243
Difficult Patients 158, 189
Dimensions 9, 71, 93, 95, 100, 108, 209-222, 224-226, 228, 234
Distress 5-6, 13-14, 16, 18-21, 25-26, 44, 48-50, 69, 71, 74-76, 78, 83, 102, 127, 145, 147, 150-153, 155-157, 161, 163, 169, 181, 191, 196-197, 202, 212, 236, 245, 249
Dysfunctional Attitude Scale 91

E

Ethnic Minority 47-49, 59
Ethnicity 47-48, 50, 67

F

Formation 95, 104, 109-110, 121, 201

G

Graduate Medical Education (GME) 41-42, 71, 145-147, 151-152, 154, 158, 160, 163, 169, 171-173, 176-177, 179, 193

H

Health Education 209, 221, 224-226, 228
Health Education Models 209, 221, 228
Health Education Theory 221, 224-226, 228
Health Promotion 9, 17, 42, 57, 213, 221, 224, 226, 228
Healthy Universities 17, 41
Help-Seeking 12, 49, 52, 122, 131-133, 195, 199, 219
Hidden Curriculum 5, 19-20, 23, 26, 69, 155, 201, 217, 219, 228
High Expectations 69, 71, 130
Higher Education 1, 3, 12-13, 15-18, 41, 128, 176
Hippocratic Oath 234, 252

I

Intern 5, 154, 158, 160, 169, 194
Interpersonal Skills 203, 208, 231
Intolerance of Uncertainty 172, 189

M

Maladaptive Perfectionism 68, 70, 73-74, 82-83, 91
Medical Academic Faculty Burnout 171
Medical Education 1-3, 5, 11, 17-19, 23, 25-26, 29, 41-42, 54, 69, 71, 73, 83, 93-94, 99-100, 102-105, 107, 110-111, 145-147, 151-152, 154, 158, 160, 163, 169, 171-177, 179-180, 182-183, 191-195, 198, 204-205, 209-211, 214-215, 219, 244, 248
Medical Educators 6, 25, 68-70, 75, 79, 83, 102, 132, 138, 183, 233
Medical Resident 145, 169
Medical School Culture 20, 22-23, 67
Medical Schools 2-4, 6, 18-23, 25-26, 28-29, 42, 44-45, 49, 51, 53-56, 58-60, 67-71, 74, 76, 79-80, 93-95, 98, 100-102, 123, 129-131, 135-138, 145-149, 151, 169, 173-175, 179, 181, 183, 189-193, 195-197, 199-206, 209-212, 214-217, 219-221, 224-226, 232, 235-237, 239, 248
Medical Student 3-6, 18, 20-21, 26, 28, 45-47, 49, 54, 58, 60, 71-72, 83, 92-93, 100-101, 111, 122-124, 130, 135, 137, 145, 149, 173, 183, 185, 190, 193, 197, 201, 203, 205-206, 210-211, 214-215, 217, 219-221, 224, 245
Medical Student Burnout 92-93
Medical Student Distress 5-6, 20, 26, 197
Medical Students 1-2, 4-6, 8, 11, 18-21, 23, 25-26, 28-29, 44-55, 57-60, 68-71, 73, 75-77, 80-83, 92-96, 99-100, 102, 108, 111-112, 122-123, 127-138, 146-149, 153, 157-159, 172-173, 175-176, 182-183, 190-192, 194-206, 209-219, 221-222, 224-226, 228, 230-232, 234-237, 240-241, 247, 249
Medical Students' Mental Health 1-2, 4-5, 19, 92
Mental Health 1-2, 4-9, 11-19, 21, 23, 26, 28-29, 41-42, 44, 46-47, 49-52, 54-59, 67-70, 72, 83, 92, 122-124, 127, 132-133, 135-138, 145-147, 151-154, 159-164, 169, 172, 176, 181-183, 191, 196, 201-202, 205, 209-210, 217, 230, 233-236, 249
Mental Health Literacy 45, 54-56, 59, 67, 122, 132-133
Mental Health Promotion 42, 57
Mental Ill Health 17, 29, 42, 235
Mental Illness 9, 11-12, 16, 22, 45, 49-52, 54-57, 136-137, 151-153, 155-159, 161-162, 169
Mentor 52, 99, 197, 199, 208, 214, 219-220, 239
Mindfulness 8, 28, 111, 146, 154, 161-162, 175-176, 179, 181-182, 189, 197, 215-218, 220, 228, 244

Morbidity 127, 159, 238, 249, 252
Mortality 133, 159, 249, 252

N

Needs Assessment 209, 215

O

Obeah 50, 67
Occupational Development 197, 200, 206, 208

P

Perception 5, 47-48, 51, 53, 58, 72, 75, 78, 91, 94-99, 105, 110-112, 154, 172, 189, 222, 232
Personality Type 69, 91
Physician Burnout 151, 153, 158-159, 164, 171-173
Physicians 1, 5-6, 18, 21, 26, 42, 72, 80, 93, 111, 146-152, 155, 157-158, 161, 164, 171-174, 176-178, 181-183, 189-191, 193-196, 200, 203, 206, 212, 224, 230-233, 237-238, 244, 246, 248-249, 252
Positive Psychology 219-220, 228
Prevention 9, 11, 26, 45, 57, 59, 132-138, 143, 164, 176, 213
Primary Prevention 133, 137, 143
Professionalism 5, 100-101, 108, 123, 150, 190, 194-195, 197, 201, 206, 208, 212
Psycho-Educational Intervention 143

R

Religious Beliefs 67
Residency 1-2, 20, 42, 145-153, 155, 159-164, 172, 176-180, 189, 191-194, 200, 204, 206, 239
Residency training 146, 149-150, 152-153, 155, 159-160, 162-164, 177, 189, 194
Resident Burnout 158, 178
Resident Physician 149, 171, 178, 189
Resident Wellness 154, 177
Resilience 8, 17, 23, 102, 111, 123, 130-131, 158, 175, 178-179, 181-182, 194, 197, 219, 235, 239, 244
Resiliency 151, 163-164, 171, 181, 183, 189

S

Secondary Prevention 133, 143
Situative Learning 104-105, 108, 121
Social Cognitive Learning Theory 107, 121
Social Skills 231, 252
Socially-Prescribed Perfectionism 91
Spirituality 46, 48-49, 67, 213, 247, 252
Stigma 16, 23, 44-48, 50-56, 58-59, 122, 130, 132, 136, 145, 147, 152, 196, 201, 235-236, 249
Stress Management 176, 178, 181, 195, 208, 212-213, 241, 244-245
Stressor 5, 149, 153, 172-173, 191-192, 197, 252
Student Success 197-198, 200
Student well-being 11, 123, 190, 201, 206
Students 1-6, 8, 11-13, 15-23, 25-26, 28-29, 41, 44-60, 68-69, 71, 73-83, 92-103, 105, 107-112, 122-123, 127-138, 146-149, 153, 157-159, 172-176, 179-180, 182-183, 190-192, 194-206, 210-226, 228, 230-237, 239-241, 245, 247-249
Studying 17, 68, 76, 79-80, 94, 97, 105, 192, 216, 218, 231
Suicide 4-5, 12, 19, 59, 68, 75, 93, 122-124, 126-127, 129-136, 138, 143, 153, 163, 173, 176, 180, 210, 235-236
Suicide Ideology 122-124, 126-127, 129-130, 132, 138, 143

T

Tertiary Prevention 134-135, 143
Trends 13, 110, 154, 209, 215

U

USMLE 148, 193, 199

V

Value Exploration 178, 189

W

Wellness 9-11, 17, 28, 57-58, 92, 154-155, 159-160, 162-163, 171, 173-178, 180-183, 190, 194-198, 200-201, 203-206, 208-210, 213-222, 224-226, 228, 233-234, 246
Wellness Curriculum 201
Wellness Dimension 214, 228
Wellness Programmes 171, 173-177, 179-181, 183, 197, 206, 209, 211-213, 215, 217, 221-222, 224-226, 228
Western Psychotherapy 49, 67
Witchcraft 50, 67

Y

Yerkes-Dodson Law 252

www.ingramcontent.com/pod-product-compliance
Lightning Source LLC
LaVergne TN
LVHW080339011026
849161LV00009B/2129